Clinical Pathology and Diagnostic Testing

Editors

MARY JO BURKHARD
MAXEY L. WELLMAN

VETERINARY CLINICS OF NORTH AMERICA: SMALL ANIMAL PRACTICE

www.vetsmall.theclinics.com

November 2013 • Volume 43 • Number 6

ELSEVIER

1600 John F. Kennedy Boulevard • Suite 1800 • Philadelphia, Pennsylvania, 19103-2899
http://www.vetsmall.theclinics.com

**VETERINARY CLINICS OF NORTH AMERICA: SMALL ANIMAL PRACTICE Volume 43, Number 6
November 2013 ISSN 0195-5616, ISBN-13: 978-0-323-26138-8**

Editor: John Vassallo; j.vassallo@elsevier.com
Developmental Editor: Susan Showalter

Veterinary Clinics of North America: Small Animal Practice (ISSN 0195-5616) is published bimonthly by Elsevier Inc., 360 Park Avenue South, New York, NY 10010-1710. Months of issue are January, March, May, July, September, and November. Business and Editorial Offices: 1600 John F. Kennedy Blvd., Ste. 1800, Philadelphia, PA 19103-2899. Customer Service Office: 3251 Riverport Lane, Maryland Heights, MO 63043. Periodicals postage paid at New York, NY and additional mailing offices. Subscription prices are $310.00 per year (domestic individuals), $500.00 per year (domestic institutions), $150.00 per year (domestic students/residents), $410.00 per year (Canadian individuals), $621.00 per year (Canadian institutions), $455.00 per year (international individuals), $621.00 per year (international institutions), and $220.00 per year (international and Canadian students/residents). To receive student/resident rate, orders must be accompanied by name of affiliated institution, date of term, and the *signature* of program/residency coordinator on institution letterhead. Orders will be billed at individual rate until proof of status is received. Foreign air speed delivery is included in all *Clinics* subscription prices. All prices are subject to change without notice. **POSTMASTER:** Send address changes to *Veterinary Clinics of North America: Small Animal Practice*, Elsevier Health Sciences Division, Subscription Customer Service, 3251 Riverport Lane, Maryland Heights, MO 63043. Customer Service (orders, claims, online, change of address): Elsevier Periodicals Customer Service, Elsevier Health Sciences Division Subscription Customer Service 3251 Riverport Lane Maryland Heights, MO 63043. Tel: 1-800-654-2452 (U.S. and Canada); 314-447-8871 (outside U.S. and Canada). Fax: 314-447-8029. E-mail: journalscustomerservice-usa@elsevier.com (for print support); journalsonlinesupport-usa@elsevier.com (for online support).

Reprints. For copies of 100 or more of articles in this publication, please contact the Commercial Reprints Department, Elsevier Inc., 360 Park Avenue South, New York, NY 10010-1710. Tel.: 212-633-3874; Fax: 212-633-3820; E-mail: reprints@elsevier.com.

Veterinary Clinics of North America: Small Animal Practice is also published in Japanese by Inter Zoo Publishing Co., Ltd., Aoyama Crystal-Bldg 5F, 3-5-12 Kitaaoyama, Minato-ku, Tokyo 107-0061, Japan.

Veterinary Clinics of North America: Small Animal Practice is covered in *Current Contents/Agriculture, Biology and Environmental Sciences, Science Citation Index, ASCA, MEDLINE/PubMed (Index Medicus), Excerpta Medica,* and *BIOSIS.*

Printed and bound by CPI Group (UK) Ltd, Croydon, CR0 4YY

Transferred to digital print 2012

Contributors

EDITORS

MARY JO BURKHARD, DVM, PhD
Diplomate, American College of Veterinary Pathologists (Clinical Pathology); Associate Professor, Department of Veterinary Biosciences, College of Veterinary Medicine, The Ohio State University, Columbus, Ohio

MAXEY L. WELLMAN, DVM, MS, PhD
Diplomate, American College of Veterinary Pathologists (Clinical Pathology); Professor, Department of Veterinary Biosciences, College of Veterinary Medicine, The Ohio State University, Columbus, Ohio

AUTHORS

KARIN ALLENSPACH, DR med vet, FVH, PhD, FHEA
Diplomate, European College of Veterinary Internal Medicine (Companion Animals); Associate Professor and Reader in Internal Medicine, Department of Clinical Sciences and Services, Royal Veterinary College, University of London, North Mymms, United Kingdom

DOROTHEE BIENZLE, DVM, PhD
Diplomate, American College of Veterinary Pathologists (Clinical Pathology); Professor and Canada Research Chair in Veterinary Pathology, Department of Pathobiology, University of Guelph, Guelph, Ontario, Canada

ANDREA A. BOHN, DVM, PhD
Diplomate, American College of Veterinary Pathologists (Clinical Pathology); Associate Professor, Department of Microbiology, Immunology, and Pathology, College of Veterinary Medicine and Biomedical Sciences, Colorado State University, Fort Collins, Colorado

MARJORY B. BROOKS, DVM
Director, Comparative Coagulation Section, Animal Health Diagnostic Center, College of Veterinary Medicine, Cornell University, Ithaca, New York

MARY JO BURKHARD, DVM, PhD
Diplomate, American College of Veterinary Pathologists (Clinical Pathology); Associate Professor, Department of Veterinary Biosciences, College of Veterinary Medicine, The Ohio State University, Columbus, Ohio

JAMES L. CATALFAMO, MS, PhD
Senior Research Associate, Comparative Coagulation Section, Animal Health Diagnostic Center, College of Veterinary Medicine, Cornell University, Ithaca, New York

SETH E. CHAPMAN, DVM, MS
Diplomate, American College of Veterinary Pathologists (Clinical Pathology); IDEXX Laboratories Inc, Worthington, Ohio

JOSHUA B. DANIELS, DVM, PhD
Diplomate, American College of Veterinary Microbiologists (Bacteriology/Mycology); Associate Professor–Clinical, Department of Veterinary Clinical Sciences, College of Veterinary Medicine, The Ohio State University, Columbus, Ohio

JOANNE HODGES, DVM
Clinical Pathologist, VDx Veterinary Diagnostics, Davis, California

MARIE K. HOLOWAYCHUK, DVM
Diplomate, American College of Veterinary Emergency and Critical Care; Assistant Professor, Department of Clinical Studies, Ontario Veterinary College, University of Guelph, Guelph, Ontario, Canada

ROGER A. HOSTUTLER, DVM, MS
Diplomate, American College of Veterinary Internal Medicine (Small Animal Internal Medicine); MedVet Medical and Cancer Centers for Pets, Worthington, Ohio

CAROLINE MANSFIELD, BSc, BVMS, PhD, MANZCVS
Diplomate, European College of Veterinary Internal Medicine-Companion Animals; Hill's Associate Professor, Head of Small Animal Medicine, Faculty of Veterinary Science, The University of Melbourne, Werribee, Victoria, Australia

ANDREA A. MONNIG, DVM
Diplomate, American College of Veterinary Emergency and Critical Care; Assistant Professor – Clinical, Department of Veterinary Clinical Sciences, College of Veterinary Medicine, The Ohio State University, Columbus, Ohio

MARK A. OYAMA, DVM
Diplomate, American College of Veterinary Internal Medicine; Specialty of Cardiology, Professor and Chief, Section of Cardiology, Department of Clinical Studies-Philadelphia, School of Veterinary Medicine, University of Pennsylvania, Philadelphia, Pennsylvania

BARRAK M. PRESSLER, DVM, PhD
Diplomate, American College of Veterinary Internal Medicine; Assistant Professor of Small Animal Medicine, Department of Veterinary Clinical Sciences, College of Veterinary Medicine, The Ohio State University, Columbus, Ohio

LESLIE C. SHARKEY, DVM, PhD
Associate Professor, Veterinary Clinical Sciences Department, University of Minnesota College of Veterinary Medicine, St Paul, Minnesota

MAXEY L. WELLMAN, DVM, MS, PhD
Diplomate, American College of Veterinary Pathologists (Clinical Pathology); Professor, Department of Veterinary Biosciences, College of Veterinary Medicine, The Ohio State University, Columbus, Ohio

Contents

Serum creatinine concentration is insensitive for detecting kidney injury and does not assist in differentiation between glomerular versus tubular damage. Advanced renal function tests, including glomerular filtration rate testing, determining fractional excretion of electrolytes, and assay of urine biomarkers, may allow earlier detection of reduced renal function mass, differentiation of renal from non-renal causes of azotemia, and assist with localization of damage. This article reviews the principles, indications, and limitations of these tests and describes their use in sample clinical scenarios.

Routine biochemical tests generally include serum enzymes, proteins, and other markers useful for identifying hepatobiliary disease in dogs and cats. Obtaining results outside the reference intervals can occur with direct hepatocellular injury, enzyme induction by hepatocytes or biliary epithelium, or decreased hepatic function. However, detection of biochemical abnormalities does not necessarily indicate clinically significant disease. For a comprehensive approach to detection and treatment of hepatobiliary disease, the laboratory results must be correlated with the history and physical examination findings, diagnostic imaging results, and other assays.

Laboratory tests are an important part of the workup of small intestinal diseases in dogs and cats. Especially in chronic cases, when extragastrointestinal causes need to be ruled out, it is important to adhere to a systematic workup. This article details the newest available data on tests to aid this diagnostic process. Once the diagnosis of a chronic enteropathy is made, there are many laboratory tests that can help in monitoring the disease and providing prognostic information. Several new tests being evaluated for clinical usefulness are discussed.

The pancreas remains a difficult organ to evaluate using laboratory methods alone. No single laboratory test is diagnostic of pancreatitis (chronic or acute) without other diagnostic modalities concurring with the diagnosis or ruling out other diseases. The diagnosis of pancreatitis is particularly difficult in cats, and pancreatitis often occurs with other diseases. The use of pancreatic cytology may be useful in diagnosing both inflammation and neoplasia. Exocrine pancreatic insufficiency (EPI) can be relatively easily diagnosed when clinically manifested by the measurement of trypsinlike immunoreactivity. Diagnosis is more difficult when EPI is subclinical.

Blood-based assays for various cardiac biomarkers can assist in the diagnosis of heart disease in dogs and cats. The two most common markers are cardiac troponin-I and N-terminal pro-B–type natriuretic peptide. Biomarker assays can assist in differentiating cardiac from noncardiac causes of respiratory signs and detection of preclinical cardiomyopathy. Increasingly, studies indicate that cardiac biomarker testing can help assess the risk of morbidity and mortality in animals with heart disease. Usage of cardiac biomarker testing in clinical practice relies on proper patient selection, correct interpretation of test results, and incorporation of biomarker testing into existing diagnostic methods.

Acid-base abnormalities are common in critically ill veterinary patients. Rapid recognition of disturbances can be helpful in identifying the underlying cause of the patient's clinical signs, directing diagnostics, and monitoring response to therapy. If acid-base disturbances are left unidentified and untreated, severe physiologic consequences can result, including cardiovascular and neurologic dysfunction, protein and enzyme dysfunction, and electrolyte derangements. Treatment of acid-base disorders is aimed at correcting the underlying disease process.

Lactate is a product of anaerobic metabolism. Lactate concentration in blood is used clinically as an indicator of tissue hypoperfusion and hypoxia to determine disease severity, assess response to therapy, and predict outcome. This article reviews lactate physiology, sample collection and processing, and interpretation of lactate concentration in clinical practice.

Hypocalcemia occurs in critically ill dogs and cats and is associated with medications, treatments, and underlying diseases such as acute kidney disease, pancreatitis, parathyroid disease, sepsis, and trauma. Possible underlying mechanisms include hypovitaminosis D, acquired or relative hypoparathyroidism, hypomagnesemia, and alterations in the ionized fraction of calcium caused by changes in chelated or protein-bound calcium. If severe or acute, hypocalcemia can cause obvious clinical signs related to muscle or neurologic hyperexcitability or more subtle signs of cardiovascular dysfunction. Emergency treatment with calcium gluconate administration is recommended when clinical signs are present or if there is moderate to severe ionized hypocalcemia.

generate practice revenue whether assessed in-house or sent to a clinical pathologist. Thorough in-house evaluation is adequate in some cases, but expert opinion is important in many cases. Specimen slides should at least be reviewed in-house for assessment of cellularity and potential artifacts before submission to a reference laboratory. Reference laboratories also provide special stains and advanced molecular diagnostics to help further characterize many neoplastic processes, search for organisms, identify pigments, and address other important aspects of the lesion.

VETERINARY CLINICS OF NORTH AMERICA: SMALL ANIMAL PRACTICE

RELATED INTEREST

Veterinary Clinics of North America: Exotic Animal Practice
January 2013, Volume 16, Number 1
Clinical and Diagnostic Pathology
Alessandro Melillo, DVM, *Editor*

THE CLINICS ARE NOW AVAILABLE ONLINE!
Access your subscription at:
www.theclinics.com

Preface

Clinical Pathology and Diagnostic Testing

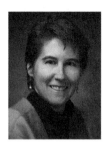 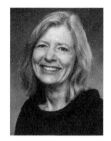

Mary Jo Burkhard, DVM, PhD, DACVP   Maxey L. Wellman, DVM, MS, PhD, DACVP

Editors

It has been our privilege to work with an outstanding group of authors to bring you this issue of *Veterinary Clinics of North America* devoted to Clinical Pathology and Diagnostic Testing. This topic was last covered in 2007 by good friends from another "OSU" (Robin Allison and Jim Meinkoth, Oklahoma State University) and we felt honored to build on their previous work.

Our goal with this issue was to focus on the diagnostic application of laboratory testing. We asked authors to provide practical application within each topic—providing our audience with material that they could read this morning and use on a case this afternoon. Even from the titles, you will see a focus on the practical.

Inside, you will find articles that help to develop a diagnostic approach to a specific organ system or a clinical conundrum. We targeted these articles around topics of recent interest in the literature—areas where there have been new findings, topical developments, or challenges in interpretation or application.

We are grateful for the hard work and expertise put into each article by our contributing authors. In addition, we hope that you enjoy reading these articles as much as we did. Not only are they informative, they are really well done!

Vet Clin Small Anim 43 (2013) xi–xii

http://dx.doi.org/10.1016/j.cvsm.2013.07.013   **vetsmall.theclinics.com**

We would also like to thank John Vassallo and Elsevier for their most excellent support and assistance during this project.

Mary Jo Burkhard, DVM, PhD, DACVP

Maxey L. Wellman, DVM, MS, PhD, DACVP
Department of Veterinary Biosciences
College of Veterinary Medicine
The Ohio State University
1925 Coffey Road
Columbus, OH, 43210, USA

E-mail addresses:
Burkhard.19@osu.edu (M.J. Burkhard)
Wellman.3@osu.edu (M.L. Wellman)

Erratum

In the July 2013 issue (Volume 43, number 4), in the article "The Use of Ultrasound for Dogs and Cats in the Emergency Room: AFAST and TFAST" by Søren R. Boysen and Gregory R. Lisciandro, on page 791, the first sentence under the header "The Future of Small Animal Lung Ultrasound," should read: "The wet (ULRs or B-lines) versus dry lung (glide sign and A-lines) concept is easily mastered by the nonradiologist veterinarian."

Vet Clin Small Anim 43 (2013) xiii
http://dx.doi.org/10.1016/j.cvsm.2013.10.001
0195-5616/13/$ – see front matter © 2013 Elsevier Inc. All rights reserved.

vetsmall.theclinics.com

Clinical Approach to Advanced Renal Function Testing in Dogs and Cats

Barrak M. Pressler, DVM, PhD

KEYWORDS

- Biomarkers • Fractional excretion • Glomerular filtration rate
- γ-Glutamyl transpeptidase • Microalbuminuria • Urine

KEY POINTS

- Advanced renal function tests may allow earlier detection of reduced renal functional mass and localization of damage to a particular nephron segment, and are required for diagnosis or exclusion of some causes of kidney injury.
- Measurement of glomerular filtration rate (GFR) allows for precise quantitative assessment of remaining filtration and excretion ability by the kidneys.
- Spot samples of simultaneously collected urine and plasma provide clinically reasonable approximations of total daily urine electrolyte excretion.
- The majority of plasma albumin is size and charge excluded from the ultrafiltrate; glomerular damage results in increased filtration of albumin and excretion into the urine. Microalbuminuria may be detected prior to positive reactions on standard urine protein dipstick pads, and before the urine protein:creatinine (UPC) ratio increases above reference range.
- Urinary N-acetyl-β-D-glucosaminidase (NAG):creatinine ratio is increased in dogs with chronic kidney disease, pyelonephritis, uncontrolled diabetes mellitus, pyometra, or X-linked hereditary nephropathy but does not differ before versus after control of hyperadrenocorticism with trilostane or transphenoidal hypophysectomy.

Serum biochemical analysis and urinalysis are the mainstay diagnostic tests for initial detection and estimation of severity of kidney disease in dogs and cats. Increased serum creatinine concentration and impaired urine concentrating ability, however, are relatively insensitive for detecting early kidney injury and do not assist in differentiation between glomerular versus proximal or distal tubular damage. Advanced renal function tests, including GFR testing, determining fractional excretion (FE) of

Funding Sources: Morris Animal Foundation, International Renal Interest Society, and The Ohio State University College of Veterinary Medicine.
Conflict of Interest: Previous funding from FAST Diagnostics.
Department of Veterinary Clinical Sciences, College of Veterinary Medicine, The Ohio State University, 601 Vernon Tharp Street, Columbus, OH 43210, USA
E-mail address: pressler.21@osu.edu

electrolytes, and assay of urine biomarkers, may allow earlier detection of reduced renal functional mass and differentiation of various renal and nonrenal differential diagnoses and assist with localization of damage. This article reviews the principles, indications, and limitations of these tests and describes their use in sample clinical scenarios.

GLOMERULAR FILTRATION RATE

Serum creatinine concentration is insensitive for detecting kidney injury. Increases in serum creatinine concentration are mild and often remain within reference range, until approximately 60% to 75% of all nephrons are no longer functional. In contrast, measurement of GFR allows for precise quantitative assessment of remaining filtration and excretion ability by the kidneys. Example situations when GFR measurement may provide critical information regarding remaining kidney function beyond serum creatinine concentration alone include diagnostic evaluation of dogs and cats with unexplained polyuria and polydipsia, to avoid overdosing of medications that are excreted by the kidneys or that have potential nephrotoxic effects, and to predict risk of overt renal failure after nephrectomy in dogs or cats with unilateral kidney disease, such as tumors or pyonephrosis.

Several methods for determination of GFR have been validated in dogs and cats, all of which report the volume of plasma, which has been cleared over a given interval of time, per kilogram of patient body weight. After injecting a substance (the marker) that is eliminated solely via filtration through the glomeruli and which then passes into the urine without being reabsorbed or further secreted by the tubules, the rate at which the concentration of marker decreases in successive blood samples allows calculation of the plasma clearance and GFR.[1] Assays that measure the rate of marker appearance in urine are more accurate than those that assay marker disappearance in plasma (because few markers are solely excreted via glomerular filtration without any tubular reuptake or secretion); however, urine assays that allow calculation of renal clearance (vs plasma clearance) are more cumbersome to perform because they require collection of all urine produced in a 24-hour period. Fortunately, plasma clearance assays using blood sampling techniques are sufficiently close to renal clearance, such that in the clinical setting urine collection is not required.[1–4]

Several markers have been validated for measurement of GFR in dogs and cats, including creatinine, cystatin C (CysC), iohexol, and radiolabeled molecules. In people, GFR is most commonly estimated (rather than measured) using serum creatinine concentration, body weight, and correction factors based on a patient's gender and race. Unfortunately, formulae for estimating GFR from serum creatinine have not proved accurate in dogs and cats due to greater individual, gender, and breed variation than occurs in people.[5,6] Intravenous administration of a sterile creatinine bolus is safe and cost effective; however, comparison of various markers suggests that exogenous creatinine GFR assays underestimate true GFR, likely due to some excretion into the gastrointestinal tract and perhaps tubular reuptake.[2,7,8] CysC is an endogenous protein produced by all nucleated cells at a constant rate that undergoes glomerular filtration without tubular secretion; however, commercial assays are limited, and comparative studies in dogs have suggested lower specificity for detection of reduced kidney function than exogenous creatinine GFR.[9–11]

Iohexol GFR measurement uses a marker that can be easily obtained by veterinarians and has been well validated for use in dogs and cats, and a commercial assay is available at a reasonable cost to owners. After intravenous bolus injection of the same iodinated contrast agent used in diagnostic imaging studies, plasma samples are collected at predetermined times (usually 2, 3, and 4 hours after injection); the volume of injection is based on concentration of elemental iodine within the iohexol.[12] Iodinated compounds are stable for long periods, and plasma samples can be frozen for extended periods of time and assayed later if indicated.[13] Intravenous iohexol can induce acute kidney injury and renal failure in people, particularly in patients with pre-existing kidney damage; however, this idiosyncratic drug reaction is rare in dogs and cats.[14,15] Iohexol GFR assays have been safely used to study renal function in healthy dogs and cats,[16–21] in dogs with gentamicin-induced acute kidney injury,[22] in dogs and cats administered various nonsteroidal anti-inflammatory drugs (NSAIDs) after anesthesia,[20,23] and in cats with untreated or post-treated naturally occurring hyperthyroidism.[24–26] The most commonly used commercial assay for iohexol concentrations is offered by the Michigan State University Diagnostic Center for Population and Animal Health (http://www.animalhealth.msu.edu/); this diagnostic laboratory reports the calculated GFR after assaying serial plasma iohexol concentrations.

Radiolabeled markers validated for measurement of GFR currently used in clinical patients include chromium-51 ethylenediaminetetraacetic acid (EDTA) and technetium-99m diethylenetriamine pentaacetic acid (DTPA). These radionucleotides undergo glomerular filtration without tubular reabsorption or excretion and are stable in dog and cat blood samples but have short half-lives in vivo; this permits storage and shipping of samples to outside laboratories for assay of plasma clearance while patients are cleared of radioactivity and able to be released to owners within 24 to 48 hours.[27] Use of radiolabeled markers is limited, however, to specialty practices that are appropriately licensed to perform nuclear medicine–based testing. Radionucleotide GFR assays have been safely used to study renal function in anesthetized dogs,[28] in cats with solid tumors administered nephrotoxic chemotherapeutic agents,[29] and in dogs and cats with naturally occurring (cats with polycystic kidney disease[30] or azotemic chronic kidney disease[31]) or induced (cats with rejection of transplanted kidneys[32] or dogs that had previously undergone renal biopsy[33]) kidney disease (**Box 1**).

Although serial measurement of plasma iohexol or radionucleotides can be used to determine total, or global, GFR, these assays cannot determine the relative contributions of the right versus left kidney (ie, per-kidney GFR) to total renal excretion. Clinical use of per-kidney GFR is most commonly recommended in dogs or cats requiring unilateral nephrectomy (for example, due to presence of a renal tumor) but which have confirmed or suspected bilateral renal dysfunction. In these animals, determining both global and per-kidney GFR allows clinicians to predict the whether removal of the right or left kidney will result in renal failure and worsened quality of life.

Global and per-kidney GFR measurement can be determined using either iohexol or radionucleotide markers, when performed in tandem with advanced diagnostic imaging studies. CT of the abdomen in conjunction with iohexol allows per-kidney uptake of marker to be compared.[17] The ratio of uptake in the right versus left kidneys can then be used to calculate the per-kidney GFR. Gamma camera imaging of the abdomen after bolus administration of radionucleotide allows a similar comparison of marker uptake by each kidney over time and estimation of per-kidney GFR (**Box 2**).[8,34,35]

URINARY FRACTIONAL EXCRETION OF ELECTROLYTES

The kidneys are the primary organs responsible for excretion of electrolytes at times of excess and conservation at times of deficiency. Nonprotein-bound electrolytes are freely filtered through the glomeruli and then reabsorbed by electrolyte-specific exchange receptors throughout the proximal convoluted tubule, loop of Henle, and distal convoluted tubule. The rate of electrolyte reabsorption depends on multiple factors,

Box 1
Clinical scenarios: measurement of glomerular filtration rate

Case 1

An 8-year-old spayed female Shetland sheepdog was evaluated for polyuria and polydipsia of 3 months' duration. The owners reported that the dog had been urinating large volumes of clear urine every 2 to 3 hours and emptying the water bowl multiple times per day; however, the urine stream appeared normal without any associated straining, and the dog was otherwise acting normal with unchanged appetite and activity level. Physical examination of the dog was unremarkable, but the bladder was distended with a large volume of urine. All values on complete blood cell count and serum biochemistry panel were within reference range, although serum creatinine concentration were at the upper end of the reference range (1.2 mg/dL; reference range, 0.3–1.4 mg/dL). Urine specific gravity was 1.009 on 2 different occasions and the remainder of the urinalysis unremarkable. Abdominal radiography revealed that the kidneys were bilaterally smaller than expected and slightly misshapen.

Differential diagnoses for a dog with polyuria and polydipsia and unremarkable physical examination and minimum database may include atypical hypoadrenocorticism, central or primary nephrogenic diabetes insipidus, hyperadrenocorticism infections with lipopolysaccharide-producing bacteria, liver dysfunction, psychogenic polydipsia, and renal insufficiency. Loss of urine concentrating ability occurs in dogs with approximately 66% loss of total nephron function. Azotemia may not be noted, however, until 75% of nephrons are lost; during the intervening period (ie, damage to approximately 66%–75% of total nephrons) dogs may be polyuric and polydipsic due to kidney injury, but serum creatinine and blood urea nitrogen concentrations remain within reference ranges. This scenario, termed *renal insufficiency*, rather than *renal failure*, is of particular concern in this dog given the repeatable isosthenuria and appearance of the kidneys on abdominal radiographs.

Plasma iohexol clearance determination of GFR was performed in this dog using 1 mL/kg of iohexol containing 300 mg/mL elemental iodine/mL (Omnipaque 300 (iohexol) injection, GE Healthcare, Princeton, New Jersey); blood samples were collected 2, 3, and 4 hours after administration. Calculated GFR result was 0.9 mL/min/kg (reference range, 2.89–8.07 mL/min/kg), supporting a presumptive diagnosis of renal insufficiency. Ultrasonographic examination of the abdomen was recommended to better characterize the dog's kidney disease; bilateral dilatation of the renal pelves was noted with echogenic debris. Aerobic bacterial culture of urine resulted in greater than 100,000 colony-forming units/mL of *Staphylococcus aureus* and a 6-week course of amoxicillin-clavulanic acid was prescribed for a presumptive diagnosis of bilateral pyelonephritis. The owners reported that after 2-weeks of therapy, the dog's polyuria and polydipsia had resolved, and 2 weeks after the end of antibiotic therapy, repeat aerobic culture of urine did not result in any growth, and repeat GFR measurement revealed plasma iohexol clearance had increased to 3.27 mL/min/kg.

Case 2

An 11-year-old castrated male Labrador retriever was evaluated for a gradual decrease in activity level over the previous year and left hind limb lameness after playing with the other dogs in the household. Orthopedic examination and radiographs of both hind limbs were consistent with moderate osteoarthritis of both stifles and hocks. Two years before the current evaluation, this dog had been diagnosed with leptospirosis-induced acute renal failure (serum creatinine concentration 5.7 mg/dL); aggressive treatment with intravenous fluids and antibiotics were successful in resolving the azotemia (current serum creatinine concentration is 1.3 mg/dL).

NSAIDs are the mainstay treatment of osteoarthritis in dogs but may induce or exacerbate kidney injury. Unfortunately, these owners declined treatment with alternative analgesics due to cost concerns. Although serum creatinine concentration is within the laboratory reference range, there is a concern that sufficient residual chronic kidney injury may be present from the previous leptospirosis infection, such that there is an increased likelihood of drug nephrotoxicity but not enough to currently result in azotemia. Samples were submitted for determination of plasma iohexol clearance, and calculated GFR was 1.4 mL/min/kg, or approximately 50% of the lower end of the laboratory reference range (2.89–8.07 mL/min/kg). The prescribed NSAID was, therefore, reduced by 50% of the recommended milligram/kilogram dosage; 2 years later, the owners reported that the dog's lameness and activity level were much improved, and serum creatinine concentration remained within reference range.

> **Box 2**
> **Clinical scenario: measurement of global and per-kidney glomerular filtration rate**
>
> An 11-year-old, spayed female domestic shorthaired cat was evaluated for gross hematuria of 2 weeks' duration. On physical examination, a midabdominal mass was palpated in the region of the left kidney, and the right kidney was slightly smaller than expected. Ultrasonographic examination of the abdomen revealed a large mass completely effacing the normal left kidney parenchyma, and several hyperechoic, wedge-shaped lesions in the right kidney extending from the renal medulla up to the cortical surface, consistent with chronic infarction. Serum creatinine concentration was 1.9 mg/dL (reference range, 0.2–1.6 mg/dL).
>
> Based on the serum creatinine concentration and ultrasonographic abnormalities, this cat likely had International Renal Interest Society stage 2 chronic kidney disease. Unilateral nephrectomy was recommended after further diagnostic evaluation failed to reveal any metastases; however, there was concern that further reduction in functional nephrons after nephrectomy would result in worsening of azotemia, uremia, and unacceptable quality of life. Global and per-kidney GFR were, therefore, measured via technetium-99m DTPA and gamma camera imaging to determine both the current total renal function and the percent contribution of the mass-containing kidney.
>
> Global GFR in this cat was 0.6 mL/min/kg (reference range, 1.15–2.73 mL/min/kg). The ratio of nucleotide uptake in the left, mass-containing kidney versus the right kidney was 1:9 (ie, 10% of total GFR vs 90% of total GFR). Based on the low contribution of the left kidney to total renal function, nephrectomy was performed. One month after surgery, the cat's serum creatinine was 2.7 mg/dL, and the owners report no abnormal clinical signs.

including dietary concentrations, renal function, various hormones (including parathyroid hormone and aldosterone), rate of ultrafiltrate flow through the nephron, and need to conserve or excrete water based on intravascular volume status.[36] Calculating the percent excretion of an electrolyte in relation to that electrolyte's serum concentration and correcting for filtration rate based excretion of creatinine is FE.

Although urine collection over a 24-hour period is most accurate for determining FE of electrolytes, spot samples of simultaneously collected urine and plasma provide clinically reasonable approximations of total daily excretion despite some variability.[37] The formula for calculating FE of a given electrolyte, E, is

$$\%FE = \frac{(\text{Urine concentration of E}) \times (\text{Plasma concentration of creatinine})}{(\text{Urine concentration of creatinine}) \times (\text{Plasma concentration of E})} \times 100$$

Because of the many factors that may influence FE, there are no definable reference ranges for dogs or cats with plasma electrolyte concentrations within reference range; however, as a general rule, FE of sodium should be low (<1%) whereas FE of potassium is high (up to 25%).[38,39]

Clinical use of electrolyte FE is limited due to the variety of influencing endogenous and exogenous factors. In select cases of increased or decreased serum electrolyte concentrations, however, FE may allow clinicians to prioritize differential diagnoses. Most laboratories that perform serum biochemical analyses are able to assay urine concentrations of creatinine and electrolytes. Dogs and cats in which FE of 1 or more electrolytes is considered should be fed a consistent diet before testing (the author suggests at least 1 week before submission of samples) to minimize food-associated fluctuations in urine electrolyte excretion. Dehydration should also be corrected and normal hydration should persist for several days, because healthy kidneys reabsorb excess sodium in an effort to restore water balance (under the influence of aldosterone). Interpretation of results requires forehand consideration of (1) serum electrolyte concentrations: animals with a given electrolyte concentration greater than reference range should have greater-than-expected FE of that electrolyte and vice versa; (2) possible endocrine diseases: several endocrine diseases alter renal excretion and reabsorption of electrolytes—for example, excess parathyroid hormone (ie, in animals with primary hyperparathyroidism) promotes calcium reabsorption from the urine and phosphorus excretion, whereas insufficient aldosterone (ie, in animals with hypoadrenocorticism) results in decreased sodium reabsorption and excessive potassium reuptake in the distal convoluted tubule; and (3) renal function: in most dogs and cats with either acute or chronic kidney failure, serum electrolyte concentrations remain within reference range despite widespread nephron injury; this likely occurs because remaining nephrons and undamaged segments of diseased nephrons are able to compensate for the increased per-nephron excretion or reabsorption requirements—a potassium-wasting nephropathy, however, has been historically reported in cats (although the prevalence of this disease is now low for unknown reasons), renal secondary hyperparathyroidism unpredictably alters FE of calcium and phosphorus, and animals with severe polyuria may be unable to appropriately reabsorb electrolytes due to high rate of ultrafiltrate flow through the nephron. Because of these many interrelated factors and the difficulty predicting total expected effect on electrolyte excretion in a given patient, the clinical use of FE is limited; nevertheless, on occasion these tests may be cost-effective when prioritizing a limited number of differential diagnoses (**Box 3**).

URINARY BIOMARKERS OF KIDNEY INJURY

Biomarkers are physiologic molecules (usually proteins) that increase or decrease in association with normal or pathologic processes.[40] As discussed previously, serum creatinine concentration is relatively insensitive for early detection of renal injury; therefore, serum and urinary biomarkers that increase with early kidney damage have been the focus of many studies in people with naturally occurring disease and laboratory animal models of nephrotoxicity. Serum and plasma biomarkers seem less sensitive and have poorer correlation with presence or severity of kidney injury than urinary biomarkers. Clinical use of these biomarker proteins requires normalization to urine creatinine (ie, urine biomarker:creatinine ratio) to correct for changes rate and volume of urine production: with changes in urine volume, biomarker and creatinine concentrations are expected to proportionally increase or decrease.[41] A few urinary biomarker assays are offered by diagnostic laboratories, although clinical validation in dogs and cats is still limited.

Commercially Available Urinary Biomarkers of Renal Injury

Urine albumin/microalbuminuria

The majority of plasma albumin is size excluded and charge excluded from the ultrafiltrate; glomerular damage results in increased passage of albumin into the urine.[42] Although conventional urine dipsticks are the standard initial screening test for detection of proteinuria, urine albumin concentration must be approximately 30 mg/dL or greater to be detected by this method. Normal urine albumin concentration in dogs and cats, however, is significantly lower than this limit of detection: although there are slight differences between these species, the upper end of the reference range is approximately 1 mg/dL.[43] The range between these numbers (1–30 mg/dL) is referred to as mALB, whereas proteinuria greater than 30 mg/dL is termed *overt proteinuria*. Detection of mALB may allow earlier diagnosis of pathologically increased urine protein excretion, which can occur with primary glomerular diseases or extrarenal inflammatory diseases that secondarily damage the kidneys. Just as with overt

---

Box 3
Clinical scenario: fractional excretion of electrolytes

A 12-year-old spayed female Persian cat was evaluated for routine dental cleaning. The owner reported that the cat was healthy and active and the appetite normal and on physical examination the body condition was appropriate, despite the owner reporting that for the previous 6 months she had been feeding a home-prepared organic, vegetarian mixture of rice, tofu, and blenderized carrots and green beans. She had been previously instructed to supplement the diet with an adult human-strength multivitamin once per day but admits that she has difficulty administering medications by mouth to the cat and has not followed this recommendation for at least 2 months. Complete blood cell count, serum biochemical analysis, and urinalysis were performed before anesthesia for the dental cleaning; the only abnormality noted was moderate hypokalemia (2.1 mEq/L, reference range, 3.2–5.3 mEq/L). Serum concentration of creatinine was within the reported reference range (0.9 mg/dL; reference range, 0.2–1.6 mg/dL), and indirect systolic blood pressure was 175 mm Hg.

Differential diagnoses for hypokalemia in cats included hyperaldosteronism (due to an aldosterone-secreting adrenal tumor), potassium wasting renal disease, diet-related causes (ie, insufficient dietary concentration), and gastric or proximal duodenal obstruction with protracted vomiting and secondary metabolic alkalosis. In a patient with diet-related hypokalemia (as was suspected in this cat) or protracted vomiting (which was unlikely given the reported history), the kidneys would be expected to maximize potassium reabsorption, resulting in a very low to negligible FE of this electrolyte. In contrast, cats with hyperaldosteronism or potassium wasting renal disease would be expected to have an inappropriate FE of potassium. Ultrasonographic examination of the abdomen was recommended to determine whether or not an adrenal mass was present, because hyperaldosteronism in cats often results in hypertension (which was noted during the initial examination). The owner was reluctant to consent to this diagnostic test, however, due to expense.

Given the primary differentials for this cat's hypokalemia (insufficient dietary concentration of potassium or primary hyperaldosteronism), FE of potassium was determined. Urine concentration of creatinine was 250 mg/dL, and urine potassium of creatinine was 15.2 mEq/L. Substituting these values into the FE formula,

$$\%FE = \frac{(\text{Urine concentration of } K^+) \times (\text{Plasma concentration of creatinine})}{(\text{Urine concentration of creatinine}) \times (\text{Plasma concentration of } K^+)} \times 100$$

$$\%FE = \frac{(15.2 \text{ mEq/L}) \times (0.9 \text{ mg/dL})}{(250 \text{ mg/dL}) \times (2.1 \text{ mEq/L})} \times 100 = 2.6\%$$

The low FE of potassium was more consistent with increased reabsorption of electrolytes by the kidneys in response to hypokalemia, and therefore, a presumptive diagnosis of insufficient dietary potassium, resulting in hypokalemia was made. Conversely, hyperaldosteronism would have been expected to result in an inappropriately high potassium FE, because this hormone induces potassium excretion in the distal convoluted tubule. The owner was advised to supplement the cat with a potassium gluconate paste (she declined to feed a more balanced diet). Reevaluation of serum potassium concentration after 3 weeks of paste administration confirmed that all electrolytes were now within the laboratory reference range.

---

proteinuria, however, mALB may be due to preglomerular, glomerular, or postglomerular causes.[43]

There are strong associations between presence and magnitude of mALB and poor outcome in people. mALB is a strong prognostic indicator for later development of renal failure in diabetic patients; presence of mALB is also correlated with cardiovascular disease and death in patients with type 1 or type 2 diabetes mellitus.[44–46] Successful therapy with angiotensin-converting ednzyme inhibitors and better glycemic control slow the progression of mALB to overt proteinuria and decreases the likelihood of eventual azotemia and end-stage renal disease.[45] Other inflammatory diseases associated with mALB in people include some neoplasms, inflammatory bowel disease, and acute inflammatory conditions, such as pancreatitis and myocardial infarction; in many of these diseases, the magnitude of mALB correlates with severity.[46] This correlation is particularly evident in people with lung or breast cancer or lymphoma, where presence and magnitude of mALB are associated with histologic subtype, tumor burden, presence or absence of metastatic disease, and median survival time.

The E.R.D.-HealthScreen (Heska, Loveland, Colorado) is a point-of-care test for detection of mALB. These assays are species specific, and separate kits must be purchased for detection of mALB in dogs versus cats. Urine samples are diluted to a standard concentration, thus correcting for urine specific gravity. Unfortunately, the E.R.D.-HealthScreen is only semiquantitative rather than providing a precise measurement of mALB: results are reported as negative, low positive, medium positive, or high positive. Additionally, these tests were developed for use in all dogs and cats, but mALB reference ranges for mALB may vary based on breed and age.[47]

mALB occurs in approximately one-third of dogs and cats presenting to veterinary teaching hospitals for a variety of conditions, and greater than 50% of critically ill dogs have urine protein in the mALB range but do not have increased urine protein:creatinine ratios.[48–50] mALB has been demonstrated to occur before overt proteinuria in dogs with hereditary X-linked nephritis[51] and in soft-coated wheaten terriers with protein-losing nephropathy.[52] Dogs with lymphoma or osteosarcoma have normal urine protein:creatinine ratios but often have mALB; whether urine protein correlates with tumor burden or remission status is unknown.[53] Dogs with heartworm disease develop mALB before overt proteinuria, and histologic evidence of glomerular disease is evident at the time of mALB development.[54] Other inflammatory conditions found in dogs with mALB include renal failure, pancreatitis, and cardiovascular disease, although it is unknown whether presence of mALB correlates with prognosis or glomerular injury.[48,55] Unlike in people, strenuous exercise does not cause transient mALB in dogs.[56] mALB is more common in cats with chronic kidney disease, hypertension, or hyperthyroidism, and presence and greater magnitude of mALB are associated with decreased survival time.[49,50,57–60]

It is still unclear when or how much further diagnostic investigation or therapeutic intervention is indicated in mALB-positive animals. Dogs and cats in which mALB has been detected should first have urine protein:creatinine ratios determined to quantitate the severity of proteinuria. Breeds known to develop hereditary glomerular diseases should likely be monitored regularly, and if magnitude of mALB increases, then further steps should be considered. In dogs or cats with unexpected, persistently positive E.R.D.-HealthScreen results, it may be advised to screen for glomerular diseases and/or extrarenal inflammatory diseases. No doubt, long-term longitudinal studies evaluating the benefit of these recommendations are still needed. It is unknown whether antiproteinuria therapies in animals with mALB are of any benefit.

Urine γ-glutamyl transpeptidase:creatinine ratio

Serum concentrations of the transmembrane amino acid transporter γ-glutamyl transpeptidase (GGT) are commonly used in the diagnostic evaluation of dogs and cats with hepatic or biliary tract disease. GGT is expressed in several other tissues, however, including the apical surface of proximal convoluted tubular epithelial cells, which release small amounts of GGT into the urine. Several studies in dogs with naturally occurring or experimentally induced kidney disease have demonstrated that the urine GGT:creatinine ratio is a sensitive early marker of tubular injury, oftentimes increasing before rises in serum creatinine concentration, decreases in GFR or urine specific gravity, or appearance of casts in urine sediment. Dogs with gentamicin-induced renal failure have increased urine GGT activity 24 hours after initial dosing, whereas serum creatinine concentration did not increase above reference range until 7 days of drug administration[61–63]; 50% of intact female dogs with pyometra have moderate to high increases in urine GGT:creatinine ratios before ovariohysterectomy, which then gradually decrease over the 10 days after surgery.[64]

Urine GGT is labile, and samples should be assayed within 24 hours or frozen. Reference range in normal dogs for urine GGT:creatinine ratio is wide (1.93–28.57 IU/g), likely due to interindividual variation rather than circadian changes in excretion.[65,66] Anecdotally, and in the personal experience of the author, baseline assay of urine GGT:creatinine in patients of interest followed by serial measurement is of greater clinical utility than comparison to the suggested reference range (**Box 4**).

Selected Investigational Urinary Biomarkers of Renal Injury

Cystatin C
CysC is an inhibitor of endogenous extracellular proteinases that is produced by all nucleated cells, freely filtered across the glomerulus, and reabsorbed by renal tubular cells. Serum concentrations of CysC increase as GFR decreases, and urine concentrations increase after tubular injury. Utility of absolute urine CysC concentrations and CysC:creatinine ratio in the prediction of presence, severity, and outcome of acute kidney injury in people is unclear, because prospective studies have yielded conflicting results. A single study in dogs with either acute kidney injury or chronic kidney disease evaluated urine CysC:creatinine ratio and confirmed greater excretion than in healthy dogs.[67] Several CysC assays are available for research studies using canine plasma or urine but not clinical patients.

Interleukin 18
Interleukin 18 (IL-18) is a proinflammatory cytokine that polarizes helper T cells toward a T_H1 phenotype, induces interferon-γ production and release, and enhances

---

Box 4
Clinical scenario: urine GGT:creatinine ratio

A 6-year-old castrated male Rottweiler was evaluated for tachypnea associated with aspiration pneumonia due to idiopathic megaesophagus. The dog had been appropriately treated for multiple episodes of bacterial pneumonia over the preceding 2 years, with antibiotic therapy guided by sensitivity testing of aerobic bacterial cultures of transtracheal washings. The most recent culture indicated infection with *Escherichia coli*, resistant to all tested antibiotics other than aminoglycosides and carbapenems. Because of cost concerns, the owners elected home subcutaneous administration of amikacin for treatment; they also voiced monetary concerns when told that repeat thoracic radiographs would be required to guide duration of antibiotic therapy.

Before the first dose of amikacin, urine GGT:creatinine ratio was 3.72 IU/g, urine specific gravity was 1.042 without any casts noted, and serum creatinine concentration was 0.9 mg/dL. Two days after the first injection, the owners reported by tachypnea had resolved; urine GGT:creatinine ratio was 4.55 IU/g with a specific gravity of 1.045 and no casts were noted. Five days after beginning treatment, urine GGT:creatinine ratio had increased further to 7.21 IU/g, urine specific gravity was 1.035, and urine sediment remained benign. Eight days after initiating antibiotic therapy, urine specific gravity was 1.039, but GGT:creatinine ratio had tripled from baseline to 10.48, so amikacin administration was discontinued. Two weeks after discontinuing treatment, a lateral thoracic radiograph revealed resolution of previously noted interstitial and alveolar radio-opacities.

production of complement-activating IgG subclasses. Serum and urinary IL-18 concentrations increase in people with acute kidney injury, chronic kidney disease, and glomerular disease.[68–72] Increased IL-18 mRNA or serum concentrations have been reported in dogs with various inflammatory diseases, including autoimmune thyroiditis,[73] immune-mediated hemolytic anemia,[74] and sinonasal aspergillosis[75]; increased serum concentrations of this cytokine are associated with greater likelihood of death in dogs with immune-mediated hemolytic anemia.[74] Although IL-18 expression has been demonstrated in Madin-Darby canine kidney cells (a commonly used laboratory cell line),[76] in vivo investigations have not been performed in dogs with experimentally induced or naturally occurring kidney disease as yet.

Kidney injury molecule-1
Kidney injury molecule-1 (KIM-1) is a transmembrane protein normally found in healthy proximal convoluted tubular cells and shed into the urine at low concentrations. KIM-1 expression is rapidly up-regulated, however, by tubular epithelium after kidney injury, and KIM-1:creatinine concentration increases. Urinary KIM-1 increases in people with ischemic, nephrotoxic, or septic renal damage, polycystic kidney disease, and renal neoplasia.[77–79] Although in vitro expression of KIM-1 has been confirmed in Madin-Darby canine kidney cells, there are as yet no published in vivo studies of KIM-1 in dogs or cats.[79] A KIM-1 assay is available for canine urine (MILLIPLEX MAP Canine Kidney Toxicity Magnet Bead Panel 1, EMD Millipore Corporation, Billerica, Massachusetts) in conjunction with CysC and clusterin (a proposed biomarker not discussed in this article) but is only marketed for research purposes.

N-acetyl-β-D-glucosaminidase
N-acetyl-β-D-glucosaminidase (NAG) is an intracellular protein that participates in glycosaminoglycan catabolism; glycoproteins reabsorbed by proximal convoluted tubular cells are degraded by NAG and other lysosomal enzymes.[80] Increased urine excretion occurs in people with proximal tubular epithelial cell damage, particularly with acute kidney injury. Urinary NAG:creatinine ratio is increased in dogs with chronic kidney disease,[81,82] pyelonephritis,[81] uncontrolled diabetes mellitus,[81] pyometra,[81] or X-linked hereditary nephropathy[83] but does not differ before versus after control of hyperadrenocorticism with trilostane or transphenoidal hypophysectomy.[84] In cats, urinary NAG:creatinine ratio increases with chronic kidney disease.[85,86] Assays for urine retinol binding protein (RBP) are marketed for research use only.

Neutrophil gelatinase–associated lipocalin
Neutrophil gelatinase–associated lipocalin (NGAL) is an intracellular protein of hepatocytes, neutrophil granules, and epithelial cells, including the tubular epithelium of the thick ascending loop of Henle and collecting ducts.[87] Expression of NGAL is low in healthy tissues but in response to inflammation is up-regulated and plays a role in stabilizing and potentiating matrix metalloproteinases and sequestering iron, thereby inhibiting bacterial growth. Urinary NGAL:creatinine ratio is more sensitive than serum creatinine concentration for detection of acute kidney injury in people, and increases with progression of chronic kidney disease.[88,89] A few studies in dogs have investigated the utility of NGAL as a biomarker of renal damage; increases before serum creatinine concentration have been reported in laboratory dogs with gentamicin nephrotoxicity[90] or X-linked hereditary nephropathy[83] and in privately owned dogs with naturally occurring acute kidney injury or chronic kidney disease.[91] A canine-specific urine NGAL assay is available for research use only (BioPorto Diagnostics, Gentofte, Denmark).

Retinol binding protein

RBPs complex with and transport retinol (vitamin A). The plasma isoenzyme–retinol complex binds to transthyretin, which prevents passage of the low-molecular-weight (21-kDa) RBP protein across the glomerular filtration barrier.[92] In the absence of retinol, RBP undergoes a conformational change that prevents binding to transthyretin, passes into the glomerular ultrafiltrate, and is reabsorbed by proximal convoluted tubule cells. Tubular epithelial injury of any cause in people impairs RBP reabsorption and increases the urine RBP:creatinine ratio. Similarly, increased urinary excretion of RBP has been demonstrated in dogs with chronic kidney disease,[82] untreated hyperadrenocorticism,[84] and X-linked hereditary nephropathy[83] and in cats with untreated hyperthyroidism.[26,93] Assays for RBP can be purchased for laboratory use but are not offered by commercial laboratories for clinical patients.

REFERENCES

1. Von Hendy-Willson VE, Pressler BM. An overview of glomerular filtration rate testing in dogs and cats. Vet J 2011;188:156–65.
2. Watson AD, Lefebvre HP, Concordet D, et al. Plasma exogenous creatinine clearance test in dogs: comparison with other methods and proposed limited sampling strategy. J Vet Intern Med 2002;16:22–33.
3. La Garreres AL, Laroute V, De La Farge F, et al. Disposition of plasma creatinine in non-azotemic and moderately azotemic cats. J Feline Med Surg 2007;9:89–96.
4. van Hoek I, Vandermeulen E, Duchateau L, et al. Comparison and reproducibility of plasma clearance of exogenous creatinine, exo-iohexol, and endo-iohexol and ^{51}Cr-EDTA in young adult and aged healthy cats. J Vet Intern Med 2007;21:950–8.
5. Lefebvre HP, Craig AJ, Braun JP. GFR in the dog: breed effect [abstract]. In: Proceedings of the 16th ECVIM-CA Congress. Munich, Germany: European College of Veterinary Internal Medicine–Companion Animals; 2006. p. 261.
6. Robinson T, Harbison M, Bovee KC. Influence of reduced renal mass on tubular secretion of creatinine in dog. Am J Vet Res 1974;35:487–91.
7. Ross LA, Finco DR. Relationship of selected clinical renal function tests to glomerular filtration rate and renal blood flow in cats. Am J Vet Res 1981;42:1704–10.
8. Uribe D, Krawiec DR, Twardock AR, et al. Quantitative renal scintigraphic determination of the glomerular filtration rate in cats with normal and abnormal kidney function, using 99mTc-diethylenetriaminepentaacetic acid. Am J Vet Res 1992;53:1101–7.
9. Antognoni MT, Siepi D, Porciello F, et al. Serum cystatin-C evaluation in dogs affected by different diseases associated or not with renal insufficiency. Vet Res Commun 2007;31:269–71.
10. Wehner A, Hartmann K, Hirschberger J. Utility of serum cystatin C as a clinical measure of renal function in dogs. J Am Anim Hosp Assoc 2008;44:131–8.
11. Miyagawa Y, Takemura N, Hirose H. Evaluation of the measurement of serum cystatin C by an enzyme-linked immunosorbent assay for humans as a marker of the glomerular filtration rate in dogs. J Vet Med Sci 2009;71:1169–76.
12. Sanderson SL. Measuring glomerular filtration rate: practical use of clearance tests. In: Bonagura JD, Twedt DC, editors. Kirk's veterinary therapy XIV. St Louis (MO): Saunders Elsevier; 2009. p. 868–71.
13. Mutzel W, Speck U. Pharmacokinetics and biotransformation of iohexol in the rat and the dog. Acta Radiol Suppl 1980;362:87–92.

14. Nossen JO, Jakobsen JA, Kjaersgaard P, et al. Elimination of the non-ionic X-ray contrast media iodixanol and iohexol in patients with severely impaired renal function. Scand J Clin Lab Invest 1995;55:341–50.

15. Rudnick MR, Goldfarb S, Wexler L, et al. Nephrotoxicity of ionic and nonionic contrast media in 1196 patients: a randomized trial. The iohexol cooperative study. Kidney Int 1995;47:254–61.

16. Goy-Thollot I, Chafotte C, Besse S, et al. Iohexol plasma clearance in healthy dogs and cats. Vet Radiol Ultrasound 2006;47:168–73.

17. O'Dell-Anderson KJ, Twardock R, Grimm JB, et al. Determination of glomerular filtration rate in dogs using contrast-enhanced computed tomography. Vet Radiol Ultrasound 2006;47:127–35.

18. Bexfield NH, Heiene R, Gerritsen RJ, et al. Glomerular filtration rate estimated by 3-sample plasma clearance of iohexol in 118 healthy dogs. J Vet Intern Med 2008;22:66–73.

19. Miyamoto K. Use of plasma clearance of iohexol for estimating glomerular filtration rate in cats. Am J Vet Res 2001;62:572–5.

20. Goodman LA, Brown SA, Torres BT, et al. Effects of meloxicam on plasma iohexol clearance as a marker of glomerular filtration rate in conscious healthy cats. Am J Vet Res 2009;70:826–30.

21. Heiene R, Reynolds BS, Bexfield NH, et al. Estimation of glomerular filtration rate via 2- and 4-sample plasma clearance of iohexol and creatinine in clinically normal cats. Am J Vet Res 2009;70:176–85.

22. Von-Hendy-Willson VE, Pressler BM, Sandoval RM, et al. Rapid determination of GFR in dogs with acute kidney injury using a portable fluorescence ratiometric analyzer [abstract N/U 5]. J Vet Intern Med 2011;25:717–8.

23. Kongara K, Chambers P, Johnson CB. Glomerular filtration rate after tramadol, parecoxib and pindolol following anaesthesia and analgesia in comparison with morphine in dogs. Vet Anaesth Analg 2009;36:86–94.

24. Becker TJ, Graves TK, Kruger JM, et al. Effects of methimazole on renal function in cats with hyperthyroidism. J Am Anim Hosp Assoc 2000;36:215–23.

25. Boag AK, Neiger R, Slater L, et al. Changes in the glomerular filtration rate of 27 cats with hyperthyroidism after treatment with radioactive iodine. Vet Rec 2007; 161:711–5.

26. van Hoek I, Lefebvre HP, Peremans K, et al. Short- and long-term follow-up of glomerular and tubular renal markers of kidney function in hyperthyroid cats after treatment with radioiodine. Domest Anim Endocrinol 2009;36: 45–56.

27. Krawiec DR, Twardock AR, Badertscher RR 2nd, et al. Use of 99mTc diethylene-triaminepentaacetic acid for assessment of renal function in dogs with suspected renal disease. J Am Vet Med Assoc 1988;192:1077–80.

28. Fusellier M, Desfontis J, Madec S, et al. Influence of three anesthetic protocols on glomerular filtration rate in dogs. Am J Vet Res 2007;68:807–11.

29. Bailey DB, Rassnick KM, Erb HN, et al. Effect of glomerular filtration rate on clearance and myelotoxicity of carboplatin in cats with tumors. Am J Vet Res 2004;65:1502–7.

30. Reichle JK, DiBartola SP, Leveille R. Renal ultrasonographic and computed tomographic appearance, volume, and function of cats with autosomal dominant polycystic kidney disease. Vet Radiol Ultrasound 2002;43:368–73.

31. Deguchi E, Akuzawa M. Renal clearance of endogenous creatinine, urea, sodium, and potassium in normal cats and cats with chronic renal failure. J Vet Med Sci 1997;59:509–12.

32. Halling KB, Graham JP, Newell SP, et al. Sonographic and scintigraphic evaluation of acute renal allograft rejection in cats. Vet Radiol Ultrasound 2003;44: 707–13.
33. Groman RP, Bahr A, Berridge BR. Effects of serial ultrasound-guided renal biopsies on kidneys of healthy adolescent dogs. Vet Radiol Ultrasound 2004;45: 62–9.
34. Barthez PY, Hornof WJ, Cowgill LD, et al. Comparison between the scintigraphic uptake and plasma clearance of Tc-99mdiethylenetriaminepentacetic acid (DTPA) for the evaluation of the glomerular filtration rate in dogs. Vet Radiol Ultrasound 1998;39:470–4.
35. Kampa N, Lord P, Maripuu E. Effect of observer variability on glomerular filtration rate measurement by renal scintigraphy in dogs. Vet Radiol Ultrasound 2006;47: 212–21.
36. Lefebvre HP, Dossin D, Trumel C, et al. Fractional excretion tests: a critical review of methods and applications in domestic animals. Vet Clin Pathol 2008; 37:4–20.
37. Finco DR, Brown SS, Barsanti JA, et al. Reliability of using random urine samples for "spot" determination of fractional excretion of electrolytes in cats. Am J Vet Res 1997;58:1184–7.
38. Adams LG, Polzin DJ, Osborne CA, et al. Comparison of fractional excretion and 24-hour urinary excretion of sodium and potassium in clinically normal cats and cats with induced chronic renal failure. Am J Vet Res 1991;52:718–22.
39. Corea M, Seeliger E, Boemke W, et al. Diurnal pattern of sodium secretion in dogs with and without chronically reduced renal perfusion pressure. Kidney Blood Press Res 1996;19:16–23.
40. Biomarkers Definitions Working Group. Biomarkers and surrogate endpoints: preferred definitions and conceptual framework. Clin Pharmacol Ther 2001;69: 89–95.
41. Waikar SS, Sabbisetti VS, Bonventre JV. Normalization of urinary biomarkers to creatinine during changes in glomerular filtration rate. Kidney Int 2010;78: 486–94.
42. Russo LM, Sandoval RM, McKee M, et al. The normal kidney filters nephrotic levels of albumin retrieved by proximal tubule cells: retrieval is disrupted in nephrotic states. Kidney Int 2007;71:504–13.
43. Grauer GF. Proteinuria: measurement and interpretation. Top Companion Anim Med 2011;26:121–7.
44. Mogensen CE, Chachati A, Christensen CK, et al. Microalbuminuria: an early marker of renal involvement in diabetes. Uremia Invest 1985–1986;9:85–95.
45. Viberti GC, Hill RD, Jarrett RJ. Microalbuminuria as a predictor of clinical nephropathy in insulin-dependent diabetes mellitus. Lancet 1982;1:1430–2.
46. Gosling P. Microalbuminuria: a marker of systemic disease. Br J Hosp Med 1995;54:285–90.
47. Radecki S, Donnelly RE, Jensen WA, et al. Effect of age and breed on the prevalence of microalbuminuria in dogs [abstract 110]. J Vet Intern Med 2003;17:406.
48. Whittemore JC, Gill VL, Jensen WA, et al. Evaluation of the association between microalbuminuria and the urine albumin-creatinine ratio and systemic disease in dogs. J Am Vet Med Assoc 2006;229:958–63.
49. Whittemore JC, Miyoshi Z, Jensen WA, et al. Association of microalbuminuria and the urine albumin-to-creatinine ratio with systemic disease in cats. J Am Vet Med Assoc 2007;230:1165–9.

50. Vaden SL, Turman CA, Harris TL, et al. The prevalence of albuminuria in dogs and cats in an ICU or recovering from anesthesia. J Vet Emerg Crit Care (San Antonio) 2010;20:479–87.

51. Hsieh OF, Lees GE, Clark SE, et al. Development of albuminuria and overt proteinuria in heterozygous (carrier) female dogs with X-linked hereditary nephropathy (XLHN) [abstract 118]. J Vet Intern Med 2005;19:432.

52. Vaden SL, Jensen WA, Longhofer S, et al. Longitudinal study of microalbuminuria in soft-coated wheaten terriers [abstract 115]. J Vet Intern Med 2001;15:300.

53. Pressler BM, Proulx DR, Williams LE, et al. Urine albumin concentration is increased in dogs with lymphoma or osteosarcoma [abstract 101]. J Vet Intern Med 2003;17:404.

54. Grauer GF, Oberhauser EB, Basaraba RJ, et al. Development of microalbuminuria in dogs with heartworm disease [abstract 103]. J Vet Intern Med 2002;16:352.

55. Pressler BM, Vaden SL, Jensen WA, et al. Detection of canine microalbuminuria using semiquantitative test strips designed for use with human urine. Vet Clin Pathol 2002;31:56–60.

56. Gary AT, Cohn LA, Kerl ME, et al. The effects of exercise on urinary albumin excretion in dogs. J Vet Intern Med 2004;18:52–5.

57. Jepson RE, Brodbelt D, Vallance C, et al. Evaluation of predictors of the development of azotemia in cats. J Vet Intern Med 2009;23:806–13.

58. Chakrabarti S, Syme H, Elliott J. Clinicopathological variables predicting progression of azotemia in cats with chronic kidney disease. J Vet Intern Med 2012;26:275–81.

59. Jepson RE, Elliott J, Brodbelt D, et al. Effect of control of systolic blood pressure on survival in cats with systemic hypertension. J Vet Intern Med 2007;21:402–9.

60. Syme HM, Markwell PJ, Pfeiffer D, et al. Survival of cats with naturally occurring chronic renal failure is related to severity of proteinuria. J Vet Intern Med 2006;20:528–35.

61. Cronin RE, Bulger RE, Southern P, et al. Natural history of aminoglycoside nephrotoxicity in the dog. J Lab Clin Med 1980;95:463–74.

62. Frazier DL, Aucoin DP, Riviere JE. Gentamicin pharmacokinetics and nephrotoxicity in naturally acquired and experimentally induced disease in dogs. J Am Vet Med Assoc 1988;192:57–63.

63. Rivers BJ, Walter PA, O'Brien TD, et al. Evaluation of urine gamma-glutamyl transpeptidase-to-creatinine ratio as a diagnostic tool in an experimental model of aminoglycoside-induced acute renal failure in the dog. J Am Anim Hosp Assoc 1996;32:323–36.

64. Heiene R, Moe L, Mølmen G. Calculation of urinary enzyme excretion, with renal structure and function in dogs with pyometra. Res Vet Sci 2001;70:129–37.

65. Brunker JD, Ponzio NM, Payton ME. Indices of urine N-acetyl-β-D-glucosaminidase and γ-glutamyl transpeptidase activities in clinically normal adult dogs. Am J Vet Res 2009;70:297–301.

66. Uechi M, Uechi H, Nakayama T. The circadian variation of urinary N-acetyl-β-D-glucosaminidase and γ-glutamyl transpeptidase in clinically healthy cats. J Vet Med Sci 1998;60:1033–4.

67. Monti P, Benchekroun G, Berlato D, et al. Initial evaluation of canine urinary cystatin C as a marker of renal tubular function. J Small Anim Pract 2012;53:254–9.

68. Lonnemann G, Novic D, Rubinstein M, et al. Interleukin-18, interleukin-18 binding protein and impaired production of interferon-γ I in chronic kidney failure. Clin Nephrol 2003;60:327–34.

69. Parikh CR, Jani A, Melnikov VY, et al. Urinary interleukin-18 is a marker of human acute tubular necrosis. Am J Kidney Dis 2004;43:405–14.
70. Parikh CR, Abraham E, Ancukiewicz M, et al. Urine IL-18 is an early diagnostic marker for acute kidney injury and predicts mortality in the intensive care unit. J Am Soc Nephrol 2005;16:3046–52.
71. Hewins P, Morgan MD, Holden N, et al. IL-18 is upregulated in the kidney and primes neutrophil responsiveness in ANCA-associated vasculitis. Kidney Int 2006;69:605–15.
72. Pressler BM, Falk RJ, Preston CA. Interleukin-18, neutrophils, and ANCA. Kidney Int 2006;69:424–5.
73. Choi EW, Shin LS, Bhang DH, et al. Hormonal change and cytokine mRNA expression in peripheral blood mononuclear cells during the development of canine autoimmune thyroiditis. Clin Exp Immunol 2006;146:101–8.
74. Kjelgaard-Hansen M, Goggs R, Wiinberg B, et al. Use of serum concentrations of interleukin-18 and monocyte chemoattractant protein-1 as prognostic indicators in primary immune-mediated hemolytic anemia in dogs. J Vet Intern Med 2011;25:76–82.
75. Peeters D, Peters IR, Clercx C, et al. Quantification of mRNA encoding cytokines and chemokines in nasal biopsies from dogs with sino-nasal aspergillosis. Vet Microbiol 2006;114:318–26.
76. Jalilian I, Spildrejorde M, Seavers A, et al. Functional expression of the damage-associated molecular pattern receptor P2X7 on canine kidney epithelial cells. Vet Immunol Immunopathol 2012;150:228–33.
77. Huang Y, Don-Wauchope AC. The clinical utility of kidney injury molecule 1 in the prediction, diagnosis, and prognosis of acute kidney injury: a systematic review. Inflamm Allergy Drug Targets 2011;10:260–71.
78. Lim AI, Tang SC, Lai KN, et al. Kidney injury molecule-1: more than just an injury marker of tubular epithelial cells? J Cell Physiol 2012;228:917–24.
79. Kotsis F, Nitschke R, Boehlke C, et al. Ciliary calcium signaling is modulated by kidney injury molecule-1 (Kim1). Pflugers Arch 2007;453:819–29.
80. Reeko S, Soeta S, Syuto B, et al. Urinary excretion of N-acetyl-β-D-glucosaminidase and its isoenzymes in cats with urinary disease. J Vet Med Sci 2002;64: 367–71.
81. Reeko S, Soeta S, Miyazaki M, et al. Clinical availability of urinary of N-acetyl-β-D-glucosaminidase index in dogs with urinary diseases. J Vet Med Sci 2002;64: 361–5.
82. Smets PM, Meyer E, Maddens BE, et al. Urinary markers in healthy young and aged dogs and dogs with chronic kidney disease. J Vet Intern Med 2010;24: 65–72.
83. Nabity MG, Lees GE, Cianciolo R, et al. Urinary biomarkers of renal disease in dogs with X-linked hereditary nephropathy. J Vet Intern Med 2012;26: 282–93.
84. Smets PM, Lefebvre HP, Meij BP, et al. Long-term follow-up of renal function in dogs after treatment for ACTH-dependent hyperadrenocorticism. J Vet Intern Med 2012;26:565–73.
85. Jepson RE, Vallance C, Syme HM, et al. Assessment of urinary N-acetyl-β-D-glucosaminidase activity in geriatric cats with variable plasma creatinine concentrations with or without azotemia. Am J Vet Res 2010;71:241–7.
86. Lapointe C, Bélanger MC, Dunn M, et al. N-acetyl-β-D-glucosaminidase index as an early biomarker for chronic kidney disease in cats with hyperthyroidism. J Vet Intern Med 2008;22:1103–10.

87. Paragas N, Qiu A, Zhang Q, et al. The Ngal reporter mouse detects the response of the kidney to injury in real time. Nat Med 2011;17:216–22.

88. Giasson J, Li GH, Chen Y. Neutrophil gelatinase-associated lipocalin (NGAL) as a new biomarker for non-acute kidney injury (AKI) diseases. Inflamm Allergy Drug Targets 2011;10:272–82.

89. Nickolas TL, Forster CS, Sise ME, et al. NGAL (Lcn2) monomer is associated with tubulointerstitial damage in chronic kidney disease. Kidney Int 2012;82:718–22.

90. Kai K, Yamaguchi T, Yoshimatsu Y, et al. Neutrophil gelatinase-associated lipocalin, a sensitive urinary biomarker of acute kidney injury in dogs receiving gentamicin. J Toxicol Sci 2013;38:269–77.

91. Lee YJ, Hu YY, Lin YS, et al. Urine neutrophil gelatinase-associated lipocalin (NGAL) as a biomarker for acute canine kidney injury. BMC Vet Res 2012;8:248.

92. Raila J, Mathews U, Schweigert FJ. Plasma transport and tissue distribution of β-carotene vitamin A and retinol-binding protein in domestic cats. Comp Biochem Physiol A Mol Integr Physiol 2001;130:849–56.

93. van Hoek I, Meyer E, Duchateau L, et al. Retinol-binding protein in serum and urine of hyperthyroid cats before and after treatment with radioiodine. J Vet Intern Med 2009;23:1031–7.

A Laboratory Diagnostic Approach to Hepatobiliary Disease in Small Animals

Seth E. Chapman, DVM, MS[a],*, Roger A. Hostutler, DVM, MS[b]

KEYWORDS

- Hepatic disease • Enzymes • Bile acids • Bilirubin • Proteins

KEY POINTS

- Liver enzymes can be classified as leakage or induction enzymes; although they are sensitive indicators for detection of disease and/or cholestasis, they often are not specific for a primary cause.
- Increased serum enzyme activities can occur in clinically normal animals, and in animals with hepatic and nonhepatic disease.
- Serum bile acids and ammonia can be measured to evaluate hepatic function.
- Detection of other biochemical abnormalities, such as hypoproteinemia, hypoglycemia, or hypocholesterolemia, may be useful. However, these analytes are often not sensitive indicators of liver disease.

TESTING AND REFERENCE INTERVALS

Understanding the limitations of laboratory diagnostic tests for hepatobiliary disease is important in avoiding misinterpretation of results. Most of these tests are quantitative assays performed on serum or plasma samples and measured on a continuous scale. Clinical interpretation of tests results is guided by reference intervals (RI), but there is inherent overlap in results between clinically healthy and diseased animals. Animals with clinically significant disease can have "normal" test results, and clinically healthy animals can have "abnormal" results.

Determination of RI varies based on the number of test subjects (minimum of 40 based on The American Society for Veterinary Clinical Pathology guidelines) and distribution of data (Gaussian vs nonparametric).[1] Intervals are often established based

Disclosures: The authors have nothing to disclose.
[a] IDEXX Laboratories Inc, 300 East Wilson Bridge Road, Suite 200, Worthington, OH 43085, USA; [b] MedVet Medical and Cancer Centers for Pets, 300 East Wilson Bridge Road, Worthington, OH 43085, USA
* Corresponding author.
E-mail address: seth-chapman@idexx.com

on results from the central 95% of the reference group. Therefore, values from 5% of the test population of clinically healthy animals will fall outside the established interval. In effect, 2.5% of the reference population will have values above or below the RI. RI for a given analyte may vary between laboratories, and comparison of results obtained from different instruments or using different methodology must be done with caution. Adherence to quality-control guidelines and instrument maintenance with proper sample collection and handling are paramount for consistently obtaining accurate results and minimizing variation attributable to instrument or operator error.

OVERVIEW OF HEPATIC ENZYMES

- Enzymes are categorized into leakage enzymes (alanine aminotransferase [ALT], aspartate aminotransferase [AST]) indicating hepatocellular injury, and induction enzymes (alkaline phosphatase [ALP], γ-glutamyltransferase [GGT]) associated with increased synthesis.
- The severity of serum-activity elevation for leakage enzymes depends on the cellular concentration and the subcellular location. Elevation of serum activity from enzymes found within the cytosol and mitochondria suggests a greater degree of cell injury than elevation of activity from enzymes found within the cytosol alone.
- Induction enzymes are typically associated with the cell membrane, and severity of the serum-activity elevation depends on the capacity for enzyme production.
- The severity of increase of serum enzyme activity may be interpreted as a fold elevation above the upper limit of the RI. A 2-fold to 3-fold elevation is often considered of mild severity. A 4-fold to 5-fold elevation and greater than 10-fold elevation may be considered of moderate and marked severity, respectively.[2]
- The finding of elevated liver enzyme activity is commonly encountered during routine biochemical testing. Detection of a single elevated liver enzyme, particularly of mild severity, may be nonspecific and insufficient for the diagnosis of hepatobiliary disease. In a study of biochemical abnormalities detected in a large population of healthy and diseased canines of various ages, elevations of serum activity for both leakage enzymes (ALT, AST) and induction enzymes (ALP, GGT) was observed in approximately 17%, 11%, 39%, and 19% of the cases, respectively.[3]
- The diagnostic utility of serum enzyme measurement for detection of hepatobiliary disease is enhanced by evaluation of both leakage and induction enzymes, as well as correlation with additional diagnostics such as hepatic function tests or histopathology.
- The duration of increase for leakage and induction enzymes depends on the rate of clearance or half-life, and on the nature and severity of the inciting cause.

Alanine Aminotransferase

ALT is found in high concentrations in the cytoplasm of canine and feline hepatocytes, and is a useful marker of hepatocellular injury in dogs and cats. This enzyme is a catalyst in a reaction resulting in deamination of alanine with production of pyruvate for entry into the Krebs cycle or gluconeogenesis pathway.[4] The enzyme is also found in cardiac and skeletal muscle cells, renal epithelial cells, and red blood cells (RBCs). The primary clinical utility of this enzyme is detection of hepatocellular injury, although enzyme distribution in other tissues can present a diagnostic challenge. Examples include differentiating elevation of serum enzyme activity due to hepatic disease from artifactual elevation (ie, in vitro hemolysis, lipemia) or extra-hepatic origin (severe muscle trauma). Enzyme activity in skeletal and cardiac muscle is substantially less (approximately 5% and 25%) than in hepatocytes, but the capacity for elevated serum activity is considerable when factoring total body muscle mass as a potential source of ALT.[5] Correlation with serum creatine kinase (CK) activity is often useful in differentiating a muscle origin from a hepatic origin for ALT. CK activity increases quickly after muscle injury, with peak levels occurring at approximately 6 to 12 hours, although activity decreases within 24 to 48 hours owing to a short half-life.[6]

Increased serum activity of this enzyme is typically associated with alterations of permeability of the hepatocellular membrane, with potential causes including toxic insult, inflammatory disease, hypoxia, tissue trauma, and neoplasia (**Box 1**). Elevations of ALT associated with corticosteroids or phenobarbital therapy may be multifactorial because of increased enzyme synthesis and cell injury.[7] Increased ALT activity is not specific for a particular disease process, and can occur with reversible or irreversible hepatocellular injury. Although the degree of serum elevation may be roughly proportional to severity of disease and hepatic mass affected, underlying abnormality may be present in the absence of elevated enzyme activity resulting from a quantitative decrease in hepatocytes (eg, advanced cirrhosis, portosystemic shunting with atrophy). Inflammatory or necrotizing disorders are often associated with the most severe serum enzyme elevations, while moderate elevations can occur with hepatic neoplasia, biliary tract disease (obstructive or nonobstructive), and cirrhosis.[8] Mild serum enzyme elevation is nonspecific and can occur with a wide spectrum of metabolic, neoplastic, vascular, and (chronic) inflammatory disorders. There are also multiple disorders or drugs that can result in elevated serum ALT activity without the presence of significant primary hepatocellular disease (**Box 2**).

Box 1
Potential causes for elevated serum activity of ALT and AST

Hepatocellular Injury or Necrosis:

Cirrhosis

Corticosteroid hepatopathy (endogenous or exogenous)

Drug toxicity/idiosyncratic reaction

> Acetaminophen, anesthetic agents, arsenical compounds, carprofen, diazepam/oxazepam, griseofulvin, itraconazole, ketoconazole, lomustine, phenobarbital, phenytoin, primidone, mebendazole, methimazole, oxibendazole-diethylcarbamazine, tetracycline, trimethoprim-sulfadiazine

Diabetes mellitus

Hepatic lipidosis

Hypoxia (cardiac insufficiency, hepatic congestion, anemia)

Hyperthyroidism (feline)

Inflammatory disease (hepatitis, cholangiohepatitis)

> Infectious: ascending enteric bacterial infection, feline infectious peritonitis virus, liver fluke, histoplasmosis, leptospirosis

> Noninfectious: copper-associated hepatopathy (Bedlington terrier, Dalmatian, Doberman Pinscher, Labrador retriever), idiopathic chronic hepatitis

Portosystemic shunt

Toxin ingestion (aflatoxin, amanita mushroom, blue-green algae, copper, herbicides or insecticides, iron, sago palm, zinc, xylitol)

Neoplasia (primary hepatobiliary or metastatic)

Trauma

Myocyte Injury or Necrosis:

Canine musculodystrophy

Ischemia

Myositis

Trauma

Data from Refs.[4,9,10]

Box 2
Nonhepatic causes for elevated serum activity of hepatic leakage enzymes (ALT and AST)

Inflammation

Pancreatitis

Enteritis

Myositis

Infection

Urinary tract infections

Endocarditis

Pneumonia

Septic peritonitis

Pyothorax

Pyometra

Endocrine Disease

Hyperthyroidism/hypothyroidism

Hyperadrenocorticism

Diabetes mellitus

Drugs

Corticosteroids (dogs)

Antiepileptic drugs

Other

Hemolysis (AST)

Following hepatocellular injury, serum ALT levels increase within 12 hours and reach peak concentration in approximately 24 to 48 hours.[4,11] Resolution of the elevated serum enzyme activity depends on the nature of disease, such as an acute toxic insult versus an ongoing inflammatory or infectious process. ALT has a half-life of approximately 40 to 61 hours in dogs, and approximately 3.5 hours in cats.[7]

Aspartate Aminotransferase

AST is an enzyme that is present in marked quantities in the mitochondria of hepatocytes. Therefore, its elevation may indicate significant hepatocellular damage, given the mitochondria are not as readily injured as the cell membrane in many disease processes. This aspect is important because AST determined in serial samples will often normalize before ALT with resolution of hepatocellular abnormality.

However, AST is not specific to the liver, and is present in significant quantities in myocytes and RBCs. Should an elevated AST be noted, a CK, ALT, and hematocrit may be useful in determining true hepatic origin. Hemolysis can be associated with significant increases in serum AST activity.[4] The causes of an elevated AST are similar to those of ALT (see **Box 1**). There are no significant causes of a decreased AST. It is important to bear in mind that other disease processes or drugs may cause elevated AST without the presence of significant primary hepatocellular disease (see **Box 2**). AST has a half-life of approximately 12 hours in dogs and 1.5 hours in cats.[7,11]

Alkaline Phosphatase

ALP is an enzyme found in the membranes of hepatocytes that line bile canaliculi and sinusoids. An increased ALP can indicate primary hepatic disease such as cholestatic liver disease, canalicular cell necrosis, and increased hepatic synthesis. An elevated ALP in cats always warrants further investigation into underlying primary hepatic disease, because cats have less hepatocellular ALP than dogs and ALP is readily excreted by the kidneys. However, in dogs ALP is not liver specific. The elevation may be due to extrahepatic sources (kidney, pancreas, brain, bone marrow, spleen, testes, lymph node, placenta, cardiac and skeletal muscle). However, it should be noted that the magnitude of elevation resulting from extrahepatic sources is likely to be minimal, or may be secondary to endogenous or exogenous glucocorticoids and other drugs such as phenobarbital. The most common drugs that cause an elevation in ALP are shown in **Box 3**. Liver-specific ALP has a serum half-life of approximately 70 hours in the dog and 6 hours in the cat.[7]

Other than drug induction, causes for an elevated ALP can be grouped into 4 primary categories: (1) primary biliary tract disease; (2) hepatic parenchymal disease; (3) systemic disease; and (4) normal for growing dogs younger than 8 months. In these individuals, the ALP typically is increased 2 to 3 times the upper end of the RI. Common causes of ALP increases associated with categories (1) to (3) for dogs and cats are shown in **Box 4**.

Given the vast array of diseases that may be associated with an elevated ALP, systemic disease should be ruled out before more invasive diagnostics such as a liver biopsy. This aspect is important because many concurrent diseases can imitate primary liver disease in presenting clinical signs or client complaints.

γ-Glutamyltransferase

GGT is a membrane-associated enzyme found in biliary epithelial cells and hepatocytes, as well as in pancreatic, renal tubular, and mammary gland epithelial cells. The enzyme acts as a catalyst for transfer of glutamyl groups to amino acids or peptides, and is involved in glutathione synthesis and degradation.[4] Elevations of serum levels are generally attributed to cholestasis or biliary hyperplasia resulting in enzyme induction. GGT may be a more sensitive indicator than ALP of hepatobiliary disease in cats, owing to the short half-life of ALP in cats. A notable exception is hepatic lipidosis, as moderate to marked elevation of ALP may be present with minimal, if any, elevation of GGT. In dogs, GGT is often considered more specific but less sensitive than ALP for

---

Box 3
Common drugs causing elevated ALP

Azathioprine

Barbiturates[a]

Cephalosporins

Cyclophosphamide

Doxycycline

Estrogens

Glucocorticoids[a]

Griseofulvin

Halothane

Ibuprofen

Methimazole (cats)

Methotrexate

Nitrofurantoin

Oxacillin

Phenobarbital[a]

Primidone[a]

Progesterone

Salicylates

Testosterone

Tetracycline

Thiabendazole

Trimethoprim-sulfamethoxazole–based drugs

   [a] Drugs that most consistently increase ALP.

---

the detection of hepatobiliary disease. Corticosteroid administration or elevated endogenous corticosteroid levels may result in increased serum GGT activity in dogs, likely due to enzyme induction. Mild to modest increases of serum GGT can also occur with anticonvulsant therapy (phenobarbital, phenytoin, primidone). GGT has a half-life of approximately 72 hours in dogs.[7]

Lactate Dehydrogenase

Lactate dehydrogenase (LDH) is an enzyme that catalyzes the conversion of lactate to pyruvate. It is non–tissue specific and can be found in liver, heart, and skeletal muscle. Therefore, there are 5 isoenzymes identified with LDH. LDH1 is found in cardiac muscle and erythrocytes in small animals, LDH2, LDH3, and LDH4 are found in all tissues, and LDH5 is found in the liver and skeletal muscle of small animals. LDH may be reported on routine serum biochemical profiles for dogs and cats. However, its diagnostic value is of limited significance because it may be found in multiple body tissues as outlined here. Artifactual elevations can be seen with excessive exercise and hemolysis. Therefore, if an elevated LDH is noted, other liver indices should be

| Box 4 |
Common diseases associated with an increased ALP
Primary Biliary Tract Disease (Dog and Cat)
Cholangitis
Pancreatitis
Cholelithiasis
Biliary neoplasia
Ruptured biliary tract
Cholecystitis
Parenchymal Disease (Dog)
Cholangiohepatitis (septic and immune mediated)
Chronic active hepatitis
Cirrhotic liver disease
Neoplasia
Lymphoma
Hepatoma
Hepatocellular carcinoma
Hemangiosarcoma
Histiocytic sarcoma
Metastatic carcinoma (secondary to localized cholestasis)
Toxins
Parenchymal Disease (Cat)
Neoplasia: lymphoma (most common), mast-cell tumor
Biliary sludging (especially in anorexic cats)
Cholangiohepatitis (septic and immune mediated)
Hepatic lipidosis (hallmark of diagnosis is an elevated ALP with a normal GGT)
Feline infectious peritonitis
Toxins
Systemic Disease (Dog)
Hyperadrenocorticism
Diabetes mellitus
Cholestasis associated with sepsis
Tick-borne disease such as ehrlichiosis
Osteomyelitis
Osteosarcoma
Hepatic entrapment as seen with diaphragmatic hernia
Right-sided heart failure
Primary and secondary hyperparathyroidism
Healing fracture
Systemic Disease (Cat)
Hyperthyroidism
Diabetes mellitus

evaluated before an extensive diagnostic workup, because inexplicable elevations of great magnitude are not uncommon. It should be noted that the isoenzymes are not routinely available, and its measurement does not provide any additional information to that provided from evaluation of CK, AST, and ALT.

Bilirubin

Bilirubin is predominantly formed during removal of senescent RBCs through the mononuclear phagocyte system, primarily through the action of intracellular microsomal heme oxygenase. This enzyme catalyzes degradation of hemoglobin to iron, carbon monoxide, globin, and biliverdin, with biliverdin further reduced to bilirubin and released from the cell for protein-bound transport (albumin) to the liver.[7] Following transfer of bilirubin into hepatocytes, mediated by the transport proteins ligandin or fatty-acid binding protein, bilirubin is conjugated with glucuronide via the enzyme uridine diphosphate glucuronyl transferase.[4,7] The conjugated water-soluble form of bilirubin is actively transported from hepatocytes across the bile canalicular membrane and, following entry into the intestine as a component of bile, is subsequently degraded by colonic bacteria into urobilogen.[4] Hyperbilirubinemia can be caused by prehepatic (hemolytic) disease, primary hepatic disease, and post-hepatic disease.

Prehepatic hyperbilirubinemia is secondary to hemolysis of RBCs. This process is easily distinguishable from other causes because marked concurrent anemia is also present. RBC morphology should be evaluated in all anemic hyperbilirubinemic patients for spherocytosis, autoagglutination, Heinz bodies, and hemotropic parasites. Common causes of hemolysis include immune-mediated disease processes, hemotropic parasites, drugs and toxins (**Box 5**), disseminated intravascular coagulation, vasculitis, and microangiopathic disease. Concurrent elevation in ALT is often noted because of hypoxic injury to hepatocytes.

Primary hepatic hyperbilirubinemia is often secondary to concurrent decreased hepatocyte function and intrahepatic cholestasis. This condition leads to decreased bilirubin uptake, conjugation, and excretion. However, significant hepatic disease must be present to result in hyperbilirubinemia. There are numerous diseases associated with hyperbilirubinemia in dogs and cats, and the most common disease processes are listed in **Box 6**.

Post-hepatic hyperbilirubinemia is secondary to obstruction of the extrahepatic bile duct. The most common causes include pancreatitis, cholelithiasis, biliary neoplasia,

---

Box 5
Common drugs and toxins that may cause hemolysis

Acetaminophen

β-Lactam antibiotics (penicillins and cephalosporins)

Lead

Macrodantin

Onions

Sulfonamides

Vitamin K (cats)

Zinc

Box 6
Common hepatic diseases causing hyperbilirubinemia

Dogs:

Chronic hepatitis with interface hepatitis with or without fibrosis (chronic active hepatitis)

Cirrhosis

Infectious disease (leptospirosis)

Hepatic necrosis (toxins)

Septicemia

Round-cell neoplasia such as lymphoma, histiocytic sarcoma, and mast-cell disease

Cholangiohepatitis

Cats:

Hepatic lipidosis

Cholangitis

Cholangiohepatitis

Feline infectious peritonitis

Round-cell neoplasia (lymphoma, mast-cell tumor)

---

and pancreatic neoplasia. With extrahepatic biliary duct obstruction there often are disproportionate increases in cholestatic enzymes (ALP and GGT) in comparison with hepatocellular enzymes (ALT and AST). In addition, serum cholesterol levels are often elevated with biliary obstruction. Imaging of the liver with ultrasonography is often helpful in confirming the diagnosis and further directing therapy.

Serum Bile Acids

Bile acids are amphipathic steroids primarily synthesized in the liver from cholesterol via the enzyme 7α-hydroxylase, with cholic acid as the predominant type in the dog and cat.[7] Through micelle formation, bile acids enhance solubilization of lipids within the intestine, facilitating digestion and absorption of fats. Serum bile acids often are used to assess hepatic function. Serum bile acids are indicated for further evaluation of persistently elevated serum liver enzyme activity, suspected portosystemic shunts or cirrhosis, and monitoring the therapy of inpatients with hepatic diseases (**Box 7**). To obtain maximum sensitivity, both a 12-hour fasting preprandial sample and a 2-hour postprandial sample should be obtained. Patients should be fed a diet that has a moderate fat density to stimulate gallbladder contraction after obtaining the preprandial sample.

Multiple factors may affect the results of bile acids testing. Hemolysis and lipemia may falsely decrease or increase serum bile acid concentrations measured by spectrophotometric methods. Therefore, one should not feed an extremely fat-dense food or use a radioimmunoassay. In addition, patients that have had a cholecystectomy or have ileal disease may have unreliable results because the ileum is the primary source of bile-acid absorption. Therefore, results may be unreliable in animals that have had ileal resection or are suspected to have significant ileal or lower gastrointestinal tract disease. Spontaneous gallbladder contraction may occur during the fasting period, and can result in a fasting value exceeding the postprandial sample. However, both values should be within the RI unless hepatic abnormality is present.

Box 7
Causes of decreased and increased serum bile acids

Decreased Bile Acids

Decreased gastric motility

Hypermotile gastrointestinal tract

Gastrointestinal malabsorption

Ileal resection

Ileal disease

Increased Bile Acids

Hepatocellular disease

- Hepatic lipidosis
- Toxic insult
- Necrosis (toxic, ischemic, heat, and so forth)
- Inflammatory (cirrhosis, immune mediated, infectious)
- Infectious, primary hepatic
- Cholangiohepatitis (septic and nonseptic)
- Infectious, nonhepatic origin
- Neoplastic

Cholestatic disease (bile acids need not be performed in patients with hyperbilirubinemia)

Portosystemic shunting

Microvascular disease

Although bile acids are an excellent indicator of hepatic function, the magnitude of the increase is not specific to an underlying particular diagnosis or prognosis. Bile acids typically are not often elevated with nonhepatic disease, antiepileptic therapy, or glucocorticoid administration.

Urine bile acids have a diagnostic utility similar to that of serum bile acids in dogs and cats. Advantages of performing urine bile acids testing include: sensitivity and specificity comparable with those of serum bile acids for detecting liver dysfunction in both dogs and cats; a nonfasted sample is acceptable; a sample may be collected at home; sampling avoids shortcomings of serum bile acids such as delayed gastric emptying, spontaneous gallbladder contraction, and delayed intestinal transit time. Urine bile acids may be beneficial for routine monitoring of patients on potentially hepatotoxic drugs such as phenobarbital.

Ammonia

Ammonia is derived mostly from colonic bacteria through digestion of dietary protein, gastrointestinal mucosa, and gastrointestinal hemorrhage. The ammonia is then transported to the liver via the portal vein. With normal liver function, the liver metabolizes most of the ammonia to urea. As with serum bile acids, ammonia levels can be a sensitive and specific indicator of liver function, and should be performed on a fasted sample. Samples must be kept in an ice bath and analyzed within 30 minutes for reliable results. Decreased ammonia levels can be seen with administration of aminoglycosides such as neomycin, lactulose, probiotics, and enemas. A decreased ammonia level in patients not on concurrent therapy is of no clinical significance.

Common causes of increased ammonia levels are shown in **Box 8**.

Indirect Markers of Hepatobiliary Disease

Hepatobiliary disease can result in decreased protein synthesis as well as altered glucose and lipid metabolism. However, a reduction of approximately 70% to 80% of hepatic function must be present before these biochemical abnormalities are detected. As such, these are typically not considered sensitive indicators for detection of disease, and fluctuations can occur with some analytes depending on the specific disease process.

Coagulation Factors
- Enzymatic and nonenzymatic coagulation factors are synthesized in the liver, and hepatic insufficiency can result in hemostatic defects caused by decreased production.
- Enzymatic factors include II (prothrombin), VII, IX, X, XI, XII, and XIII.
- Nonenzymatic factors include I (fibrinogen), V, and VIII.
- Prolongation of activated clotting time, prothrombin time, and activated partial thromboplastin time can occur with severe hepatic insufficiency; thromboelastography may reveal tracings consistent with a hypocoagulable state.
- Cholestasis rarely results in hemostatic defects, attributed to maldigestion with decreased absorption of fat-soluble vitamins, and diminished vitamin K–dependent carboxylation of factors II, VII, IX, and X.
- Investigation for a coagulopathy should always be performed before fine-needle aspiration or biopsy of the liver, given the potential complication of hemorrhage.

Albumin and Globulins:
- Hypoalbuminemia can occur as a result of decreased protein synthesis.
- Hyperalbuminemia has rarely been reported with hepatocellular carcinoma.[12]
- α- and β-globulin hepatic synthesis may be decreased; γ-globulin production is primarily dependent on B lymphocytes and plasma cells.
- Hyperglobulinemia can potentially occur as a result of diminished filtration and clearance of toxins and microbial agents from the portal circulation. This process can occur with vascular anomalies (eg, shunts) or with decreased hepatic mass resulting in fewer Kupffer cells.

Blood Urea Nitrogen (BUN) and Ammonia:
- Altered circulation or hepatic insufficiency can result in decreased delivery of ammonia from the portal circulation for entry into the urea cycle, resulting in hyperammonemia and decreased serum BUN.

Box 8
Causes of increased ammonia levels

High-protein meals

Excessive exercise

Improper sample handling or delayed submission

Hepatic insufficiency

Inherited disorders of the urea cycle

Drugs: narcotics, diuretics leading to alkalosis

Glucose:
- Hypoglycemia can occur as a result of reduction of hepatic glycogen stores, delayed insulin clearance, or decreased gluconeogenesis.
- Hyperglycemia can potentially occur as a result of decreased absorption from the portal circulation or hyperglucagonemia associated with hepatocutaneous syndrome.

Cholesterol:
- Hypercholesterolemia can occur as a result of cholestasis.
- Hypocholesterolemia can occur from diminished synthesis associated with decreased hepatic function or portosystemic shunts.

HEMATOLOGY

There are relatively few abnormalities specific for hepatobiliary disease that can be detected on a complete blood count with a blood smear review.

- Microcytosis can occur with portosystemic shunts or potentially with severe hepatic insufficiency, likely due to altered iron transport or metabolism.
- Acanthocytes can occur with lipid disorders and disruption of normal vasculature (eg, hemangiosarcoma).
- Ovalocytes (elliptocytes) can occur in cats with hepatic lipidosis.

URINALYSIS ABNORMALITIES SECONDARY TO HEPATIC DISEASE

One of the most common, and earliest, clinical signs of liver disease is polyuria and polydipsia. Therefore, the specific gravity of urine in patients with liver disease is often markedly decreased. Bilirubinuria and urate urolithiasis or crystalluria are also indicators that hepatic disease may be present.

For bilirubin to be excreted in the urine, it must be conjugated. Bilirubinuria greater than 2+ in a urine dipstick in a dog, and any bilirubinuria in cats, should raise the index of suspicion for underlying hepatic disease. Bilirubinuria may be seen in dogs without hepatic or hemolytic disease, owing to loss of unconjugated bilirubin (in patients with proteinuric renal disease) or conjugation and production of bilirubin in renal tubular cells (primarily in males). Cats have a much higher renal threshold for bilirubin than dogs, and any degree of bilirubinuria warrants investigation into hepatic or hemolytic disease.

Urate urolithiasis or crystalluria is seen in approximately 40% to 70% of patients with portosystemic shunts (both intrahepatic and extrahepatic); this may also be breed related in Dalmatians, English bulldogs, miniature schnauzers, Shih Tzus, and Yorkshire terriers, in which no underlying portosystemic shunt is present. Acidic urine may lead to urate urolithiasis in both dogs and cats.

CYTOLOGY

Fine-needle aspiration cytology can be useful in the diagnosis of several hepatic diseases, but there are other disorders or lesions that typically require histopathology for diagnosis. The greatest utility is typically for metabolic or neoplastic disorders with multifocal or diffuse distribution throughout the liver. Multiple studies have been performed comparing the accuracy of fine-needle aspiration cytology of the liver with histopathology.

In a study by Roth[13] comparing liver cytology and biopsy diagnoses, 56 cases (25 canine, 31 feline) were reviewed, with complete agreement noted in approximately 60% of the cases, partial agreement in approximately 20% of the cases, and disagreement in the remaining 20%. Agreement was most common with lipidosis, lymphoma, and epithelial neoplasia. Disagreement was most common for cases of hepatitis, although disagreement was also observed in cases of fibrosis, amyloidosis, lymphoma, and hemangiosarcoma.

Another study by Wang and colleagues[14] compared accuracy of ultrasound-guided fine-needle aspiration cytology with histopathology in 97 cases (56 canine, 41 feline). Overall agreement was observed in approximately 30% of the canine cases and 51% of the feline cases. A cytologic diagnosis of vacuolar change was confirmed by histopathology as a predominant disease process in approximately 64% and 83% of the canine and feline cases, respectively. Vacuolar change was also reported as the disorder most often misdiagnosed cytologically. Such misdiagnosis was partially attributed to cases of vacuolar change occurring as a secondary process, and the limitation of cytology in detecting the primary underlying disorder (such as metabolic or nutritional disease, hypoxia, inflammation). Inflammatory disease was accurately identified cytologically in approximately 25% and 27% of canine and feline cases.

A large study by Bahr and colleagues[15] was conducted on the accuracy of ultrasound-guided fine-needle aspiration cytology of focal liver lesions in dogs. In comparison with histology, cytology had the highest sensitivity for detection of vacuolar change (58%) and neoplasia (52%). Cytology had lower sensitivity for detection of inflammation (31%), necrosis (20%), and hyperplasia (14%). Within the category of neoplasia, cytology had the highest sensitivity for detection of round-cell tumors (60%), and lowest sensitivity for detection of sarcomas (17%). The sensitivity for detection of carcinomas varied based on tumor type, with higher sensitivity for identification of nonhepatocellular carcinoma (55%) than for hepatocellular carcinoma (35%). Cytology carried the highest positive predictive value (87%) for neoplasia, and although limited in detection of disease (depending on tumor type), a cytologic diagnosis of neoplasia could be interpreted with a high degree of confidence. Regarding inflammatory disease, cytology had limited sensitivity for detection of nonsuppurative inflammation (31%), with poor sensitivity for identification of suppurative (14%) or mixed-cell inflammation (8%).

Neoplasia

Diagnosis of round-cell neoplasia is often possible, including lymphoma, histiocytic sarcoma, plasma cell neoplasia, and mast-cell disease. In some cases, distinction between the various tumor types can be difficult if the cells are poorly differentiated. Regarding lymphoma, cytology is often useful when there is a predominance of large lymphocytes or large granular lymphocytes (**Figs. 1** and **2**). Small-cell or intermediate-cell predominant forms of lymphoma can be cytologically indistinguishable from hyperplastic or inflammatory populations, requiring collection of samples for histopathology or polymerase chain reaction for clonality.

For epithelial neoplasia, aspiration of solitary nodules for the purpose of differentiating nodular hyperplasia from neoplasia may be of limited value. There can be considerable overlap in the cytologic appearance of hepatocellular hyperplasia and neoplasia (hepatoma, well-differentiated hepatocellular carcinoma). A diagnosis of carcinoma can be made cytologically, particularly in cases when there is moderate to marked cellular anaplasia (**Fig. 3**). However, correlation with other clinical findings and imaging results is often necessary to help differentiate a primary hepatobiliary tumor from a metastatic lesion. Similarly, a cytologic diagnosis of neuroendocrine neoplasia is possible in some cases, but specific tumors in this category can be cytologically indistinguishable, thus limiting the differentiation of a primary tumor (hepatic or biliary neuroendocrine carcinoma) from a metastatic process (eg, insulinoma,

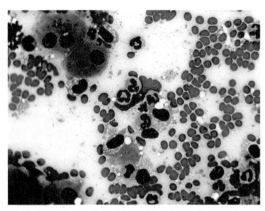

Fig. 1. Fine-needle aspiration biopsy (FNA) from the liver of a cat shows lymphoma of large granular lymphocytes (Diff-Quik, original magnification ×100).

gastrinoma, pheochromocytoma). Mesenchymal neoplasms often do not exfoliate well, and cytology may be poorly sensitive for detection of these lesions. For hemangiosarcoma in particular, fine-needle aspiration may be of limited utility because definitive cytologic diagnosis is often not achieved, and there may be considerable risk of complication with sample collection (eg, rupture of cavitated mass, hemorrhage due to thrombocytopenia).

Lipid and Nonlipid Vacuolar Change

Cytology is useful in identifying vacuolar change such as occurs with feline hepatic lipidosis (**Fig. 4**), although a cause is often not identified. Canine nonlipid vacuolar hepatopathy (**Fig. 5**) is a common finding, but this is a nonspecific process that can occur with a variety of metabolic disorders, hypoxia, toxin ingestion, inflammation, nodular hyperplasia, and neoplasia.

Infectious and Inflammatory Disease

Lesions such as a bacterial abscess or fungal infection (eg, histoplasmosis) are often amenable to cytologic diagnosis. Diagnosis of viral disease (eg, feline infectious

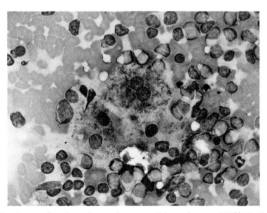

Fig. 2. FNA from the liver of a dog shows large-cell lymphoma (Diff-Quik, original magnification ×100).

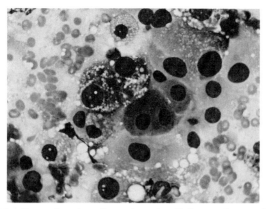

Fig. 3. FNA from the liver of a dog shows hepatocellular carcinoma (Diff-Quik, original magnification ×100).

peritonitis, infectious canine hepatitis), protozoal disease (eg, toxoplasmosis, neosporosis), leptospirosis, mycobacteriosis, and parasitic disease often requires additional diagnostics such as serology, polymerase chain reaction, and/or histopathology with special stains.

HISTOPATHOLOGY

Histopathology is necessary in many cases for the differentiation of benign from malignant lesions, identification of vascular anomalies (eg, microvascular dysplasia, portosystemic shunts) or cirrhosis, diagnosis of inflammatory conditions, and detection of storage disorders (eg, glycogen storage disease, copper hepatopathy). Additional stains may necessary for diagnosis (eg, rhodanine for copper, immunohistochemistry for tumor identification). Collection of a wedge biopsy via exploratory laparotomy or laparoscopic biopsy is preferred over ultrasound-guided Tru-Cut biopsy. Tru-Cut biopsy may be useful in cases with diffuse disease (eg, lymphoma, lipidosis), but microscopic evaluation may be limited by small sample size or because of

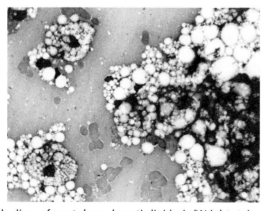

Fig. 4. FNA from the liver of a cat shows hepatic lipidosis (Wright stain, original magnification ×100).

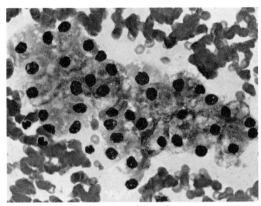

Fig. 5. FNA from the liver of a dog shows nonlipid vacuolar change (Diff-Quik, original magnification ×100).

fragmentation. Collection of samples containing a minimum of 15 portal triads has been recommended to help ensure the tissue is representative of acinar units.[10]

In a study by Cole and colleagues,[16] morphologic diagnosis from liver samples obtained by needle biopsy from dogs and cats were compared with those obtained by wedge biopsy, with the diagnosis obtained from the wedge biopsy considered the definitive diagnosis. The morphologic diagnosis from the needle-biopsy specimen was in agreement with the diagnosis from the wedge biopsy in 40% of animals with hepatic disease, and in 48% of all animals in the study (including 33 animals without hepatic disease). The results of this study suggest that caution must be exercised when interpreting histopathologic findings from needle-biopsy specimens.

REFERENCES

1. Friedrichs KR, Harr KE, Freeman KP, et al. ASVCP reference interval guidelines: determination of de novo reference intervals in veterinary species and other related topics. Vet Clin Pathol 2012;41(4):441–53.
2. Bunch SE. Diagnostic tests for the hepatobiliary system. In: Nelson RW, Couto CG, editors. Small animal internal medicine. 3rd edition. St. Louis, Missouri: Mosby; 2003. p. 483–505.
3. Comazzi S, Pieralisi C, Bertazzolo W. Haematological and biochemical abnormalities in canine blood: frequency and associations in 1022 samples. J Small Anim Pract 2004;45(7):343–9.
4. Stockham SL, Scott MA. Fundamentals of veterinary clinical pathology. Ames, Iowa: Iowa State Press; 2002. p. 435–86.
5. Lassen ED. Laboratory evaluation of the liver. In: Thrall MA, editor. Veterinary hematology and clinical chemistry. Baltimore, Maryland: Lippincott Williams & Wilkins; 2004. p. 355–75.
6. Steinberg J. Creatine Kinase. In: Vaden SL, Knoll JS, Smith FW, et al, editors. Blackwell's five minute veterinary consult: laboratory tests and diagnostic procedures: canine and feline. Ames, Iowa: Wiley-Blackwell; 2009. p. 196–7.
7. Meyer DJ, Harvey JW. Veterinary laboratory medicine. 2nd edition. Philadelphia, Pennsylvania: W. B. Saunders and Co.; 1998. p. 157–86.
8. Washbau RJ, Day MJ. Canine and feline gastroenterology. St. Louis, Missouri: Elsevier Saunders; 2013. p. 849–957.

9. Bain PJ. Alanine aminotransferase. In: Vaden SL, Knoll JS, Smith FW, et al, editors. Blackwell's five minute veterinary consult: laboratory tests and diagnostic procedures: canine and feline. Ames, Iowa: Wiley-Blackwell; 2009. p. 32–3.

10. Center SA. Hepatic disease in small animals. In: The Merck veterinary manual. Available at: http://www.merckmanuals.com/vet/digestive_system/hepatic_disease_in_small_animals/overview_of_hepatic_disease_in_small_animals.html.   Accessed June 1, 2013.

11. Bain PJ. Liver. In: Latimer KS, editor. Duncan and Prasse's veterinary laboratory medicine clinical pathology. 5th edition. Ames, Iowa: Wiley-Blackwell; 2011. p. 211–30.

12. Cooper ES, Wellman ML, Carsillo ME. Hyperalbuminemia associated with hepatocellular carcinoma in a dog. Vet Clin Pathol 2009;38(4):516–20.

13. Roth L. Comparison of liver cytology and biopsy diagnoses in dogs and cats: 56 cases. Vet Clin Pathol 2001;30(1):35–8.

14. Wang KY, Panciera DL, Al-Rukibat RK, et al. Accuracy of ultrasound-guided fine-needle aspiration of the liver and cytologic findings in dogs and cats: 97 cases (1990-2000). J Am Vet Med Assoc 2004;224(1):75–8.

15. Bahr KL, Sharkey LC, Murakami T, et al. Accuracy of US-guided FNA of focal liver lesions in dogs: 140 cases (2005-2008). J Am Anim Hosp Assoc 2013;49(3): 190–6.

16. Cole TL, Center SA, Flood SN, et al. Diagnostic comparison of needle and wedge biopsy specimens of the liver in dogs and cats. J Am Vet Med Assoc 2002; 220(10):1483–90.

Diagnosis of Small Intestinal Disorders in Dogs and Cats

Karin Allenspach, Dr med vet, FVH, DECVIM-CA, PhD, FHEA

KEYWORDS

- Diagnostic workup • Chronic diarrhea • Small intestine • Laboratory tests

KEY POINTS

- A serum albumin concentration of less than 2 g/L is an indicator of poor prognosis in dogs with inflammatory bowel disease (IBD).
- Cobalamin should be supplemented in all cases with decreased serum cobalamin concentrations.
- Increased canine pancreatic lipase in dogs with IBD is associated with a worse outcome.
- In cases of suspected intestinal lymphoma, polymerase chain reaction for antigen receptor rearrangements and immunophenotyping by flow cytometry or immunohistochemistry should be used in conjunction with clinical signs to help establish a diagnosis.
- Evaluation of intestinal biopsies for expression of CD11c using immunofluorescence may be a helpful diagnostic test for IBD in dogs.
- Genetic testing for mutations in innate immunity receptors is available for German Shepherd dogs, and could become a useful test for other breeds of dogs in the future.

INTRODUCTION: DIAGNOSTIC WORKUP OF SMALL INTESTINAL DISORDERS

The last decade has brought numerous advances in our knowledge about the pathogenesis of chronic intestinal disorders in people, particularly regarding inflammatory bowel disease (IBD), which comprises Crohn disease and ulcerative colitis. Specifically, the interplay of innate immunity receptors with commensals of the intestinal microbiome plays an important role in the disease pathogenesis. Molecular studies have identified specific disbalances in the microbiome of people with IBD. In addition, genetic polymorphisms that are associated with an increased risk of development of IBD have been identified. These data promise to be helpful in the development of new diagnostic options and targeted molecular treatment strategies for IBD. New findings

Current Funding Sources: Morris Animal Foundation, British Biotechnology and Bioscience Research Fund, Probiotics Ltd UK, Laboklin GmbH Germany.
Conflict of Interests: None.
Department of Clinical Sciences and Services, Royal Veterinary College, University of London, Hawkshead Lane, North Mymms, Hatfield AL9 7PT, UK
E-mail address: kallenspach@rvc.ac.uk

Vet Clin Small Anim 43 (2013) 1227–1240
http://dx.doi.org/10.1016/j.cvsm.2013.07.001
0195-5616/13/$ – see front matter © 2013 Elsevier Inc. All rights reserved.

vetsmall.theclinics.com

in chronic enteropathies in dogs and cats suggest a pathogenesis similar to that in people with IBD. Recent studies have detected disbalances in expression of innate immunity receptors (so-called toll-like receptors [TLRs]) in the intestines of dogs with IBD[1,2] that are similar to those seen in people with IBD. The expression of some of these receptors also has been correlated with severity of clinical disease in dogs with IBD, which makes it likely that they are causally implicated in the pathogenesis.[3] In addition, disbalances in the microbiome (so-called dysbiosis) have been identified using molecular methods in dogs and cats with IBD.[4–6] These findings point toward a pathogenesis of IBD in dogs and cats similar to that in people, even if the clinical manifestations of these diseases are different. There is hope that similar advances regarding diagnostic options and new therapeutic modalities will be made for canine and feline IBD as has been done for IBD in humans.

A thorough history is important in the evaluation of small animal patients exhibiting signs of intestinal disorder. The first differentiation should be to establish whether the disease is acute or chronic. Diarrhea, vomiting, dehydration, weight loss, lethargy, and melena all can be signs of small intestinal disease. The disease is acute if clinical signs have been present for only a few days. However, if clinical signs persist for more than 3 weeks or are intermittently present for more than 3 weeks, the disease is defined as chronic.

If the animal has diarrhea, the next step is to determine whether it has small intestinal, large intestinal, or a combination of small and large intestinal diarrhea (**Table 1**).

Differential Diagnoses for Acute Small Intestinal Diseases

Systemically well

- Dietary indiscretion
- Intestinal parasites (*Ancylostoma caninum*, *Toxocara*, *Giardia*, *Tritrichomonas fetus*)

Systemically unwell, abnormal abdominal palpation, severe diarrhea with hematochezia, melena, and frequent vomiting

- Dietary indiscretion
- Toxicity
- Viral infection (parvovirus, coronavirus, distemper, feline leukemia virus [FeLV]/feline immunodeficiency virus [FIV])
- Bacterial infection (*Salmonella*, *Campylobacter*, *Clostridium*)
- Intestinal parasites (*Giardia*, *Tritrichomonas*)

Table 1 Differentiation of small-bowel and large-bowel diarrhea	Small	Large
Volume	+++	+
Mucus	−	+++
Frequency	+	+++
Tenesmus	−	+++
Dyschezia	−	+
Weight loss	++	+
Vomiting	+	+
General condition	+	−

- Acute pancreatitis
- Intestinal obstruction
- Hypoadrenocorticism (Addison disease)

DIAGNOSTIC WORKUP OF CHRONIC SMALL INTESTINAL DIARRHEA

Once clinical signs persist for more than 3 weeks, additional workup is required to establish the diagnosis. In chronic cases it is more common for systemic, nongastrointestinal problems to cause the signs, and therefore the first diagnostic steps must be directed at excluding these extragastrointestinal causes.

Causes of Chronic Small Intestinal Disease

Extragastrointestinal (Metabolic) Causes
- Hepatic disease (portosystemic shunt)
- Hyperthyroidism (cats)
- Hypoadrenocorticism (Addison disease) (dogs)
- Renal insufficiency
- Pancreatitis (acute or chronic)
- Exocrine pancreatic insufficiency (EPI)

Gastrointestinal Causes
- Intestinal parasites (*Giardia* infection, *Tritrichomonas* infection) (cats)
- Chronic partial obstruction of the small intestine
- Lymphangiectasia
- Neoplasia: lymphosarcoma
- Food intolerance/food allergy
- Chronic enteropathies/IBD
  - Eosinophilic enteritis
  - Lymphoplasmacytic enteritis

The diagnosis of chronic gastrointestinal causes is one of exclusion, and a full diagnostic workup needs to be done first to rule out all known causes of extragastrointestinal inflammation. This workup commonly involves a complete blood cell count, serum biochemical analysis, urinalysis, and fecal analysis for helminth and protozoal parasites (*Giardia* and *Tritrichomonas* in cats). Further tests are indicated if none of these tests are abnormal: trypsin-like immunoreactivity to exclude EPI, canine pancreatic lipase immunoreactivity (cPLI) to assess the possibility of pancreatitis or pancreatic tumors, corticotropin stimulation test or basal cortisol concentration to exclude hypoadrenocorticism, and cobalamin concentrations to assess the absorptive function of the distal small intestine. Total thyroxine (T4) and FeLV/FIV infection also should be assessed in cats. Abdominal ultrasonography will be more helpful than endoscopy in determining whether the small and/or large intestine is affected and whether there are mass lesions that need surgical intervention. If the results of these tests do not determine the cause for the clinical signs and the patient is stable (ie, has a normal appetite, is not lethargic, there is no or minimal weight loss, the serum protein concentration is normal, and there is no intestinal thickening on diagnostic imaging), a well-conducted therapeutic trial with an elimination diet or hydrolyzed diet for at least 2 weeks can be performed. If there is no response to a well-conducted dietary trial within 2 weeks after starting the diet, it is unlikely that the patient is suffering from food-responsive disease (FRD) (food allergy or food intolerance).[7] If the dietary trial is unsuccessful, antimicrobials (metronidazole, 10–15 mg/kg by mouth twice a day or tylosin, 10 mg/kg by mouth once to twice a day) for 2 to 3 weeks can be administered. Intestinal biopsies for histopathology are collected from those patients that either fail to respond to empiric therapy or have worsening of their clinical signs. Most patients with chronic enteropathies can be diagnosed by obtaining endoscopic biopsies, as long as at least 12 to 15 biopsies from the small intestine are taken (**Fig. 1**). In rare cases, a diagnosis of lymphoma can be missed if no full-thickness biopsies are obtained, especially in cats, and if the ileum has not been sampled.

INTERPRETATION OF LABORATORY TESTS TO AID THE DIAGNOSIS OF CHRONIC SMALL INTESTINAL DIARRHEA
Serum Albumin Concentrations

Dogs
Decreased serum albumin concentration has been described as a negative prognostic indicator in retrospective and prospective studies of IBD in dogs. Protein-losing enteropathy (PLE) accounts for the loss of albumin through the gut mucosa in severely affected dogs with IBD. PLE in dogs can be associated with severe lymphoplasmacytic IBD, intestinal lymphoma, or, rarely, primary lymphangiectasia. In one study of dogs with IBD, 12 of 80 (16%) dogs had hypoalbuminemia and 4 of 80 (5%) had panhypoproteinemia.[8] Seven of 12 dogs with hypoalbuminemia had to be euthanized for intractable IBD, identifying decreased serum albumin concentration as a major risk factor associated with a worse outcome. In another recent prospective study of dogs with IBD, 12 of 58 (21%) dogs initially presented with hypoalbuminemia.[7] Of these 12 dogs, 7 were panhypoproteinemic with severe hypoalbuminemia (mean albumin level 11 g/L), and 3 of these dogs eventually had to be euthanized. However, it must be noted that relatively mild reductions in serum albumin (<2 g/L) previously

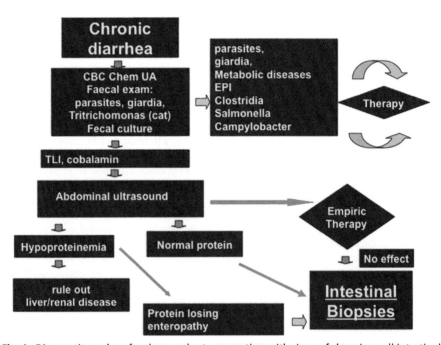

Fig. 1. Diagnostic workup for dogs and cats presenting with signs of chronic small intestinal disease. CBC, complete blood cell count; Chem, serum biochemical profile; EPI, exocrine pancreatic insufficiency; UA, urinalysis.

had been associated with an increased risk of refractoriness to treatment. At this level, most patients will not yet show any clinical signs of hypoalbuminemia, such as ascites, peripheral edema, or pleural effusion.

Furthermore, another study found that severely hypoalbuminemic dogs that failed to improve on immunosuppressive doses of steroids were successfully treated with cyclosporine.[9] This finding suggests that early aggressive treatment in hypoalbumine-mic dogs may potentially decrease mortality rates in severely ill animals. Serum albumin concentration also can be used to monitor patients, as improvement of serum albumin concentrations higher than 2 g/L usually indicates treatment success, even if clinical improvement can be seen earlier in some cases. It is therefore recommended to evaluate serum albumin concentrations every 2 to 3 weeks to assess when treatment can be tapered off or discontinued.

Cats

There is not much published information regarding serum albumin concentrations in cats with chronic intestinal disease. PLE as a clinical syndrome does not exist in cats, as clinical signs such as ascites and peripheral edema do not usually occur in cats with hypoalbuminemia caused by intestinal disease. In addition, the hypoalbumine-mia seen in such cases is usually mild. In cats with IBD, the prevalence of hypoalbu-minemia ranged from 5% to 24%.[10–12] However, there is evidence that cats with chronic intestinal disease and decreased serum albumin concentrations may have concurrent pancreatic disease.

In one recent retrospective study, cats with IBD and serum feline pancreatic lipase (fPLI) concentrations of 2.0 µg/L or higher had a lower median serum albumin concentration than cats with IBD and a normal fPLI.[13] However, hypoalbuminemia was not a negative predictor of survival in this study. Another study found that cats with moderate to severe pancreatitis were significantly more likely to be hypoalbuminemic than were healthy cats and cats with mild pancreatitis.[14]

Therefore, hypoalbuminemia in cats with chronic intestinal disease should prompt the clinician to measure fPLI concentrations and/or to perform abdominal ultrasonographic examination to determine if there is concurrent pancreatitis. Depending on the severity of the hypoalbuminemia, the clinician's approach to treatment might be altered.

Serum Cobalamin Concentrations in Dogs and Cats

Serum cobalamin concentrations should be measured in any small animal patient with chronic small intestinal disease. Cobalamin absorption is receptor-mediated in the ileum, and decreased serum cobalamin concentrations are most commonly seen when this part of the small intestine is affected. However, absorption of cobalamin also involves intrinsic factor, which in dogs and cats is produced primarily in the pancreas. For this reason most small animals with EPI have low serum cobalamin concentrations (**Fig. 2**). The author's group[7] has shown recently that serum cobalamin also is very important for prognosis in dogs with chronic enteropathies. If cobalamin serum concentration is below the reference interval, the risk for later euthanasia increases by a factor of 10. It is therefore important to supplement dogs with hypoco-balaminemia while they undergo treatment of IBD, as this "risk of euthanasia" can be reversed by cobalamin supplementation.

Cats

Serum cobalamin concentration has long been known to be an important negative prognostic factor in cats with chronic enteropathies.[15] The prevalence of decreased serum cobalamin concentrations in cats with chronic gastrointestinal signs has

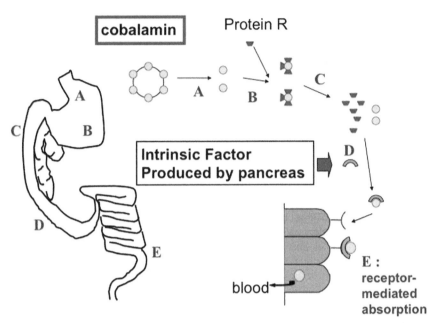

Fig. 2. Absorption of cobalamin is a complex process involving several steps. Cobalamin is released from food protein in the stomach (A) and immediately bound to R-binder proteins (B). In the proximal small intestine, the cobalamin-R-binder complex is cleaved after digestion of the R-binder by pancreatic proteases (C). Free cobalamin can now bind to intrinsic factor (IF) (D), the majority of which is secreted by the pancreas in cats and dogs. This cobalamin-IF complex is subsequently absorbed by specialized receptors in the ileum (E).

been reported to be up to 16.5%.[16] In cats, it has also been reported that cobalamin supplementation can improve clinical signs regardless of the underlying diagnosis, and even if given as the sole treatment for their disease.[15] It is therefore recommended that cats with chronic intestinal disease are supplemented with cobalamin regardless of whether a specific cause for the disease can be identified.

Supplementation recommendations for dogs and cats

Supplementation of cobalamin should be given parenterally (subcutaneously) as a weekly injection for at least 6 weeks. Exact dosages are not reported, as it is a water-soluble vitamin and cannot be overdosed. For tested recommendations, please visit the Web site of the Texas GI Laboratory (http://vetmed.tamu.edu/gilab).

Canine Pancreatic Lipase

cPLI has recently become available as a commercial test and is useful in the assessment of pancreatitis in dogs.[17] However, cPLI also can be elevated in dogs with chronic enteropathy. In a retrospective study of 50 dogs with IBD, the author's group[18] evaluated clinical signs, age, serum lipase and amylase activities, albumin and cobalamin concentrations, abdominal ultrasonography results, histopathologic review of intestinal biopsies, management of IBD, and follow-up in dogs with IBD, either with or without concurrent chronic pancreatitis. Sixteen dogs with increased cPLI and 32 dogs with normal cPLI values were compared. No significant differences were found for clinical activity score, serum amylase activity, serum lipase activity, serum cobalamin concentration, serum albumin concentration, abdominal ultrasonography scores, and histopathology scores for IBD. There was no difference in the frequency of steroid treatment between the groups. Dogs with IBD and concurrent elevated cPLI were significantly older than dogs without elevated cPLI. Moreover, dogs with elevated cPLI had a higher risk of a poor follow-up score and were significantly more likely to be euthanized at follow-up. These data show that elevated cPLI in canine IBD may indicate that a subset of these patients could also have chronic subclinical pancreatitis. In patients that have been diagnosed with IBD and also have elevated cPLI without overt imaging evidence of acute pancreatitis, it is recommended to discuss treatment options for IBD that also will treat possible autoimmune pancreatitis. The author has had anecdotal success with cyclosporine at 5 mg/kg daily for 8 weeks in such cases.

C-Reactive Protein

C-reactive protein (CRP) is a serum acute-phase protein that can be elevated in many different diseases. In people with IBD, several calculated indices of clinical activity of disease incorporate measurements of CRP.[19] In dogs, a similar correlation between the canine IBD activity index (CIBDAI) and serum CRP concentration has been found in one large study of 58 dogs.[20] CRP was elevated in the 28 dogs with CIBDAI scores greater than 5 (which comprises mild to moderate disease activity) in comparison with normal dogs, and CRP decreased significantly after treatment.[20]

In the author's experience, CRP is not very helpful when assessing dogs with chronic enteropathies. CRP was measured in 21 dogs with IBD before treatment and in 18 dogs after treatment.[7] CRP was elevated in only 6 of 21 dogs before treatment, and did not correlate with CIBDAI or histologic scoring.

A large percentage of dogs with IBD do not show any elevations in CRP. Interpretation of elevated levels also may be hampered by increases related to diseases other than IBD.

Fecal α_1-Proteinase Inhibitor

Fecal α_1-proteinase inhibitor (α_1-PI) can be used as a test for dogs in which the clinician suspects PLE although the clinical signs are not yet overtly visible. α_1-PI is a plasma protein similar in size to albumin. If the intestinal mucosal barrier is compromised and loss of protein into the intestinal lumen occurs, α_1-PI is lost at approximately the same rate as albumin. Unlike albumin, however, its proteinase inhibitor properties protect α_1-PI from degradation by intestinal proteases, and can be measured in feces. The test recently has been validated for dogs.[21]

Prompt diagnosis of PLE in a patient with IBD is important because hypoalbuminemia is a risk factor for negative outcome,[7] and the cause should be treated aggressively to improve survival. The α_1-PI assay is especially valuable in patients with intestinal disease that have concurrent renal or hepatic disease. In these patients, measurement of fecal α_1-PI can help assess which portion, if any, of the protein loss can be attributed to the intestine. This test is available only at the Texas GI Laboratory. Ideally, 3 consecutive fresh fecal samples should be submitted to improve test accuracy, which means that fecal α_1-PI is not a useful test for practitioners outside North America.

Histology and World Small Animal Veterinary Association (WSAVA) Scoring of Intestinal Biopsies

Sampling of intestinal biopsies is an essential step in the evaluation of small intestinal disorders, to exclude neoplastic causes and confirm the presence of intestinal inflammation. However, interpretation of intestinal biopsies is difficult and subject to controversy. In several recent studies looking at conventional histologic interpretation of intestinal biopsies, there was no correlation between clinical activity and histologic grading either before or after therapy.[7,20,22] In addition, total lymphocyte counts as well as the number of infiltrating CD3 cells in the lamina propria cannot be used as markers for clinical activity of disease, as there is no difference in cell counts before and after treatment.[23] These findings suggest that the type and degree of histologic infiltrates in canine IBD may not be as helpful as in human medicine, in which clinical scores correlate very well with histologic grading. Therefore, a new grading scheme for the histologic interpretation of endoscopically obtained biopsies from dogs and cats with IBD has recently been published by the WSAVA Working Group.[24] The findings in this study suggest that microarchitectural changes seem to be much more important than cellular infiltrates when assessing histologic severity. However, there is limited information on how well this new grading system correlates with clinical disease. In one retrospective study, the interpathologist variability was still very high even when using the picture guide from the original publication.[25] In addition, it is of concern that the only parameter that correlated with clinical disease was the presence of lymphangiectasia and hypoalbuminemia. Further prospective studies are warranted before the WSAVA scoring can be adopted as a useful tool for clinicians.

PARR in Intestinal Biopsies

The polymerase chain reaction for antigen receptor rearrangements (PARR) amplifies the highly variable T- or B-cell antigen receptor genes, and is used to detect the presence of a clonally expanded population of lymphocytes. This test has been advocated as useful when applied on endoscopically sampled biopsies if a diagnosis of intestinal lymphoma is suspected but not confirmed by conventional histopathology. In a study at the Royal Veterinary College, the author prospectively evaluated the accuracy of PARR for the diagnosis of intestinal lymphoma in biopsies obtained endoscopically from dogs in a comparison with the gold standard of histopathology and clinical outcome determined by follow-up information of at least 2 years. Samples from 39 dogs were included. PARR results indicated a clonal expansion in 7 of 36 dogs. However, these dogs were clinically healthy after dietary treatment 2 years after the endoscopy, so they clearly did not have lymphoma. The data from this study indicate a false-positive rate of almost 20% for PARR when performed on endoscopic biopsies. Another recent study has confirmed these findings, showing that in dogs with IBD, PARR results showed at least one oligoclonal pattern in 38% of dogs, and an immunoglobulin (7 of 47; 14.9%) or T-cell receptor (1 of 47: 2.1%) monoclonal pattern in 17% of dogs.[26] The conclusion that a positive PARR test on an endoscopic biopsy means a diagnosis of lymphoma must therefore be made cautiously in a clinical situation, and clinical signs, response to treatment, and immunohistochemistry must also be taken into account.

Perinuclear Antineutrophilic Cytoplasmic Antibodies

Perinuclear antineutrophilic cytoplasmic antibodies (pANCA) have been useful in the diagnosis of human IBD for decades.[27] These antibodies are serum autoantibodies similar to antinuclear antibodies (ANA), but seem to be more specific for intestinal disease than for ANA. pANCA are detected by immunofluorescence by visualizing a typical pattern of perinuclear staining.

In the first study to assess the clinical usefulness of pANCA in dogs with IBD, sensitivity for pANCA was 0.51 and specificity ranged between 0.56 and 0.95. pANCA proved to be a highly specific marker for IBD in dogs when the group of dogs with chronic diarrhea of other causes were tested against dogs with IBD (specificity 0.95).[28] This finding is in agreement with reports from human medicine that show a specificity of up to 94% for pANCA when distinguishing between IBD and healthy controls, as well as patients with non–IBD-related diarrhea from other causes.[29] When pANCA were tested in a group of dogs with FRD and compared with pANCA in dogs with steroid-responsive disease, a positive pANCA titer was significantly associated with FRD.[30]

The pANCA assay might be helpful in differentiating dogs with chronic diarrhea caused by FRD or IBD: If the result is positive, a food-responsive chronic enteropathy is highly likely, however, if the result is negative, IBD cannot be excluded.

pANCA also may be associated with the syndrome of familial PLE in soft-coated wheaten terriers (SCWT).[31] pANCA were detectable in the serum of dogs an average 1 to 2 years before the onset of clinical disease, and were highly correlated with hypo-albuminemia. This test could be a useful screening test for this specific disease in SCWT.

Care must be taken in interpreting a positive pANCA test result if other inflammatory or immune-mediated diseases are present. A recent study showed that many dogs with various vector-borne diseases or immune-mediated hemolytic anemia were positive for pANCA.[32]

Calprotectin and S100A12

Calprotectin and S100A12 are calcium-binding proteins that are abundant in the granules of neutrophils and macrophages. In people with IBD, serum and fecal concentrations of these proteins are increased in comparison with healthy people. In addition, fecal concentrations of calprotectin correlate very well with clinical disease activity in children with IBD.[33]

An immunoassay for measurement of canine calprotectin in serum and fecal samples is available.[34] A serum calprotectin concentration of 296.0 μg/L or higher has sensitivity of 82.4% and specificity of 68.4% for distinguishing dogs with idiopathic IBD from healthy dogs. However, calprotectin concentrations were not significantly correlated with clinical severity, serum CRP concentration, or severity of histopathologic changes. The clinical usefulness of this test needs further evaluation.

Immunohistochemistry for P-Glycoprotein on Intestinal Biopsies

P-glycoprotein (P-gp) is a transmembrane protein that functions as a drug-efflux pump in the intestinal epithelium. Human patients with IBD who fail to respond to treatment with glucocorticosteroids express high levels of P-gp in lamina propria lymphocytes.[35] Two research groups have evaluated P-gp expression in biopsies of dogs with IBD. In one study,[36] duodenal biopsies from 48 dogs were evaluated by immunohistochemistry. Biopsies were evaluated after treatment with prednisolone in 15 dogs and after dietary therapy alone in 16 dogs. Dogs treated with prednisolone showed significantly higher P-gp expression in lamina propria lymphocytes after treatment compared with expression before treatment. By contrast, the group treated solely with an elimination diet showed no difference in P-gp scores before and after treatment. Moreover, a statistically significant association between refractoriness to steroid treatment and high P-gp expression was found in the glucocorticosteroid-treated group.[36] In another recent study, P-gp expression was higher in duodenal epithelial cells of dogs with IBD compared with healthy control dogs.[37] However, there was no difference in P-gp expression in colonic epithelial cells between IBD and control groups. These results indicate that epithelial and lamina propria lymphocyte expression of P-gp is upregulated in dogs with IBD, and they are even higher after prednisolone treatment. In addition, high P-gp expression could indicate possible multidrug resistance and should be taken into account when managing dogs that have failed steroid treatment previously.

Immunohistochemistry for CD11c in Intestinal Biopsies

CD11c is a marker of human and murine dendritic cells (DCs), and cells expressing this marker have been shown to have similar morphologic and functional characteristics in dogs. DCs are important in determining the outcome of an immune reaction in the gut, that is, whether a pathogen will elicit a massive immune response or whether a commensal will induce tolerance.[38] Specific subsets of inducible DCs are decreased in the diseased tissues of people with IBD.[39] It is plausible that the number of DCs in the intestine could be used as a surrogate marker of inflammation in dogs with IBD. In one recent study, endoscopic biopsies from the duodenum, ileum, and colon were obtained from dogs with IBD and healthy dogs.[40] CD11c expression was assessed by immunofluorescence using a canine monoclonal antibody (**Fig. 3**). The number of CD11c-positive cells in the duodenum, ileum, and colon of dogs with IBD was significantly reduced in comparison with controls. There was a significant negative correlation between the number of CD11c-positive cells in the colon of dogs with IBD and clinical severity. This marker therefore holds promise as a useful test to assess histologic samples. However, additional prospective studies are needed to evaluate the clinical utility of this test.

Genetic Testing

Over the last decade, numerous genes have been associated with an increased risk of development of IBD in humans, many of them implicated in the innate immune response in the intestine.[41] Dogs with IBD may have a similar genetic component, especially because there are breeds predisposed to certain forms of IBD. Boxers are predisposed to histiocytic ulcerative colitis, and German shepherd dogs (GSD) are predisposed to lymphoplasmacytic IBD.[42] The author's group[43] recently performed a mutational analysis of the canine genes for TLR2, TLR4, TLR5, and NOD2 in GSD with IBD, and then further evaluated these in a case-control study with more than 50 cases and healthy GSD controls. Several mutations in TLR4 and TLR5 were found to be significantly associated with an increased risk of development of IBD. Moreover, these results were replicated in 38 other non-GSD breeds for the TLR5 mutation.[44] A follow-up study showed that peripheral blood cells of dogs carrying

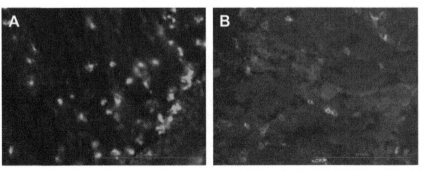

Fig. 3. Immunofluorescence for CD11c on intestinal biopsies from (*A*) a healthy dog and (*B*) a dog with IBD. CD11c expression in the intestinal mucosa is more abundant in healthy dogs than in dogs with IBD (original magnification ×100).

the mutation are hyperresponsive to flagellin, which is the natural ligand for TLR5.[45] This finding proves for the first time that a genetic mutation implicated in the pathogenesis of dogs with IBD has functional consequences at the protein level. Taken together, these findings make it very likely that TLR5 mutations are causally associated with canine IBD. Genetic testing for these polymorphisms currently is available only at the Royal Veterinary College. Such tests could become important for breeders and practitioners in the future. However, it is likely that in a multifactorial disease such as IBD in dogs, other genetic mutations and environmental factors also play a role in the pathogenesis. With the advent of genome-wide association studies, it is possible that more causative mutations will be identified.

SUMMARY

Many laboratory tests are available to aid the diagnostic workup of cats and dogs with chronic small intestinal disorders. Some of these have been available for many years, such as serum albumin and cobalamin concentrations, as well as canine pancreatic lipase, and new data now show that these tests also may be prognostic indicators in animals with chronic enteropathy. Other tests have only relatively recently become available to practitioners, such as serum CRP, fecal α_1-PI, WSAVA standardization of histopathology readings, and PARR. The value of these tests needs to be evaluated in every clinical situation. New tests that are not yet widely available, such as pANCA, calprotectin, CD11c immunofluorescence, and genetic testing, may become very useful tests in the future.

REFERENCES

1. Burgener IA, Konig A, Allenspach K, et al. Upregulation of toll-like receptors in chronic enteropathies in dogs. J Vet Intern Med 2008;22:553–60.
2. Allenspach K, House A, Smith K, et al. Evaluation of mucosal bacteria and histopathology, clinical disease activity and expression of Toll-like receptors in German shepherd dogs with chronic enteropathies. Vet Microbiol 2010;146: 326–35.
3. McMahon LA, House AK, Catchpole B, et al. Expression of Toll-like receptor 2 in duodenal biopsies from dogs with inflammatory bowel disease is associated with severity of disease. Vet Immunol Immunopathol 2010;135:158–63.
4. Janeczko S, Atwater D, Bogel E, et al. The relationship of mucosal bacteria to duodenal histopathology, cytokine mRNA, and clinical disease activity in cats with inflammatory bowel disease. Vet Microbiol 2008;128:178–93.
5. Xenoulis PG, Palculict B, Allenspach K, et al. Molecular-phylogenetic characterization of microbial communities imbalances in the small intestine of dogs with inflammatory bowel disease. FEMS Microbiol Ecol 2008;66:579–89.
6. Suchodolski JS, Camacho J, Steiner JM. Analysis of bacterial diversity in the canine duodenum, jejunum, ileum, and colon by comparative 16S rRNA gene analysis. FEMS Microbiol Ecol 2008;66(3):567–78.
7. Allenspach K, Wieland B, Grone A, et al. Chronic enteropathies in dogs: evaluation of risk factors for negative outcome. J Vet Intern Med 2007;21:700–8.
8. Craven M, Simpson JW, Ridyard AE, et al. Canine inflammatory bowel disease: retrospective analysis of diagnosis and outcome in 80 cases (1995-2002). J Small Anim Pract 2004;45:336–42.
9. Allenspach K, Rufenacht S, Sauter S, et al. Pharmacokinetics and clinical efficacy of cyclosporine treatment of dogs with steroid-refractory inflammatory bowel disease. J Vet Intern Med 2006;20:239–44.

10. Jergens AE. Feline idiopathic inflammatory bowel disease: What we know and what remians to be unraveled. J Fel Med Surg 2012;14(7):445–58.
11. Dennis JS, Kruger JM, Mullaney TP. Lymphocytic/plasmacytic colitis in cats: 14 cases (1985-1990). J Am Vet Med Assoc 1993;202:313–8.
12. Baez JL, Hendrick MJ, Walker LM, et al. Radiographic, ultrasonographic, and endoscopic findings in cats with inflammatory bowel disease of the stomach and small intestine: 33 cases (1990-1997). J Am Vet Med Assoc 1999;215: 349–54.
13. Bailey S, Benigni L, Eastwood J, et al. Comparisons between cats with normal and increased fPLI concentrations in cats diagnosed with inflammatory bowel disease. J Small Anim Pract 2010;51:484–9.
14. Forman MA, Marks SL, De Cock HE, et al. Evaluation of serum feline pancreatic lipase immunoreactivity and helical computed tomography versus conventional testing for the diagnosis of feline pancreatitis. J Vet Intern Med 2004;18: 807–15.
15. Ruaux CG, Steiner JM, Williams DA. Early biochemical and clinical responses to cobalamin supplementation in cats with signs of gastrointestinal disease and severe hypocobalaminemia. J Vet Intern Med 2005;19:155–60.
16. Reed N, Gunn-Moore D, Simpson K. Cobalamin, folate and inorganic phosphate abnormalities in ill cats. J Feline Med Surg 2007;9:278–88.
17. Mansfield C. Acute panceatitis in dogs: Advances in understanding, diagnostics and treatment. Top Compan Anim Med 2012;27(3):123–32.
18. Kathrani A, Steiner JM, Suchodolski J, et al. Elevated canine pancreatic lipase immunoreactivity concentration in dogs with inflammatory bowel disease is associated with a negative outcome. J Small Anim Pract 2009;50:126–32.
19. Nielsen OH, Vainer B, Madsen SM, et al. Established and emerging biological activity markers of inflammatory bowel disease. Am J Gastroenterol 2000;95: 359–67.
20. Jergens AE, Schreiner CA, Frank DE, et al. A scoring index for disease activity in canine inflammatory bowel disease. J Vet Intern Med 2003;17:291–7.
21. Heilmann RM, Paddock CG, Ruhnke I, et al. Development and analytical validation of a radioimmunoassay for the measurement of alpha1-proteinase inhibitor concentrations in feces from healthy puppies and adult dogs. J Vet Diagn Invest 2011;23:476–85.
22. Garcia-Sancho M, Rodriguez-Franco F, Sainz A, et al. Evaluation of clinical, macroscopic, and histopathologic response to treatment in nonhypoproteinemic dogs with lymphocytic-plasmacytic enteritis. J Vet Intern Med 2007;21:11–7.
23. Schreiner NM, Gaschen F, Grone A, et al. Clinical signs, histology, and CD3-positive cells before and after treatment of dogs with chronic enteropathies. J Vet Intern Med 2008;22:1079–83.
24. Day MJ, Bilzer T, Mansell J, et al. Histopathological standards for the diagnosis of gastrointestinal inflammation in endoscopic biopsy samples from the dog and cat: a report from the World Small Animal Veterinary Association Gastrointestinal Standardization Group. J Comp Pathol 2008;138(Suppl 1):S1–43.
25. Willard M, Mansell J. Correlating clinical activity and histopathologic assessment of gastrointestinal lesion severity: current challenges. Vet Clin North Am Small Anim Pract 2011;41:457–63.
26. Olivero D, Turba ME, Gentilini F. Reduced diversity of immunoglobulin and T-cell receptor gene rearrangements in chronic inflammatory gastrointestinal diseases in dogs. Vet Immunol Immunopathol 2011;144:337–45.

27. Vermeire S, Peeters M, Rutgeerts P. Diagnostic approach to IBD. Hepatogastroenterology 2000;47:44–8.
28. Allenspach K, Luckschander N, Styner M, et al. Evaluation of assays for perinuclear antineutrophilic cytoplasmic antibodies and antibodies to *Saccharomyces cerevisiae* in dogs with inflammatory bowel disease. Am J Vet Res 2004;65:1279–83.
29. Dubinsky MC, Ofman JJ, Urman M, et al. Clinical utility of serodiagnostic testing in suspected pediatric inflammatory bowel disease. Am J Gastroenterol 2001;96:758–65.
30. Luckschander N, Allenspach K, Hall J, et al. Perinuclear antineutrophilic cytoplasmic antibody and response to treatment in diarrheic dogs with food responsive disease or inflammatory bowel disease. J Vet Intern Med 2006;20:221–7.
31. Allenspach K, Lomas B, Wieland B, et al. Evaluation of perinuclear antineutrophilic cytoplasmic autoantibodies as an early marker of protein-losing enteropathy and protein-losing nephropathy in soft coated wheaten terriers. Am J Vet Res 2008;69:1301–4.
32. Karagianni AE, Solano-Gallego L, Breitschwerdt EB, et al. Perinuclear antineutrophil cytoplasmic autoantibodies in dogs infected with various vector-borne pathogens and in dogs with immune-mediated hemolytic anemia. Am J Vet Res 2012;73:1403–9.
33. Aadland E, Fagerhol MK. Faecal calprotectin: a marker of inflammation throughout the intestinal tract. Eur J Gastroenterol Hepatol 2002;14:823–5.
34. Heilmann RM, Jergens AE, Ackermann MR, et al. Serum calprotectin concentrations in dogs with idiopathic inflammatory bowel disease. Am J Vet Res 2012;73:1900–7.
35. Farrell RJ, Menconi MJ, Keates AC, et al. P-glycoprotein-170 inhibition significantly reduces cortisol and cyclosporin efflux from human intestinal epithelial cells and T lymphocytes. Aliment Pharmacol Ther 2002;16:1021–31.
36. Allenspach K, Bergman PJ, Sauter S, et al. P-glycoprotein expression in lamina propria lymphocytes of duodenal biopsy samples in dogs with chronic idiopathic enteropathies. J Comp Pathol 2006;134:1–7.
37. Van der Heyden S, Vercauteren G, Daminet S, et al. Expression of P-glycoprotein in the intestinal epithelium of dogs with lymphoplasmacytic enteritis. J Comp Pathol 2011;145:199–206.
38. Ng SC, Benjamin JL, McCarthy NE, et al. Relationship between human intestinal dendritic cells, gut microbiota, and disease activity in Crohn's disease. Inflamm Bowel Dis 2011;17:2027–37.
39. Ng SC, Kamm MA, Stagg AJ, et al. Intestinal dendritic cells: their role in bacterial recognition, lymphocyte homing, and intestinal inflammation. Inflamm Bowel Dis 2010;16:1787–807.
40. Kathrani A, Schmitz S, Priestnall SL, et al. CD11c+ cells are significantly decreased in the duodenum, ileum and colon of dogs with inflammatory bowel disease. J Comp Pathol 2011;145:359–66.
41. Lees CW, Barrett JC, Parkes M, et al. New IBD genetics: common pathways with other diseases. Gut 2011;60:1739–53.
42. Kathrani A, Werling D, Allenspach K. Canine breeds at high risk of developing inflammatory bowel disease in the south-eastern UK. Vet Rec 2011;169:635.
43. Kathrani A, House A, Catchpole B, et al. Polymorphisms in the TLR4 and TLR5 gene are significantly associated with inflammatory bowel disease in German shepherd dogs. PLoS One 2010;5:e15740.

44. Kathrani A, House A, Catchpole B, et al. Breed-independent toll-like receptor 5 polymorphisms show association with canine inflammatory bowel disease. Tissue Antigens 2011;78:94–101.

45. Kathrani A, Holder A, Catchpole B, et al. TLR5 Risk-associated haplotype for canine inflammatory bowel disease confers hyper-responsiveness to flagellin. PLoS One 2012;7:e30117.

Practical Interpretation and Application of Exocrine Pancreatic Testing in Small Animals

Caroline Mansfield, BSc, BVMS, PhD, MANZCVS, DECVIM

KEYWORDS

- Specific canine pancreatic lipase (spec-cPL) • SNAP®-cPL™
- Trypsinlike immunoreactivity (TLI) • Pancreatic elastase (PE-1)

KEY POINTS

- A positive specific canine pancreatic lipase (spec-cPL) or SNAP-cPL in dogs should be considered in conjunction with other clinical signs and diagnostic imaging to ensure acute pancreatitis is the main cause of the clinical presentation.
- A negative spec-cPL or SNAP-cPL result means acute pancreatitis is unlikely to be the cause of the dog's presenting signs.
- Serum canine pancreatic elastase-1 (cPE-1) has a high specificity (92%) for the diagnosis of pancreatitis; increases in serum cPE-1 are more likely to be seen in severe acute pancreatitis.
- Feline acute pancreatitis is best diagnosed by a combination of clinical signs, feline pancreatic lipase immunoreactivity, and abdominal ultrasound.
- Close evaluation of cats with pancreatitis for concurrent disease is essential.
- Chronic pancreatitis is difficult to diagnose with laboratory testing.
- Pancreatic cytology may be of benefit in diagnosing pancreatic neoplasia.

INTRODUCTION

The assessment of the pancreas can be difficult in clinical situations because the pancreas is located adjacent to many other abdominal organs (**Fig. 1**). As a result, disease located within the abdomen can cause bystander pancreatic inflammation. The clinical signs of primary acute pancreatitis are indistinguishable from other acute abdominal crises, such as septic peritonitis or intestinal obstruction. The diagnosis of acute pancreatitis generally relies on a combination of investigations rather than one single test. Chronic inflammation of the pancreas is even more difficult to

Disclosures: The author received no incentive or payment from a commercial company in the preparation of this article.
Faculty of Veterinary Science, The University of Melbourne, 250 Princes Highway, Werribee, Victoria 3030, Australia
E-mail address: cmans@unimelb.edu.au

Vet Clin Small Anim 43 (2013) 1241–1260
http://dx.doi.org/10.1016/j.cvsm.2013.07.014
0195-5616/13/$ – see front matter © 2013 Elsevier Inc. All rights reserved.

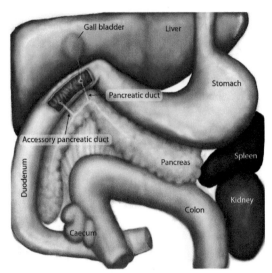

Fig. 1. The regional anatomy of the cranial abdomen in the dog. (*From* Mansfield C. Acute pancreatitis in dogs: advances in understanding, diagnostics and treatment. Top Companion Anim Med 2012;27:125; with permission.)

diagnose because there is often an association with other abdominal disease and biochemical testing is less useful. A strong index of suspicion, ideally pancreatic histology, and evaluation for intestinal or hepatic disease is generally required for a diagnosis of chronic pancreatitis.

The clinical assessment of exocrine pancreatic insufficiency is more straightforward, with most clinical cases capable of being diagnosed readily. There is a subset of animals whereby there are equivocal results of pancreatic function testing that can pose a diagnostic challenge.

ACUTE PANCREATITIS IN THE DOG

Dogs with acute pancreatitis generally present with a sudden onset of anorexia, abdominal pain, and vomiting, as detailed in **Table 1**.[1-3] The onset of pancreatic inflammation and/or necrosis can set up a wide array of inflammatory pathways, which may progress to cause hypovolemia, systemic inflammatory response syndrome (SIRS), or multiple organ dysfunction.[4] Even in very severe cases, the clinical signs of acute pancreatitis in dogs are not pathognomonic. It is essential, therefore, to ensure that differential diagnoses for acute pancreatitis, such as intestinal obstruction, closed pyometron, or septic peritonitis, that all are life threatening and require surgical intervention, are eliminated as a priority (**Box 1**). The next essential step is to eliminate diabetes ketoacidosis, liver disease, uremia and other metabolic causes of vomiting that require specific intervention. A typical diagnostic algorithm for acute pancreatitis is shown in **Fig. 2**.

Routine Clinical Pathology

Because of the need to rule out metabolic disease and to establish the baseline clinical status before treatment, routine clinical pathology (complete blood count, serum biochemical profile, urinalysis) should be obtained. Most laboratory abnormalities in dogs with pancreatitis result from hypovolemia or inflammation and are, therefore,

Table 1
Summary of clinical findings of 60 dogs with fatal acute pancreatitis

Historical Finding	Number of Cases	Percentage (%)
Anorexia	64	91
Vomiting	63	90
Weakness	55	79
Diarrhea	23	33
Polyuria/polydipsia	35	50
Neurologic abnormalities	14	20
Melena	11	16
Weight loss	8	11
Hematemesis	7	10
Hematochezia	3	4

Data from Hess RS, Saunders HM, Van Winkle TJ, et al. Clinical, clinicopathologic, radiographic, and ultrasonographic abnormalities in dogs with fatal acute pancreatitis: 70 cases (1986–1995). J Am Vet Med Assoc 1998;213:665–70.

not specific for pancreatitis.[5,6] Many of the differential diagnoses for pancreatitis, such as uremia or gastrointestinal inflammation, will also result in similar laboratory changes. In brief, these changes include leucocytosis, azotemia, and increased liver enzymes (eg, alanine transferase, alkaline phosphatase). Decreased calcium has also been documented in dogs with acute pancreatitis and has been suggested to carry a poorer prognosis.[7,8] Many dogs with acute pancreatitis have gross lipemia, whether as a cause or consequence of the disease (**Fig. 3**). However, the exact percentage of dogs with acute pancreatitis that have lipemia is not known.

Fluid Cytology

Because one of the major differential diagnoses for acute pancreatitis in dogs is septic peritonitis, the evaluation of free fluid should be performed early in the investigation. Fluid can be obtained by abdominocentesis using a 22- to 25-G needle or by using ultrasound guidance. In cases of small-volume free fluid, the areas between the bladder and the abdominal wall and between liver lobes seem to be frequent sites of initial fluid accumulation. Once fluid has been obtained, it should be stained and assessed for the presence of bacteria as well as having routine fluid analysis

Box 1
Suggested criteria for diagnosis of acute pancreatitis in dogs

- Absence of surgical disease on abdominal radiographs or analysis of abdominal fluid **AND**
- Abdominal ultrasound with evidence of primary pancreatitis **AND**
- One or more of the following:
  - Spec-cPL greater than 400 μg/L
  - Positive SNAP-cPL
  - Gross lipemia
  - Serum PE-1 greater than 17.24 ng/mL
  - Total lipase greater than 3 times the upper reference interval

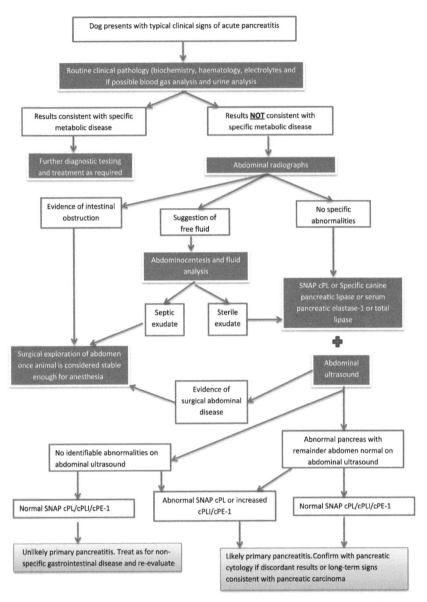

Fig. 2. A diagnostic algorithm for the diagnosis of acute pancreatitis in the dog. cPE-1, canine pancreatic elastase; cPL, canine pancreatic lipase; cPLI, canine pancreatic-lipase immunoreactivity.

(**Fig. 4**). Fluid from dogs with acute pancreatitis will also be a neutrophilic exudate (see **Fig. 4**), but bacteria are not present cytologically or on culture.

Serum Lipase and Amylase

Serum lipase and amylase concentrations have been shown to increase in experimental and naturally occurring canine pancreatitis.[5,8,9] However, neither enzyme is specific to the pancreas because they also originate from gastrointestinal mucosa

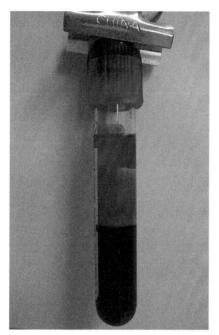

Fig. 3. A blood sample obtained from a dog with acute pancreatitis following centrifugation. The serum sits on top of a lipid layer, indicating gross lipemia.

and are excreted by the kidneys. It has been shown that serum lipase activity is markedly increased in dogs with acute enteritis, gastroenteritis, liver disease, and in renal failure.[10–12] Lipase concentration can also be elevated up to 5 times by the administration of dexamethasone in dogs with no pancreatic inflammation.[13] Serum lipase and amylase concentrations can also be normal in dogs that do have pancreatitis. In one retrospective review by Hess and colleagues,[1] (1998) less than 50% of dogs with acute fatal pancreatitis had increased lipase concentrations, whereas only 30.8% had increased amylase concentrations. Other estimates place the value more conservatively at 15% to 20% of dogs with acute pancreatitis having normal serum lipase and amylase concentrations.[10,14]

Trypsinogen Activation Peptide

Trypsinogen activation peptide (TAP) is the cleavage peptide produced when trypsinogen is cleaved to trypsin (**Fig. 5**). Theoretically, in pancreatitis, TAP will be released into the abdominal cavity and then the circulation in high concentrations and subsequently be cleared through the kidneys.[15] Several studies in people showed a high correlation between the severity of pancreatitis and urinary TAP concentration and a high degree of specificity and sensitivity for diagnosis.[16,17] A reference interval for the measurement of TAP in healthy dogs was established, and its utility as a diagnostic test for canine pancreatitis was assessed.[10] Unfortunately, TAP measurement was specific but not highly sensitive for the diagnosis of pancreatitis in dogs; because it is not readily available for routine clinical use, it cannot be recommended.

Trypsin-like Immunoreactivity

Serum trypsin-like immunoreactivity (TLI) is an accurate and specific indicator of pancreatic function and is thought to be entirely pancreatic in origin.[18] Serum TLI

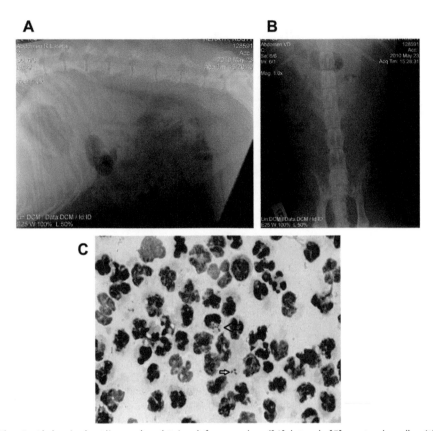

Fig. 4. Abdominal radiographs obtained from a dog ([A] lateral, [B] ventrodorsal) with abdominal pain. There is decreased contrast, suggesting effusion within the abdomen. Abdominocentesis should be performed. Septic peritoneal fluid (C) would have large numbers of activated neutrophils, with both free (*small solid arrow*) and intracellular (*large open arrow*) bacteria (Wright's stain, ×100 magnification).

has been shown in experimental canine models of acute pancreatitis to increase early in the course of the disease, followed by a rapid decrease.[19] In acute pancreatitis, the TLI concentration is often decreased by the time of sampling, so it is seldom useful clinically.[10,20] This reason, along with an often-lengthy delay in receiving results, makes the usefulness of TLI for the diagnosis of pancreatitis questionable.

Canine Pancreatic Lipase

Canine pancreatic lipase (cPL) is one of the most recently established laboratory tests in veterinary medicine, and its use is now widespread. The premise of this test is that it measures lipase that originates solely in the pancreas, and so it will only be increased in pancreatic inflammation.[21] Immunolocalization studies showed pancreatic lipase was present only within pancreatic tissue of dogs, and serum concentrations in dogs with absent exocrine pancreatic function were decreased.[22,23] The pancreatic lipase assay itself (first a radioimmunoassay and then an enzyme immunoassay) has been well validated.[24,25]

The canine pancreatic-lipase immunoreactivity (cPLI) assay was further developed into a commercially available specific canine pancreatic lipase (spec-cPL) sandwich

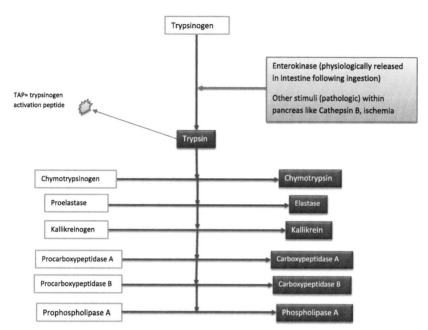

Fig. 5. Trypsin activating the pancreatic cascade and then perpetuating the activation of inert pancreatic zymogens (*blue boxes*) to active digestive pancreatic enzymes (*blue boxes*). TAP is one of the small peptides cleaved during the normal activation of trypsinogen, which normally should only occur within the intestine mediated by enterokinase; however, in pancreatitis, it occurs within the acinar cells themselves.

enzyme-linked immunosorbent assay (ELISA), using a recombinant peptide as the antigen and monoclonal antibody for measurement. This new commercially available assay shows a good correlation to the original assay as well as high reproducibility.[26] The newer assay has caused a change in the reference intervals for the diagnosis of pancreatitis, with results less than 200 µg/L expected in healthy dogs, and results more than 400 µg/L considered consistent with a diagnosis of pancreatitis.[27] A new in-clinic rapid semiquantitative assay (SNAP-cPL; Iddex Laboratories, Westbrook, ME) has also been developed and shows good alignment and reproducibility with the laboratory-based fully quantitative assay.[28] The current manufacturer recommendations are to follow up an in-house SNAP-cPL with a quantitative spec-cPL in order to be able to monitor the response to treatment. However, there are no studies to show that following pancreatic enzymes alters clinical management.

There have been several studies of cPLI and cPL, with most relying on histologic evidence of pancreatic inflammation as their gold standard. The results of these studies are summarized in **Table 2**. The sensitivity of cPLI/cPL for diagnosing pancreatic inflammation in dogs ranges from 21% to 88%.[29–33] The sensitivity of pancreatic lipase is greatly increased when more severely affected dogs are assessed.

The specificity of pancreatic lipase has been reported to range from to 80.0% to 97.5%, which is greater than for total lipase in some studies but comparable in others.[30,32–34] Again, studies assessing the specificity of pancreatic lipase have largely been based on histologic evaluation. Most of these samples were obtained at post mortem, but the primary cause of death was seldom reported. Therefore, it is important to bear in mind that the high specificities relate to histologic evidence of pancreatitis and not a primary clinical diagnosis of acute pancreatitis.

Table 2
Summary of sensitivity and specificity for various laboratory testing in dogs from various studies

Study	Number of Dogs	Method of Diagnosis	Analyte Assessed	Sensitivity (%)	Specificity (%)
McCord et al,[32] 2012	n = 84 AP = 57 Non-AP = 27	Combination of clinical and imaging results	Spec-cPL >400 µg/L Lipase Amylase	71.7–77.8 43.4–53.6 52.4–56.0	80.5–88.0 89.3–92.5 76.7–80.6
Trivedi et al,[33] 2011	n = 70 Mild AP = 56 Moderate-severe AP = 7 Normal pancreas = 7	Histology	Spec-cPL >400 µg/L cTLI Lipase Amylase	21 (mild) 71 (moderate-severe) 30 (mild) 29 (moderate-severe) 54 (mild) 71 (moderate-severe) 7 (mild) 14 (moderate-severe)	100 100 43 100
Mansfield et al	n = 32 Minimal/no inflammation = 20	Histology	Spec-cPL >400 µg/L	NA	90
Mansfield et al	n = 61 AP = 41 CP = 3 Pancreatic carcinoma = 5 Nonpancreatitis = 12	Histology	cPE-1 >17.24 ng/mL	61.4 (all) 66 (AP) 78 (severe AP)	91.7

Study	n	Gold standard	Test		
Steiner et al	n = 11 (Severe AP)	Clinical findings and histology	Spec-cPL >400 µg/L	88	NA
Steiner et al	n = 22	Gross evidence at post mortem	Spec-cPL >400 µg/L	63.6	NA
			Lipase	31.8	NA
			Amylase	40.9	NA
Neilson-Carley et al,[34] 2011	n = 64 AP = 20 Other disease = 17 Healthy = 27	Histology	Spec-cPL >400 µg/L	NA	95
Haworth et al,[36]	n = 38 AP = 11 Non-AP = 26	Clinical evaluation of dogs presenting with acute abdominal disease	SNAP-cPL	82	59
			Spec-cPL >400 µg/L	70	77
Mansfield & Jones,[10] 2000	n = 42 AP = 15 Non-AP = 27	Clinical findings and histology	Lipase >3 × RI	63.6	54.6
			Amylase >3 × RI	22.7	78.1
			TLI >100 µL	37.5	89.3

Abbreviations: AP, acute pancreatitis; CP, chronic pancreatitis; cPE-1, serum canine pancreatic-elastase-1; cPL, canine pancreatic lipase (or canine pancreatic lipase immunoreactivity in earlier studies); NA, not assessed; RI, reference interval.
Data from Refs.[10,29–34,36,45]

In many of the initial studies of pancreatic lipase, dogs with renal failure were not expressly evaluated. However, one study that assessed dogs with experimentally induced chronic renal failure showed no increase in pancreatic lipase.[35] Further evaluation in animals with an acute decline in glomerular filtration rate is required.

One recent study showed a poor correlation between a positive SNAP-cPL test and a primary presentation of AP in dogs presenting with acute abdomen ($\kappa = 0.33$).[36] This study assessed dogs presenting to an emergency center with signs of acute abdominal disease and found a sensitivity of 82% but a specificity of 59% for SNAP-cPL. Another way of interpreting this is that approximately 40% of dogs with a positive SNAP-cPL had disease other than pancreatitis as their primary presenting problem. The conditions most commonly associated with this false-positive finding were small intestinal foreign-body obstruction, septic peritonitis, and hepatic disease (**Box 2, Fig. 6**). As previously discussed, it is possible that those dogs indeed did have histologic pancreatic inflammation that occurred secondary to the primary problem. However, failure to correctly identify the primary cause of the presentation would lead to inadequate treatment and management. Indeed, when assessing the specificity of pancreatic laboratory testing using histology as the gold standard, the presence of pancreatic bystander inflammation obscures the clinical relevance of such results. This idea is borne out in one study of dogs undergoing postmortem examination at a referral center that determined that 92% had pancreatic inflammation of some sort,[37] which is likely a gross overestimation of pancreatitis as the clinical cause of death.

A negative result for SNAP-cPL, on the other hand, seems to have a good correlation to dogs having disease other than acute pancreatitis.[36] This correlation is also demonstrated in a multicenter study that used Bayesian statistics to overcome the need for pancreatic histology as a gold standard, which also determined that dogs with Spec-cPL of 200 µg/L or less and/or a negative SNAP-cPL were unlikely to have clinical acute pancreatitis.[32]

Serum Pancreatic Elastase

Pancreatic elastase (PE-1) is released immediately after trypsin activation and also plays a role in perpetuating inflammation (see **Fig. 5**).[38] In a study in people, a sensitivity

---

Box 2
Case study

Tiny, a 5-year-old male neutered Australian cattle dog, was referred with a history of vomiting and abdominal pain. He had shown similar clinical signs 2 weeks before the referral and was diagnosed with pancreatitis based on a positive SNAP-cPL test. Routine clinical pathology was also consistent with pancreatitis. Nonspecific treatment (fluid, antibiotics, and analgesia) resulted in improvement, but he had deteriorated clinically in the last 2 days.

Physical examination findings: Tiny was moribund, had poor systolic blood pressure, was tachycardic, and had prolonged capillary refill time (>3 seconds). There was abdominal pain and free abdominal fluid.

Further testing: An abdominal ultrasound was performed that showed distended loops of bowel, large volume of abdominal effusion, and a foreign body within the small intestine.

Diagnosis: Septic peritonitis secondary to perforated small intestine was the diagnosis.

Outcome: After stabilization, Tiny underwent exploratory surgery, whereby a tennis ball was removed from his small intestine. Extensive parts of the small intestine required resection, and recovery was prolonged.

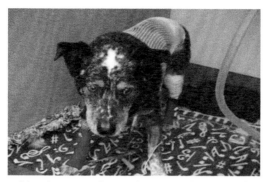

Fig. 6. Tiny, a 5-year-old male neutered Australian cattle dog, was referred with a history of vomiting and abdominal pain.

of 100% and specificity of 96% for the measurement of serum PE-1 to diagnose acute pancreatitis was reported.[39] These results were similar to a larger study that found that people with acute pancreatitis had significantly increased concentrations.[40]

Early medical studies used a radioimmunoassay that detected polyclonal elastase (bound to 1-α-antitrypsin complex) with a half-life of 2.2 days. The ELISA that has been more recently developed detects free or unbound elastase and has a half-life of 0.4 days.[41] The use of the ELISA narrows the window of opportunity for the detection of increased serum PE-1; there is a reasonable variation in the reference interval in healthy people.[42]

The canine PE-1 (cPE-1) assay used in these studies is an ELISA (ScheBo Elastase 1-Canine, ScheBo Biotech AG, Netanyastrasse 3, D-35394, Giessen, Germany), but it is less readily available than the fecal test. One study of dogs reported a serum cPE-1 interval of 32.1 to 659.3 ng/mL (median 55.8 ng/mL) in 16 healthy dogs; 24 to 1720 ng/mL (median 160 ng/mL) in 14 dogs with pancreatitis; and 5 to 182 ng/mL (median 43.3 ng/mL) in 6 dogs with renal disease.[43] A further study from the same investigators assessed the measurement of serum cPE-1, along with amylase, lipase, and TLI in 7 healthy beagles after endoscopic retrograde pancreatography, a procedure that is commonly associated with the development of pancreatic inflammation.[44] There was no difference between the baseline and any subsequent measurement of cPE-1 in any dog, although there was in the other 3 enzymes. Additionally, the range at baseline for the 7 healthy dogs was quite wide (0.1–411.6 ng/mL) with a median of 5.5 ng/mL. It is possible that the wide variation in normal dogs was caused by hemolysis, or the storage of blood samples in temperatures greater than 8°C for more than 72 hours caused a false increase in some samples, as advised by the assay manufacturer.

A later study that assessed 61 dogs that all had pancreatic histology determined overall a sensitivity of 61.4% and specificity of 91.7% when using a cutoff value for cPE-1 of 17.24 ng/mL.[45] The sensitivity of this test increased to 78.26% when only dogs with severe acute pancreatitis were assessed. Therefore, this assay seems to have a high positive likelihood ratio and low negative likelihood ratio.

There is a strong suggestion that serum PE-1 is not affected by renal clearance, as compared with many other pancreatic enzymes.[46] The proposed reason for this is that elastase circulates in the serum bound to inhibitor proteins, such as α-macroglobulin, and is too large to pass through the glomeruli, relying on extrarenal metabolic pathways for clearance. Again, in the larger cPE-1 study, there were 3 dogs with severe renal failure (urea 70.4 mmol/L, reference <12; creatinine 804 μmol/L, reference <120), and none had increased cPE-1.

Determining Severity

Early detection of severe pancreatitis is considered particularly important in people because this enables rapid transfer to intensive care units and improves outcome.[47] A similar conclusion could be made for canine acute pancreatitis. However, extrapolating from the studies that have been performed extensively in people, and to some extent in dogs, there is unlikely to be a single laboratory test that can differentiate severe from mild disease. Indeed, in the largest human study (more than 18,000 people in more than 200 centers), it was determined that SIRS, age greater than 60 years, and the presence of pleural effusion were most associated with prognosis.[48] This concept is similar to a severity score developed in dogs using clinical and laboratory data that could easily be obtained in general practice within 24 hours of admission.[3] The poor prognostic indicators identified in that study are outlined in **Table 3**. It is likely that other critical care parameters may be added to this scheme once further validation of the criteria is undertaken in larger cohorts of dogs.

Table 3
Factors contributing to clinical severity index as published for canine acute pancreatitis.[3] A higher combined score (>3) is associated with significantly higher mortality. This index has yet to be validated in a larger animal population

Parameter	Point Allocation	Criteria
Cardiac	0	No abnormalities
	1	<60 ventricular premature complexes per 24-h period or heart rate >180 beats per min
	2	Paroxysmal or sustained ventricular tachycardia
Respiratory	0	No abnormalities
	1	Clinical evidence of dyspnea or tachypnea (>40 breaths per min)
	2	Clinical evidence of pneumonia or acute respiratory distress syndrome
Intestinal integrity	0	No abnormalities
	1	Intestinal sounds not detected during >3 auscultations in 24-h period
	2	Hematochezia, melena, or regurgitation
	3	No enteral food intake for >3 d
	4	No enteral food intake for >3 d and at least 2 of the following: hematochezia, melena, and regurgitation
Vascular forces	0	No abnormalities
	1	Systolic arterial blood pressure <60 or >180 mm Hg or serum albumin concentration <18 g/L
	2	Systolic arterial blood pressure <60 or >180 mm Hg and serum albumin concentration <18 g/L

Data from Mansfield CS, James FE, Robertson ID. Development of a clinical severity index for dogs with acute pancreatitis. J Am Vet Med Assoc 2008;233:936–44.

ACUTE PANCREATITIS IN THE CAT

Cats have been increasingly reported to develop acute pancreatitis similar to dogs, with necrosis of the peripancreatic fat region being a predominant feature. A high index of suspicion for acute pancreatitis in the cat is required for a rapid diagnosis because the clinical signs are not pathognomonic (**Table 4**). Additionally, approximately two-thirds of cats with acute pancreatitis have concurrent disease, especially

Table 4
Summary of clinical findings from 3 studies of cats with acute pancreatitis and chronic pancreatitis

Clinical Sign	Hill & Van Winkle,[77] 1993	Kimmel et al,[50] 2001	Ferreri et al,[51] 2003	
Case numbers	n = 40 AP (necropsy based)	n = 46 AP	n = 30 ANP	n = 33 CP
Lethargy (%)	100	83	50	52
Anorexia (%)	97	96	63	70
Dehydration (%)	92	NR	33	51
Hypothermia (%)	68	NR	NR	NR
Vomiting (%)	35	43	43	39
Abdominal pain (%)	25	17	10	
Palpable abdominal mass (%)	23	4	3	
Diarrhea (%)	15	11	NR	NR
Dyspnea (%)	20	NR	16	
Ataxia (%)	15	NR	NR	NR
Weight loss (%)	NR	39	40	21
Jaundice (%)	NR	22	16	24
Pallor (%)	NR	NR	30	30

Abbreviations: ANP, acute necrotizing pancreatitis; AP, acute pancreatitis; CP, chronic pancreatitis; NR, not recorded.
Data from Refs.[50,51,77]

hepatic lipidosis,[49] which makes it likely that there will be nonspecific changes in routine clinical pathology, such as increased bilirubin and other liver enzymes. Cats with large-volume effusion may have hypoalbuminemia and variably increased or decreased white cell counts. Similarly, glucose may be increased either because of concurrent diabetes mellitus/diabetes ketoacidosis or because of stress hyperglycemia. The presence of hypocalcemia has been shown to be a poor prognostic indicator in cats, even in the absence of clinical signs associated with hypocalcemia.[50] However, another study showed no difference in ionized calcium between cats with acute pancreatitis and cats with chronic pancreatitis.[51]

Serum lipase concentration has been shown to increase in cats with experimentally induced acute pancreatitis, although serum amylase remained normal.[52] Unfortunately, serum lipase and amylase are seldom diagnostic in their own right in cats.[53,54]

A feline trypsin-like immunoreactivity (fTLI) assay is also available and has been shown to increase in experimentally induced pancreatitis.[55] There is a range of reported sensitivity for fTLI from 33% to 80% in acute pancreatitis, again sensitivity increasing with disease severity,[53,54,56,57] often dependent on the diagnostic cutoff value used. The concentration of fTLI may also be increased by other diseases, such as renal failure, inflammatory bowel disease, lymphosarcoma, and starvation. Unfortunately, the measurement of trypsinogen activation peptide (a by-product cleaved by trypsin activation) is no more sensitive or specific than the measurement of fTLI; because it is not readily available, it is of little benefit in diagnosing this disease.[57]

A species-specific pancreatic lipase immunoreactivity (fPLI) radioimmunoassay has also been developed, with a reference interval established of 1.2 to 3.8 μg/L.[58] One study showed a very high sensitivity (100%) in 5 cats with acute pancreatitis.[54] Overall, the specificity of fPLI in that study (compared with 8 healthy cats and 3 symptomatic cats with normal pancreatic histopathology) was 91%, which shows there may be minimal effects from other diseases. Once larger studies have been published, the true sensitivity and specificity of this test can be established. However, it does seem as if the sensitivity of fPLI will likely be greater in more severely affected animals.

CHRONIC PANCREATITIS

Chronic pancreatitis is increasingly being recognized in both dogs and cats and is defined as the presence of both fibrosis and active (generally lymphoplasmacytic) inflammation.[59] Chronic pancreatitis may be a prequel to the development of exocrine pancreatic insufficiency or diabetes mellitus.[60] In cats, there is a very high association between chronic pancreatitis and other disease, particularly cholangiohepatitis and inflammatory bowel disease.[51]

In general, all the laboratory tests discussed for acute pancreatitis may be of some use in diagnosing chronic pancreatitis in both dogs and cats. However, the sensitivity of these tests is low for chronic pancreatitis, and so diagnosis generally relies on pancreatic biopsy along with compatible historical and clinical findings. Because of the high incidence of concurrent disease in cats, concurrent histologic assessment of the liver and small intestine as a minimum is recommended.

PANCREATIC NEOPLASIA

Primary pancreatic exocrine neoplasia is rare. Clinical signs in cats are nonspecific and can include anorexia, vomiting, jaundice, and infrequently alopecia; whereas, in dogs, the clinical signs are similar to that of acute pancreatitis albeit extending over a longer period of time.[61] Some dogs with pancreatic neoplasia have been reported with multifocal steatitis.[62] Typical clinicopathologic findings reflect the accompanying pancreatic inflammation or necrosis as well as involvement with other abdominal organs.

Pancreatic Cytology

Fine-needle aspiration of the pancreas is a relatively safe procedure to do, particularly when ultrasound guided.[63] Recent work at the author's institution suggests that 25-G needles are effective for cytologic evaluation and potentially cause fewer traumas than larger-gauge needles. Fine-needle aspirates should be obtained using a 3-mL syringe with some ethylenediaminetetraacetic acid drawn into it and then, with the needle attached, be directed into the area for sampling. The needle should be moved backwards and forwards along the same line several times (but should not be redirected while in the pancreas). No negative pressure is required during sampling, and gentle squash preparation onto glass slides should then be performed. This degree of trauma to the pancreas is minimal and extremely unlikely to cause any direct inflammation.

Cytologic evaluation of the pancreas may be difficult, especially if artifacts occur (**Box 3**). However, pancreatic cytology may be of some benefit in differentiating malignant pancreatic diseases from inflammation[64]; some examples are shown in **Fig. 7**. However, because the characteristics of inflammation (neutrophils, cellular atypia, and anisocytosis) overlap considerably with neoplasia, caution must be exercised regarding overinterpretation.

EXOCRINE PANCREATIC INSUFFICIENCY

The diagnosis of exocrine pancreatic insufficiency (EPI) is usually made once more than 90% of exocrine function has been lost. Animals with EPI typically show signs

---

Box 3
Potential complications or artifacts from pancreatic fine-needle aspiration

- Hemodilution
- Overlap between inflammatory atypia and neoplasia
- Nonrepresentative lesion sampled
- Uneven distribution of disease within the pancreas
- Ruptured cells caused by sampling technique, squash preparation technique, or innate fragility of pancreatic cells
- Inclusion of cells from other abdominal organs
- Contamination with reactive mesothelial cells

---

of weight loss, have fatty, foul-smelling feces (steatorrhea), and polyphagia.[65] EPI is generally caused by pancreatic acinar atrophy but may also be a consequence of end-stage pancreatic inflammation and fibrosis or autoimmune destruction.[60,65] German shepherd dogs and Rough collies seem to be predisposed to EPI,[66] with

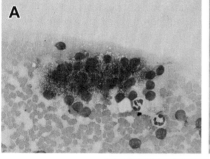
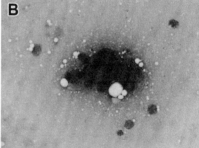
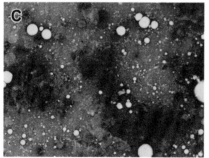

Fig. 7. Pancreatic cytology normal versus neoplasia. (*A*) A fine-needle aspirate obtained from the pancreas of a cat (H&E staining, original magnification ×100). This aspirate shows normal exocrine appearance, with little anisocytosis or anisokaryosis, small round nucleoli, and a single small nucleolus. (*B*) A fine-needle aspirate obtained from a dog (H&E staining, original magnification ×100) that shows features consistent with malignancy: binucleation, nuclear molding, and multiple nuclei. There is abundant granular cytoplasm. (*C*) A fine-needle aspirate (H&E staining, original magnification ×100) from the same dog as in (*B*), showing moderate anisocytosis and anisokaryosis, variability in the nuclear/cytoplasmic ratio, and large nucleoli. There is abundant granular cytoplasm. (*Courtesy of* S Connolly, DVM DACVP, University of Melbourne, Melbourne, Australia.)

inheritance mediated by polygenic autosomal recessive traits.[67] EPI has been considered a rare disease of cats but is being increasingly recognized.[68]

Routine clinical pathology, including total serum amylase and lipase concentration, is not helpful in diagnosing EPI. Animals may have concurrent diabetes mellitus, which can cause hyperglycemia. Because of concurrent dysbiosis in the small intestine, serum cobalamin and folate may be abnormal; but this is not pathognomonic for EPI. However, failure to recognize the potential for hypocobalaminemia may result in suboptimal treatment, particularly in cats.[68] Fecal analysis, assessing proteolytic or fat content, is unreliable and nonspecific.[65]

The most sensitive and specific test for EPI is the measurement of TLI, which is a highly specific indicator of pancreatic mass and function developed as canine or feline specific.[68,69] A serum TLI concentration of less than 2.5 μg/L is considered diagnostic of EPI in dogs, whereas a result of 8 μg/L (as measured by radioimmunoassay at the Gastrointestinal Laboratory, Texas A&M University) is considered diagnostic in cats.[65,70]

In one longitudinal study, Wiberg and colleagues[71] followed dogs that had serum TLI concentrations between 2.5 μg/L and 5.0 μg/L (5 being the lower reference interval for normal dogs). Approximately 50% of these dogs did not develop any signs of EPI, and their TLI rebounded back to more than 5.0 μg/L consistently, whereas the other 50% had repeatedly low TLI concentrations but no clinical signs of EPI. This latter group of dogs were German shepherds or Rough collies, suggesting that there may have been pancreatic acinar atrophy but with enough functional secretory reserves to be perceived as normal. This original study, combined with a later one, demonstrated that a single equivocal result of TLI cannot be used to predict the onset of EPI, that there is large variation in TLI concentrations, and that dogs with persistent results between 2.5 μg/L and 5.0 μg/L likely had a degree of subclinical EPI.[72]

The most widely used application of pancreatic elastase in human medicine is the measurement of the enzyme in feces as a determinant of exocrine pancreatic function.[73] Fecal measurement of cPE-1 seems to be of limited use in dogs for the diagnosis of EPI. A concentration of more than 20 μg/g in feces can be considered a result that excludes EPI, but values less than this are only suggestive of EPI.[74–76]

Unfortunately, no single test seems to be able to diagnose dogs with subclinical EPI or to be able to predict which dog will go on to develop EPI, even with advanced dynamic testing.[65]

REFERENCES

1. Hess RS, Saunders HM, Van Winkle TJ, et al. Clinical, clinicopathologic, radiographic, and ultrasonographic abnormalities in dogs with fatal acute pancreatitis: 70 cases (1986-1995). J Am Vet Med Assoc 1998;213:665–70.
2. Watson P. Pancreatitis in the dog: dealing with a spectrum of disease. In Practice 2004;64–77.
3. Mansfield CS, James FE, Robertson ID. Development of a clinical severity index for dogs with acute pancreatitis. J Am Vet Med Assoc 2008;233:936–44.
4. Mansfield CS. Pathophysiology of acute pancreatitis: potential application from experimental models and human medicine to dogs. J Vet Intern Med 2012;26: 875–87.
5. Whitney MS. The laboratory assessment of canine and feline pancreatitis. Vet Med 1993;85:1045–52.
6. Williams DA. Diagnosis and management of pancreatitis. J Small Anim Pract 1994;35:445–54.

7. Holowaychuk MK, Hansen BD, DeFrancesco TC, et al. Ionized hypocalcemia in critically ill dogs. J Vet Intern Med 2009;23:509–13.
8. Jacobs RM, Murtaugh RJ, DeHoff WD. Review of the clinicopathological findings of acute pancreatitis in the dog: use of an experimental model. J Am Anim Hosp Assoc 1985;21:795–800.
9. Akuzawa M, Morizono M, Nagata K, et al. Changes of serum amylase, its isozyme fractions and amylase-creatinine clearance ratio in dogs with experimentally induced acute pancreatitis. J Vet Med Sci 1994;56:269–73.
10. Mansfield CS, Jones BR. Plasma and urinary trypsinogen activation peptide in healthy dogs, dogs with pancreatitis and dogs with other systemic diseases. Aust Vet J 2000;78:416–22.
11. Rallis TS, Koutinas AF, Kritsepi M, et al. Serum lipase activity in young dogs with acute enteritis or gastroenteritis. Vet Clin Pathol 1996;25:65–8.
12. Walter GL, McGraw P, Tvedten HW. Serum lipase determination in the dog: a comparison of a titrimetric method with an automated kinetic method. Vet Clin Pathol 1992;21:23–7.
13. Parent J. Effects of dexamethasone on pancreatic tissue and on serum amylase and lipase activities in dogs. J Am Vet Med Assoc 1982;180:743–6.
14. Stewart AF. Pancreatitis in dogs and cats: cause, pathogenesis, diagnosis, and treatment. Compend Contin Educ Vet 1994;16:1423–30.
15. Hurley PR, Cook A, Jehanli A, et al. Development of radioimmunoassays for free tetra-L-aspartyl-L-lysine trypsinogen activation peptides (TAP). J Immunol Methods 1988;111:195–203.
16. Gudgeon AM, Hurley P, Jehanli A, et al. Trypsinogen activation peptide assay in the early prediction of severity of acute pancreatitis. Lancet 1990;335:4–8.
17. Neoptolemos JP, Kemppainen E, Mayer JM, et al. Early prediction of severity in acute pancreatitis by urinary trypsinogen activation peptide: a multicentre study. Lancet 2000;355:1955–60.
18. Batt RM. Exocrine pancreatic insufficiency. Vet Clin North Am Small Anim Pract 1993;23:595–608.
19. Simpson KW, Batt RM, McLean L, et al. Circulating concentrations of trypsin-like immunoreactivity and activities of lipase and amylase after pancreatic duct ligation in dogs. Am J Vet Res 1989;50:629–32.
20. Ruaux CG, Atwell RB. Levels of total alpha-macroglobulin and trypsin-like immunoreactivity are poor indicators of clinical severity in spontaneous canine acute pancreatitis. Res Vet Sci 1999;67:83–7.
21. Steiner JM, Williams DA. Purification of classical pancreatic lipase from dog pancreas. Biochimie 2002;84:1245–53.
22. Steiner JM, Berridge BR, Wojcieszyn J, et al. Cellular immunolocalization of gastric and pancreatic lipase in various tissues obtained from dogs. Am J Vet Res 2002;63:722–7.
23. Steiner JM, Rutz GM, Williams DA. Serum lipase activities and pancreatic lipase immunoreactivity concentrations in dogs with exocrine pancreatic insufficiency. Am J Vet Res 2006;67:84–7.
24. Steiner JM, Teague SR, Williams DA. Development and analytic validation of an enzyme-linked immunosorbent assay for the measurement of canine pancreatic lipase immunoreactivity in serum. Can J Vet Res 2003;67:175–82.
25. Steiner JM, Williams DA. Development and validation of a radioimmunoassay for the measurement of canine pancreatic lipase immunoreactivity in serum of dogs. Am J Vet Res 2003;64:1237–41.

26. Huth SP, Relford R, Steiner JM, et al. Analytical validation of an ELISA for measurement of canine pancreas-specific lipase. Vet Clin Pathol 2010;39:346–53.
27. Steiner JM. Diagnosis of pancreatitis. Vet Clin North Am Small Anim Pract 2003; 33:1181–95.
28. Beall MJ, Cahill R, Pigeon K, et al. Performance validation and method comparison of an in-clinic enzyme-linked immunosorbent assay for the detection of canine pancreatic lipase. J Vet Diagn Invest 2011;23:115–9.
29. Steiner JM, Newman S, Xenoulis P, et al. Sensitivity of serum markers for pancreatitis in dogs with macroscopic evidence of pancreatitis. Vet Ther 2008;9: 263–73.
30. Mansfield CS, Anderson GA, O'Hara AJ. Association between canine pancreatic-specific lipase and histologic exocrine pancreatic inflammation in dogs: assessing specificity. J Vet Diagn Invest 2012;24:312–8.
31. Steiner JM, Broussard J, Mansfield CS, et al. Serum canine pancreatic lipase immunoreactivity (cPLI) concentrations in dogs with spontaneous pancreatitis [abstract]. J Vet Intern Med 2001;15:274.
32. McCord K, Morley PS, Armstrong J, et al. A multi-institutional study evaluating the diagnostic utility of the spec cPL™ and SNAP® cPL™ in clinical acute pancreatitis in 84 dogs. J Vet Intern Med 2012;26:888–96.
33. Trivedi S, Marks SL, Kass PH, et al. Sensitivity and specificity of canine pancreas-specific lipase (cPL) and other markers for pancreatitis in 70 dogs with and without histopathologic evidence of pancreatitis. J Vet Intern Med 2011;25:1241–7.
34. Neilson-Carley SC, Robertson JE, Newman S, et al. Specificity of a canine pancreas-specific lipase assay for diagnosing pancreatitis in dogs without clinical or histologic evidence of the disease. Am J Vet Res 2011;72:302–7.
35. Steiner JM, Finco D, Williams DA. Serum lipase activity and canine pancreatic lipase immunoreactivity (cPLI) concentration in dogs with experimentally induced chronic renal failure. Vet Research 2010;3:58–63.
36. Haworth M, Hosgood G, Swindells K, et al. Diagnostic accuracy of the SNAP and spec canine pancreatic lipase (cPL) tests for pancreatitis in privately-owned dogs presenting with clinical signs of acute abdominal disease. J Vet Emerg Crit Care, in press.
37. Newman SJ, Steiner JM, Woosley K, et al. Histologic assessment and grading of the exocrine pancreas in the dog. J Vet Diagn Invest 2006;18:115–8.
38. Hartwig W, Kolvenbach M, Hackert T, et al. Enterokinase induces severe necrosis and rapid mortality in cerulein pancreatitis: characterization of a novel noninvasive rat model of necro-hemorrhagic pancreatitis. Surgery 2007;142:327–36.
39. Malfertheiner P, Buchler M, Stanescu A, et al. Serum elastase 1 in inflammatory pancreatic and gastrointestinal diseases and in renal insufficiency. A comparison with other serum pancreatic enzymes. Int J Pancreatol 1987;2:159–70.
40. Lesi C, Ruffilli E, De Mutiis R, et al. Serum elastase 1 in clinical practice. Pancreas 1988;3:444–9.
41. Millson CE, Charles K, Poon P, et al. A prospective study of serum pancreatic elastase-1 in the diagnosis and assessment of acute pancreatitis. Scand J Gastroenterol 1998;33:664–8.
42. Buchler M, Malfertheiner P, Uhl W, et al. Diagnostic and prognostic value of serum elastase 1 in acute pancreatitis. Klin Wochenschr 1986;64:1186–91.
43. Spillman T, Korrell J, Wittker A, et al. Serum canine pancreatic elastase and canine C-reactive protein for the diagnosis and prognosis of acute pancreatitis in dogs. ECVIM Congress (abstract) 2002.

44. Spillmann T, Happonen I, Sankari S, et al. Evaluation of serum values of pancreatic enzymes after endoscopic retrograde pancreatography in dogs. Am J Vet Res 2004;65:616–9.
45. Mansfield CS. Specificity and sensitivity of serum canine pancreatic elastase-1 concentration in the diagnosis of pancreatitis. J Vet Diagn Invest 2011;23:691–7.
46. Seno T, Harada H, Ochi K, et al. Serum levels of six pancreatic enzymes as related to the degree of renal dysfunction. Am J Gastroenterol 1995;90:2002–5.
47. Al Mofleh I. Severe acute pancreatitis: pathogenic aspects and prognostic factors. World J Gastroenterol 2008;14:675–84.
48. Wu BU, Johannes RS, Sun X, et al. The early prediction of mortality in acute pancreatitis: a large population-based study. Gut 2008;57:1698–703.
49. de Cock HE, Forman MA, Farver T, et al. Prevalence and histopathologic characteristics of pancreatitis in cats. Vet Pathol 2007;44:39–49.
50. Kimmel SE, Washabau RJ, Drobatz KJ. Incidence and prognostic value of low plasma ionized calcium concentration in cats with acute pancreatitis: 46 cases (1996–1998). J Am Vet Med Assoc 2001;219:1105–9.
51. Ferreri JA, Hardam E, Kimmel SE, et al. Clinical differentiation of acute necrotizing from chronic nonsuppurative pancreatitis in cats: 63 cases (1996-2001). J Am Vet Med Assoc 2003;223:469–74.
52. Kitchell BE, Strombeck DR, Cullen J, et al. Clinical and pathologic changes in experimentally induced acute pancreatitis in cats. Am J Vet Res 1986;47:1170–3.
53. Swift N, Marks SL, MacLachlan NJ, et al. Evaluation of serum feline trypsin-like immunoreactivity for the diagnosis of pancreatitis in cats. J Am Vet Med Assoc 2000;217:37–42.
54. Forman MA, Marks SL, de Cock HE, et al. Evaluation of serum feline pancreatic lipase immunoreactivity and helical computed tomography versus conventional testing for the diagnosis of feline pancreatitis. J Vet Intern Med 2004;18:807–15.
55. Steiner JM, Williams DA, Moeller EM, et al. Development and validation of an enzyme-linked immunosorbent assay for feline trypsin-like immunoreactivity. Am J Vet Res 2000;61:620–3.
56. Gerhardt A, Steiner JM, Williams DA, et al. Comparison of the sensitivity of different diagnostic tests for pancreatitis in cats. J Vet Intern Med 2001;15:329–33.
57. Allen HS, Steiner J, Broussard J, et al. Serum and urine concentrations of trypsinogen-activation peptide as markers for acute pancreatitis in cats. Can J Vet Res 2006;70:313–6.
58. Steiner J, Wilson BW, Williams DA. Development and analytical validation of a radioimmunoassay for the measurement of feline pancreatic lipase immunoreactivity in serum. Can J Vet Res 2004;68:309–14.
59. Watson PJ, Archer J, Roulois AJ, et al. Observational study of 14 cases of chronic pancreatitis in dogs. Vet Rec 2010;167:968–76.
60. Watson PJ. Exocrine pancreatic insufficiency as an end stage of pancreatitis in four dogs. J Small Anim Pract 2003;44:306–12.
61. Seaman RL. Exocrine pancreatic neoplasia in the cat: a case series. J Am Anim Hosp Assoc 2004;40:238–45.
62. Brown PJ, Mason KV, Merrett DJ, et al. Multifocal necrotising steatites associated with pancreatic carcinoma in three dogs. J Small Anim Pract 1994;35:129–32.
63. Bjorneby JM, Kari S. Cytology of the pancreas. Vet Clin North Am Small Anim Pract 2002;32:1293–312.

64. Bennett P, Hahn K, Toal R, et al. Ultrasonographic and cytopathological diagnosis of exocrine pancreatic carcinoma in the dog and cat. J Am Anim Hosp Assoc 2001;37:466–73.
65. Westermarck E, Wiberg M. Exocrine pancreatic insufficiency in the dog: historical background, diagnosis and treatment. Top Companion Anim Med 2012;27: 96–103.
66. Batchelor DJ, Noble PJ, Cripps PJ, et al. Breed associations for canine exocrine pancreatic insufficiency. J Vet Intern Med 2007;21:207–14.
67. Westermarck E, Saari SA, Wiberg M. Heritability of exocrine pancreatic insufficiency in German shepherd dogs. J Vet Intern Med 2010;24:450–2.
68. Steiner JM. Exocrine pancreatic insufficiency in the cat. Top Companion Anim Med 2012;27:113–6.
69. Williams DA, Batt RM. Sensitivity and specificity of radioimmunoassay of serum trypsin-like immunoreactivity for the diagnosis of canine exocrine pancreatic insufficiency. J Am Vet Med Assoc 1988;11:191–5.
70. Steiner JM, Williams DA. Serum feline trypsin-like immunoreactivity in cats with exocrine pancreatic insufficiency. J Vet Intern Med 2000;14:627–9.
71. Wiberg M, Nurmi AK, Westermarck E. Serum trypsinlike immunoreactivity measurement for the diagnosis of subclinical exocrine pancreatic insufficiency. J Vet Intern Med 1999;13:426–32.
72. Wiberg ME, Westermarck E. Subclinical exocrine pancreatic insufficiency in dogs. J Am Vet Med Assoc 2002;220:1183–7.
73. Pezzilli R, Talamini G, Gullo L. Behaviour of serum pancreatic enzymes in chronic pancreatitis. Dig Liver Dis 2000;32:233–7.
74. Wiberg ME, Westermarck E, Spillman T, et al. Canine faecal pancreatic elastase (cE1) for the diagnosis of subclinical exocrine pancreatic insufficiency in dogs. Eur J Comp Gastroenterol 2000;5:21–5.
75. Spillmann T, Wittker A, Teigelkamp S, et al. An immunoassay for canine pancreatic elastase 1 as an indicator for exocrine pancreatic insufficiency in dogs. J Vet Diagn Invest 2001;13:468–74.
76. Spillman T, Wiberg M, Teigelkamp S, et al. Canine faecal pancreatic elastase (CE 1) in dogs with clinical exocrine pancreatic insufficiency, normal dogs and dogs with chronic enteropathies. Eur J Comp Gastroenterol 2001;2:5–10.
77. Hill RC, Van Winkle TJ. Acute necrotizing pancreatitis and acute suppurative pancreatitis in the cat. A retrospective study of 40 cases (1976-1989). J Vet Intern Med 1993;7:25–33.

Using Cardiac Biomarkers in Veterinary Practice

Mark A. Oyama, DVM

KEYWORDS

- Natriuretic peptide • BNP • Troponin • Cardiac biomarkers • Heart disease

KEY POINTS

- Blood-based assays for cardiac biomarkers can assist in the diagnosis of heart disease in dogs and cats.
- The most established applications are differentiation of cardiac versus noncardiac causes of respiratory signs and the detection of preclinical cardiomyopathy.
- Cardiac biomarkers are best used as part of the overall clinical cardiac workup that includes the medical history, physical examination, electrocardiogram, thoracic radiographs, and echocardiography.
- The selection of proper patient populations in which to test is key to obtaining reliable results.
- Future applications might include the use of cardiac biomarkers to help guide therapy and improve patient outcomes.

INTRODUCTION: NATURE OF THE PROBLEM

The evaluation of cardiac disease in small animals can be challenging. The patient history is often nonspecific; the presence or intensity of a heart murmur on physical examination is not always a reliable measure of disease severity; concurrent pulmonary disease can confound the interpretation of thoracic radiographs; and other diagnostics, such as echocardiography, are relatively expensive and might not be readily available. For these reasons, blood-based biomarkers that are capable of detecting and staging cardiac disease are a subject of considerable interest.

A biomarker is a substance that is
- Specific to the organ or tissue under study
- Released in proportion to injury or disease

Disclosures: The author consults for and has received funding for clinical trials from IDEXX Laboratories, Westbrook, ME.
Section of Cardiology, Department of Clinical Studies-Philadelphia, School of Veterinary Medicine, University of Pennsylvania, 3900 Delancey Street, Philadelphia, PA 19104, USA
E-mail address: maoyama@vet.upenn.edu

Vet Clin Small Anim 43 (2013) 1261–1272
http://dx.doi.org/10.1016/j.cvsm.2013.07.010

In order to be clinically useful, the biomarker should provide information regarding diagnosis, prognosis, or response to treatment that is otherwise not readily available using conventional testing. The use of blood-based biomarkers for noncardiac organ systems, such as the use of gamma-glutamyl transferase to detect cholestasis or the use of creatinine to detect renal disease, is a familiar concept; cardiac biomarkers act in much the same fashion for the heart. The 2 cardiac biomarkers with the most extensive evaluation in small animals are cardiac troponin-I (cTnI) and 2 forms of B-type natriuretic peptide (BNP), namely, the C-terminal fragment (C-BNP) and the N-terminal fragment (NT-proBNP).

CARDIAC TROPONIN

The cardiac biomarker cTnI, along with troponin-T (cTnT) and troponin-C, form a conglomeration of 3 myocardial proteins that is bound to the actin backbone within myocardiocytes. The troponin complex regulates calcium binding and subsequent interaction between actin and myosin filaments. Damage to the myocardiocyte and to the sarcolemmal membrane dissociates troponin from the actin and allows leakage of troponin into the extracellular space where it then enters into the circulation. The cardiac isoforms of cTnI and cTnT are specific to cardiac tissue and are specific markers of myocardial cell injury or necrosis. In healthy patients, little to no cardiac troponin is detectable blood. Because of its high specificity for cardiac tissue, detection of either circulating cTnI or cTnT is one of the primary diagnostic tools used by emergency department clinicians to diagnose acute myocardial infarction in human patients. Cardiac troponin is also elevated in patients with chronic heart disease, although not to the extent that is seen in acute myocardial infarction; circulating concentrations of cTnI also are a fraction of those seen in acute myocardial infarction. There are 2 commercially available veterinary cardiac troponin assays (i-Stat Cardiac Troponin assay, Abaxis, Union City, CA; Troponin-I, IDEXX Laboratories, Westbrook, ME), both of which test for cTnI. Current veterinary tests are plagued by a relatively low limit of detection of approximately 0.2 ng/mL, whereas circulating cTnI concentrations in dogs with mild to moderate myxomatous mitral valve disease (MMVD) are often less than 0.03 ng/mL and can be detected only using newer high-sensitivity assays.[1] Despite these relatively modest elevations, cTnI concentrations are predictive of the outcome in human patients with chronic heart failure as well as in dogs with MMVD.[2] The troponin molecules are highly conserved across species, and many high-sensitivity assays designed for human testing can be used to detect canine and feline cTnI. Thus, cardiac troponin assays have the potential to provide both diagnostic and prognostic information. In a meta-analysis of more than 6800 human patients with stable chronic heart failure, patients with elevated cTnI or cTnT were 2.9 times more likely to die during the study follow-up period than those patients with lower values.[3] Acute myocardial infarction in dogs and cats is rare. However, chronic heart diseases, such as MMVD and dilated cardiomyopathy (DCM) in dogs and hypertrophic cardiomyopathy (HCM) in cats, are relatively common; the diagnostic and prognostic value of cardiac troponin is a subject of interest. There are several factors that potentially limit the usefulness of cardiac troponin in veterinary patients. Although elevated cardiac troponin is sensitive for the presence of myocardial injury, it is not specific to any one underlying cause. Moreover, animals with mild disease can have normal cTnI concentrations. Thus, the utility of the test to screen for specific heart diseases in various populations is limited. Cardiac troponin is partially excreted through renal mechanisms, and cardiac injury in the presence of chronic or acute kidney disease can result in false elevations.[4] Finally, cTnI concentrations increase slightly but significantly with age; additional studies establishing age-related reference ranges are needed (**Box 1**).[5]

NATRIURETIC PEPTIDES

BNP and its parent protein proBNP along with A-type natriuretic peptide (ANP) and its parent protein proANP are the main natriuretic hormones produced by myocardial tissue. Both proBNP and proANP are constitutively produced by atrial and to a lesser extent ventricular myocardiocytes. Stress or stretch of the myocardium (for instance, in response to volume overload) increases the production of proBNP and proANP, particularly within ventricular myocardiocytes. On release, these substances are quickly cleaved into separate N-terminal and C-terminal fragments. C-BNP and C-terminal ANP (C-ANP) elicit vasodilation and diuresis through binding of specific natriuretic receptors found in vascular and renal tissue. Their actions provide a counterbalance to those of the renin-angiotensin-aldosterone system. In humans, C-BNP and NT-proBNP assays are primarily used to help discriminate between cardiac causes (ie, congestive heart failure [CHF]) and noncardiac causes of respiratory clinical signs as well as to help estimate the risk of morbidity and mortality in patients with chronic heart disease. C-BNP and C-ANP have short half-lives, whereas NT-proBNP and NT-proANP are more stable and make more attractive targets for assay detection. There are 3 commercially available assays in the United States for natriuretic peptides, all involving various plasma forms of BNP: one for C-BNP in dogs (Cardio-BNP, Antech Diagnostics, Chesterfield, MO) and 2 for NT-proBNP, one each for dogs (CardioPet proBNP-Canine, IDEXX Laboratories, Westbrook, ME) and cats (CardioPet proBNP-Feline, IDEXX Laboratories, Westbrook, ME). Both the C-BNP and NT-proBNP assays require special blood-collection techniques to slow degradation during collection and transport to the reference laboratory. C-BNP and NT-proBNP are elevated in a variety of cardiac conditions, including MMVD, DCM, and HCM.[6–8] Increased concentrations also are present in noncardiac disease conditions that secondarily affect the heart, such as hyperthyroidism and systemic and pulmonary hypertension.[9,10] In both dogs and cats, concentrations are positively correlated with radiographic and echocardiographic measures of disease severity, and the ability of C-BNP and NT-proBNP assays to provide diagnostic and prognostic information is a subject of considerable interest. Most of the studies investigating the clinical utility of BNP in veterinary patients involve testing for NT-proBNP, and comparatively little is known about specific guidelines and cut points using the C-BNP assay (**Box 2**).

INDICATIONS FOR C-BNP AND NT-PROBNP TESTING

There are several indications for C-BNP or NT-proBNP testing, including differentiating cardiac versus noncardiac causes of respiratory signs, detection of occult

---

Box 1
Key points regarding cTnI

- Marker of myocardial cell injury and necrosis.
- Specific for cardiac muscle injury but not specific as to the underlying cause.
- Elevated in dogs and cats with a variety of heart and systemic diseases.

Box 2
Key points regarding C-BNP and NT-proBNP

- Parent molecule, proBNP, is produced in myocardiocytes in response to mechanical stress.
- Both are formed from the cleavage of the parent molecule proBNP.
- Both are released into circulation in a variety of heart diseases in dogs and cats.
- Both are positively correlated to clinical, radiographic, and echocardiographic measures of disease severity.

DCM in Doberman pinschers and occult HCM in cats, and as a prognostic tool in dogs with MMVD or DCM.

Differentiation of Cardiac Versus Noncardiac Causes of Respiratory Signs

Dogs and cats with respiratory signs represent a considerable diagnostic challenge because, for many cases, the cause of the clinical signs is not immediately clear. Most potential causes can be classified as either cardiac in origin (ie, CHF) or noncardiac (primary airway or parenchymal diseases, such as asthma, chronic bronchitis, pneumonia, and so forth). Studies have demonstrated the utility of C-BNP and NT-proBNP assay in distinguishing the cause of respiratory signs in dogs[6,11,12] and the utility of the NT-proBNP assay in distinguishing the cause of respiratory signs in cats.[13,14] A low NT-proBNP concentration is most consistent of a noncardiac cause, whereas an elevated concentration is more suggestive of CHF. In human medicine, NT-proBNP is best used as a test to help rule out CHF because patients with low or normal NT-proBNP are highly unlikely to have CHF. The diagnostic value of an elevated NT-proBNP concentration is less than that of a low concentration because patients with symptomatic respiratory disease and concurrent asymptomatic heart disease could have elevated concentrations. For this reason, the recommended cutoff values suggestive of a cardiac cause of respiratory signs in dogs and cats are more than the upper reference value for healthy animals. NT-proBNP and C-BNP assays are not stand-alone tests; their results should be evaluated in the context of the medical history, physical examination, and other diagnostic testing, such as radiography and echocardiography. In cases for which traditional diagnostic testing reveals the cause of the respiratory signs, BNP testing adds little additional value to the already apparent diagnosis. In cases for which the diagnosis is uncertain, the addition of the NT-proBNP assay to the diagnostic workup improved the accuracy and confidence of diagnosis in cats with respiratory signs (**Box 3**).[15]

Box 3
Guidelines for differentiation of cardiac versus noncardiac causes of respiratory signs in dogs and cats using NT-proBNP assay

- Low or normal NT-proBNP concentration is most consistent with a noncardiac cause of the current signs, whereas elevated NT-proBNP is more suggestive of a cardiac cause, such as CHF.
- In animals with asymptomatic heart disease, an increased NT-proBNP concentration can confound the diagnosis of a noncardiac cause of the respiratory signs.
- Results should be viewed in context of the medical history, physical examination, and traditional diagnostics, such as thoracic radiography.

Detection of Occult Cardiomyopathy in Doberman Pinschers and in Cats

Cardiomyopathy is common in particular breeds of dogs and cats. For instance, the lifetime incidence of DCM in Doberman pinschers is as high as 60%, and the Maine coon, ragdoll, and Persian breeds of cats, among others, are highly predisposed to HCM.[16,17] Both DCM and HCM are characterized by a long preclinical (occult) phase during which clinical signs of disease are absent despite the presence of underlying cardiac dysfunction. In animals with occult cardiomyopathy, the first clinical sign of disease can be sudden death or life-threatening CHF; thus, the detection of preclinical disease using preliminary tests is a subject of interest. The gold standard for the diagnosis of occult DCM in Doberman pinschers is the detection of ventricular premature beats via in-hospital electrocardiogram (ECG) or Holter monitoring and/or the detection of left ventricular systolic dysfunction via echocardiography. Some dogs with occult DCM will demonstrate both abnormalities, whereas others will have only one or the other. Three studies have investigated the ability to detect occult DCM in Doberman pinschers, 2 involving NT-proBNP[18,19] and one involving C-BNP.[20] C-BNP has a high sensitivity (95.2%) but a low specificity (61.9%), resulting in a high number of false-positive results. The studies involving NT-proBNP yielded similar results; the NT-proBNP assay was good at detecting dogs with systolic dysfunction whether or not they also had arrhythmias, but was poor at detecting dogs whose sole criterion for occult DCM was ventricular arrhythmias. Thus, NT-proBNP cannot be used as a stand-alone test to detect occult DCM. However, the combination of an NT-proBNP assay with Holter monitoring was 94.5% sensitive and 87.8% specific for detecting all dogs with occult disease.[19] From these studies, NT-proBNP assay does not replace the current gold standards for diagnosis. In instances when echocardiography is not immediately accessible, an elevated NT-proBNP or C-BNP concentration would support the pursuit of echocardiographic examination. Thus, BNP assesses the likelihood of finding significant abnormalities on gold standard testing rather than being a diagnostic test in and of itself. This distinction is subtle but important if the number of false-positive and negative results inherent in the BNP assays are to be avoided.

Feline cardiomyopathy has a long preclinical phase similar to canine DCM, and detection of underlying heart disease in apparently healthy cats can be challenging. Unlike the situation in the dog, wherein the presence of a heart murmur is a reliable sign of underlying heart disease, cats commonly have heart murmurs of benign origin. Moreover, not all cats with cardiomyopathy will have a heart murmur; this further confounds the ability to readily detect heart disease on physical examination. The gold standard for the diagnosis of feline cardiomyopathy is echocardiography. In instances when heart disease is suspected because of a murmur, gallop, or arrhythmia, NT-proBNP has a sensitivity of 70% to 100% and a specificity of 67% to 100% to indicate the presence of significant echocardiographic abnormalities.[8,21–23] The exact sensitivity and specificity depends on the cutoff values used, with lower cutoff values resulting in higher sensitivity but lower specificity, and higher cutoff values resulting in lower sensitivity but higher specificity (**Table 1**). The NT-proBNP assay is best suited to identify cats with moderate to severe echocardiographic changes, and it is these cats that likely benefit from additional monitoring or treatment. NT-proBNP testing has been studied only in cats that have risk factors for cardiomyopathy (ie, murmur, gallop, arrhythmia, and so forth), and the clinical usefulness of NT-proBNP assay to detect cardiomyopathy in the general population is unknown (**Box 4**). For this reason, indiscriminate testing of cats is not recommended, particularly in instances when the likelihood of significant disease is very low (ie, young cats undergoing neutering). The

Table 1
Diagnostic uses of cardiac biomarker tests in dogs and cats

Indication	Marker	Cutoff Values	Sensitivity (%)	Specificity (%)	Comments
Differentiating cardiac vs noncardiac causes of respiratory signs in cats	NT-proBNP[13,14]	220, 265 (pmol/L)	90–94	88	Low values indicate cardiac causes are unlikely, high values suggest CHF
Differentiating cardiac vs noncardiac causes of respiratory signs in dogs	NT-proBNP[12,38]	1158, 1400 (pmol/L)	86–92	81	Low values indicate cardiac causes are unlikely, high values suggest CHF
	C-BNP[6,11]	17.4, 6.0 (pg/mL)	86–90	78–81	Low values indicate cardiac causes are unlikely, high values suggest CHF
Detection of cardiomyopathy in at-risk cats	cTnI[33,34]	0.157, 0.20 (ng/mL)	85–87	84–97	Elevated values not specific for primary heart disease
	NT-proBNP[21–23]	95, 99, 100 (pmol/L)	71–92	94–100	Studies were performed in populations with clinical suspicion for heart disease (ie, those with murmur, gallop, arrhythmias, and so forth)
Detection of cardiomyopathy in Doberman pinschers	NT-proBNP[18,19]	457, 550 (pmol/L)	70–79	81–90	NT-proBNP poor at detecting dogs with arrhythmias only, sensitivity and specificity improved if used in tandem with Holter monitoring
	C-BNP[20]	6.2 (pg/mL)	95	62	Low specificity results in large number of false positives

The reported cutoff values and range of respective sensitivities and specificities for various indications are presented. Cardiac biomarker assays indicate risk of a particular condition being present, and additional diagnostics are often needed to obtain a definitive diagnosis. Cardiac biomarker assays are not stand-alone diagnostic assays. When interpreting results, values that far exceed cutoff values provide more reliable information than those at or near the cutoff value.

> **Box 4**
> **Guidelines for detection of occult cardiomyopathy in Doberman pinschers and in cats using NT-proBNP assay**
>
> - Testing should be done on selected patients that are at high risk for cardiac disease, such as adult Doberman pinschers and Maine coon cats and cats with a heart murmur or arrhythmia.
> - Elevated concentrations increase the likelihood of clinically significant echocardiographic abnormalities, and further diagnostics should be pursued.
> - Elevated concentrations could help assess the need or urgency to pursue more costly or time-consuming diagnostic tests if the presence of clinically significant disease is initially unclear.
> - Elevated concentrations are not diagnostic of any one particular disease, and results should be interpreted in the context of the medical history, physical examination, and traditional diagnostic testing.

likelihood of a test result being either false positive or false negative is partly dependent on the prevalence of the disease condition in the population being tested. The less prevalent the disease, the less likely a patient has the disease, even if a test result is positive. As an example, in a dog living in Alaska, there is a high likelihood that a positive heartworm antigen test is actually a false-positive result simply because of the very low prevalence of disease in this region, whereas a positive heartworm antigen test from a dog living in the Mississippi River Valley is almost certainly a true positive. Thus, clinicians must select the appropriate patient population in which to test in order to optimize the reliability of the assay.

Predicting Morbidity and Mortality in Dogs with Heart Disease

Aside from their role in the diagnosis of heart disease, whether BNP assays can predict the risk of CHF in dogs with preclinical disease or predict the risk of cardiovascular mortality is a subject of interest. The use of the NT-proBNP assay to predict the first-onset of CHF in dogs with preclinical MMVD has been studied. In one study, baseline NT-proBNP concentration was 80% sensitive and 76% specific for identifying dogs that developed CHF within the subsequent 12 months.[24] Another study in dogs with preclinical MMVD reported that those with NT-proBNP greater than 1500 pmol/L were approximately 6 times more likely to develop CHF over the subsequent 3 to 6 months than dogs with lower values.[25] The predictive value of NT-proBNP was best when combined with measures of radiographic or echocardiographic left side of the heart size, and NT-proBNP should be used alongside traditional diagnostic methods.

Several studies have revealed an association between NT-proBNP and survival in dogs with MMVD.[2,24,26] In the most recent studies, increases in NT-proBNP, high sensitivity cTnI, and echocardiographic heart size were negatively associated with survival.[2] For each incremental increase of 100 pmol/L in NT-proBNP, the risk of death caused by cardiac disease increased by 7%. Two studies have investigated NT-proBNP and the survival of dogs with DCM. In one study, Doberman pinschers with DCM and elevated NT-proBNP had a median survival time that was 6 times shorter than those with lower values[19]; in another study, NT-proBNP predicted the survival of dogs with DCM 60 days after the initial examination.[27]

The use of the NT-proBNP assay to help predict the risk of either CHF or survival has several important limitations, and further studies are needed before the assay becomes part of the standard workup for dogs with MMVD (**Box 5**). Firstly, sensitivity and specificity are performance indices that apply to populations of individuals; the

---

Box 5
Guidelines for stratification of risk in dogs with MMVD

- Dogs with preclinical MMVD, radiographic or echocardiographic heart enlargement, and NT-proBNP greater than 1500 pmol/L are likely at an increased risk for the development of CHF.
- In dogs at an increased risk of morbidity or mortality, increased vigilance for subtle signs of heart failure and more frequent monitoring is recommended.
- There are no clinical studies assessing the value of treatment decisions based on NT-proBNP concentrations.

---

accuracy of the diagnostic test in any one individual is not 100%. Secondly, elevated NT-proBNP concentrations specify the risk, not the certainty, of morbidity or mortality. Elevated NT-proBNP, especially in dogs with radiographic or echocardiographic cardiomegaly, likely warrants heightened vigilance for early signs of CHF. In animals at high risk for CHF, owners can be counseled about how to obtain the animal's resting respiratory rate. In healthy dogs, the average sleeping respiratory rate is 13 breaths per minute and rarely exceeds 30 breaths per minute.[28] Respiratory rates of more than 41 breaths per minute have been shown to be a sensitive indicator for the detection of CHF.[29] Finally, there are no data indicating that NT-proBNP concentrations can be used to guide therapy decisions, such as when to initiate or alter existing drugs, such as diuretics or angiotensin converting enzyme inhibitor. In human patients with heart failure, 2 meta-analyses[30,31] indicated that BNP-guided therapy resulted in better outcomes, although these results are controversial. In one study of dogs being treated for CHF, dogs with NT-proBNP less than 965 pmol/L following therapy survived longer than those dogs with NT-proBNP concentrations more than 965 pmol/L,[32] suggesting the possibility that therapeutic targets of NT-proBNP could be useful. These data require specifically designed prospective studies for validation.

INDICATIONS FOR CARDIAC TROPONIN TESTING

Specific guidelines for cardiac troponin testing are not well established. Circumstances that might warrant testing include suspected myocarditis or cardiomyopathy or as a prognostic tool in dogs with MMVD or DCM. Troponin testing has also been used to detect myocardial injury in babesiosis, gastric dilatation and volvulus, brachycephalic airway syndrome, sepsis, racing and sled-dog athletes, heartworm disease, dogs receiving doxorubicin, and cases of respiratory distress with unknown cause. In general, cardiac troponin concentrations reflect the severity of cardiac injury and are inversely associated with morbidity and mortality[1,2,5]; however, more studies are needed before specific treatment guidelines can be made using specific concentrations.

Cats with HCM have higher cTnI concentrations than healthy cats; in 2 small studies, elevated cTnI was 85% to 87% sensitive and 84% to 97% specific for the detection of disease.[33,34] Comparatively, the diagnostic ability of cTnI to detect preclinical (occult) DCM in dogs is poor.[20] The cTnI concentrations are higher in cats and dogs with respiratory signs secondary to CHF, but the overlap between these animals and animals with respiratory signs caused by noncardiac causes is wide enough to limit clinical usefulness.[11,35] Elevated cTnI is not specific to primary cardiac disease because any systemic condition that causes hypoxemia and myocardial ischemia could result in elevated cTnI. In the author's experience, some of the highest cTnI concentrations observed have been from dogs with severe pulmonary parenchymal disease and resultant hypoxemia.

In dogs with MMVD, a serum cTnI concentration more than 0.025 ng/mL was associated with a 1.9 times risk for death compared with lower concentrations.[2] Animals with elevated troponin concentrations might benefit from further diagnostic tests, such as ECG, thoracic radiography, and echocardiography (**Box 6**). Whether cardiac troponin concentrations can be used to help guide therapy is an intriguing possibility but requires well-designed prospective trials. In the author's experience, serial troponin measurements in dogs with suspected myocarditis offer some prognostic information; declining values often signify a one-time insult and myocardial recovery, whereas persistently elevated or increasing concentrations are a poor prognostic indicator.

LIMITATIONS OF CARDIAC BIOMARKERS

There are important limitations to the use of cardiac biomarkers in veterinary patients. These limitations involve technical issues, such as failure to properly collect and transport samples, as well as biologic issues, such as the effect of systemic disease on the production or excretion of cTnI and NT-proBNP. Both NT-proBNP and C-BNP assays require special sample collection procedures using manufacturer-supplied blood-collection tubes designed to prevent degradation of BNP during shipping. Improper collection techniques, extended storage at room temperature, or multiple freeze-thaw cycles likely produce inaccurate results. Both NT-proBNP and C-BNP are excreted via renal filtration and can be elevated in animals with acute or chronic kidney disease.[36,37] These elevations are relatively modest in patients with mild disease but increase as renal function worsens. Many clinical studies of NT-proBNP excluded patients with renal disease, highlighting the need to interpret cutoff values in these patients with caution. Other conditions associated with increased NT-proBNP include pulmonary hypertension[10] and feline hyperthyroidism,[9] and results from animals with these diseases should be interpreted with similar caution. Since the introduction of the canine NT-proBNP assay in 2006, there have been several revisions to the assay, the most recent involving the introduction of special blood-collection tubes in 2008. Earlier clinical studies, including those investigating the detection of occult DCM in Doberman pinschers and the discrimination of cardiac versus noncardiac causes of respiratory signs in dogs were performed using the pre-2008 version of the canine assay. Ideally, these studies should be repeated using the most current version of the assay.

Box 6
Guidelines for cardiac troponin testing

- Consider testing in animals with suspected myocarditis or myocardial injury.
- Concentrations generally reflect the magnitude of myocardial injury.
- Serial evaluations that reveal declining values suggest a one-time insult and myocardial recovery, whereas persistently elevated or increasing values suggest ongoing myocardial injury.
- Consider testing as an adjunctive diagnostic test to detect cats with a high likelihood for HCM.
- It is not useful as a test to differentiate cardiac versus noncardiac causes of respiratory signs in dogs and cats.

SUMMARY

Cardiac biomarkers are an exciting and growing science. Much data regarding their clinical use in dogs and cats have been generated; however, many questions remain unanswered. The most established applications involve use of cTnI to help detect myocarditis and feline cardiomyopathy and the use of NT-proBNP to help detect occult cardiomyopathy and differentiate cardiac versus noncardiac causes of respiratory signs. Compared with NT-proBNP, there is relatively little data regarding C-BNP. However, applications of the C-BNP assay are likely similar to those involving NT-proBNP. Both cTnI and NT-proBNP assays help predict the risk of cardiovascular mortality in dogs with MMVD, but additional study is needed to better understand how to use these data in everyday clinical practice. Cardiac biomarker tests are complementary to existing cardiac diagnostic testing and should be interpreted in the context of the overall clinical picture rather than being used as a stand-alone test. Future studies will help determine whether cardiac biomarker assays can help guide therapy and lead to improved outcomes in dogs and cats with cardiac disease.

REFERENCES

1. Ljungvall I, Hoglund K, Tidholm A, et al. Cardiac troponin I is associated with severity of myxomatous mitral valve disease, age, and C-reactive protein in dogs. J Vet Intern Med 2010;24(1):153–9.
2. Hezzell MJ, Boswood A, Chang YM, et al. The combined prognostic potential of serum high-sensitivity cardiac troponin I and N-terminal pro-B-type natriuretic peptide concentrations in dogs with degenerative mitral valve disease. J Vet Intern Med 2012;26(2):302–11.
3. Nagarajan V, Hernandez AV, Tang WH. Prognostic value of cardiac troponin in chronic stable heart failure: a systematic review. Heart 2012;98(24):1778–86.
4. Sharkey LC, Berzina I, Ferasin L, et al. Evaluation of serum cardiac troponin I concentration in dogs with renal failure. J Am Vet Med Assoc 2009;234(6):767–70.
5. Oyama MA, Sisson DD. Cardiac troponin-I concentration in dogs with cardiac disease. J Vet Intern Med 2004;18(6):831–9.
6. DeFrancesco TC, Rush JE, Rozanski EA, et al. Prospective clinical evaluation of an ELISA B-type natriuretic peptide assay in the diagnosis of congestive heart failure in dogs presenting with cough or dyspnea. J Vet Intern Med 2007;21(2): 243–50.
7. Oyama MA, Fox PR, Rush JE, et al. Clinical utility of serum N-terminal pro-B-type natriuretic peptide concentration for identifying cardiac disease in dogs and assessing disease severity. J Am Vet Med Assoc 2008;232(10):1496–503.
8. Connolly DJ, Magalhaes RJ, Syme HM, et al. Circulating natriuretic peptides in cats with heart disease. J Vet Intern Med 2008;22(1):96–105.
9. Menaut P, Connolly DJ, Volk A, et al. Circulating natriuretic peptide concentrations in hyperthyroid cats. J Small Anim Pract 2012;53(12):673–8.
10. Kellihan HB, Mackie BA, Stepien RL. NT-proBNP, NT-proANP and cTnI concentrations in dogs with pre-capillary pulmonary hypertension. J Vet Cardiol 2011;13(3): 171–82.
11. Prosek R, Sisson DD, Oyama MA, et al. Distinguishing cardiac and noncardiac dyspnea in 48 dogs using plasma atrial natriuretic factor, B-type natriuretic factor, endothelin, and cardiac troponin-I. J Vet Intern Med 2007;21(2):238–42.
12. Oyama MA, Rush JE, Rozanski EA, et al. Assessment of serum N-terminal pro-B-type natriuretic peptide concentration for differentiation of congestive heart failure

from primary respiratory tract disease as the cause of respiratory signs in dogs. J Am Vet Med Assoc 2009;235(11):1319–25.

13. Connolly DJ, Soares Magalhaes RJ, Fuentes VL, et al. Assessment of the diagnostic accuracy of circulating natriuretic peptide concentrations to distinguish between cats with cardiac and non-cardiac causes of respiratory distress. J Vet Cardiol 2009;11(Suppl 1):S41–50.

14. Fox PR, Oyama MA, Reynolds C, et al. Utility of plasma N-terminal pro-brain natriuretic peptide (NT-proBNP) to distinguish between congestive heart failure and non-cardiac causes of acute dyspnea in cats. J Vet Cardiol 2009;11(Suppl 1):S51–61.

15. Singletary GE, Rush JE, Fox PR, et al. Effect of NT-pro-BNP assay on accuracy and confidence of general practitioners in diagnosing heart failure or respiratory disease in cats with respiratory signs. J Vet Intern Med 2012;26(3):542–6.

16. O'Grady MR, O'Sullivan ML. Dilated cardiomyopathy: an update. Vet Clin North Am Small Anim Pract 2004;34(5):1187–207.

17. Trehiou-Sechi E, Tissier R, Gouni V, et al. Comparative echocardiographic and clinical features of hypertrophic cardiomyopathy in 5 breeds of cats: a retrospective analysis of 344 cases (2001-2011). J Vet Intern Med 2012;26(3):532–41.

18. Wess G, Butz V, Mahling M, et al. Evaluation of N-terminal pro-B-type natriuretic peptide as a diagnostic marker of various stages of cardiomyopathy in Doberman pinschers. Am J Vet Res 2011;72(5):642–9.

19. Singletary GE, Morris NA, O'Sullivan ML, et al. Prospective evaluation of NT-proBNP assay to detect occult dilated cardiomyopathy and predict survival in Doberman pinschers. J Vet Intern Med 2012;26:1330–6.

20. Oyama MA, Sisson DD, Solter PF. Prospective screening for occult cardiomyopathy in dogs by measurement of plasma atrial natriuretic peptide, B-type natriuretic peptide, and cardiac troponin-I concentrations. Am J Vet Res 2007;68(1):42–7.

21. Fox PR, Rush JE, Reynolds CA, et al. Multicenter evaluation of plasma N-terminal probrain natriuretic peptide (NT-pro BNP) as a biochemical screening test for asymptomatic (occult) cardiomyopathy in cats. J Vet Intern Med 2011;25(5):1010–6.

22. Wess G, Daisenberger P, Mahling M, et al. Utility of measuring plasma N-terminal pro-brain natriuretic peptide in detecting hypertrophic cardiomyopathy and differentiating grades of severity in cats. Vet Clin Pathol 2011;40(2):237–44.

23. Tominaga Y, Miyagawa Y, Toda N, et al. The diagnostic significance of the plasma N-terminal pro-B-type natriuretic peptide concentration in asymptomatic cats with cardiac enlargement. J Vet Med Sci 2011;73(8):971–5.

24. Chetboul V, Serres F, Tissier R, et al. Association of plasma N-terminal pro-B-type natriuretic peptide concentration with mitral regurgitation severity and outcome in dogs with asymptomatic degenerative mitral valve disease. J Vet Intern Med 2009;23(5):984–94.

25. Reynolds CA, Brown DC, Rush JE, et al. Prediction of first onset of congestive heart failure in dogs with degenerative mitral valve disease: the PREDICT cohort study. J Vet Cardiol 2012;14(1):193–202.

26. Moonarmart W, Boswood A, Luis F, et al. N-terminal pro B-type natriuretic peptide and left ventricular diameter independently predict mortality in dogs with mitral valve disease. J Small Anim Pract 2010;51(2):84–96.

27. Noszczyk-Nowak A. NT-pro-BNP and troponin I as predictors of mortality in dogs with heart failure. Pol J Vet Sci 2011;14(4):551–6.

28. Rishniw M, Ljungvall I, Porciello F, et al. Sleeping respiratory rates in apparently healthy adult dogs. Res Vet Sci 2012;93(2):965–9.

29. Schober KE, Hart TM, Stern JA, et al. Detection of congestive heart failure in dogs by Doppler echocardiography. J Vet Intern Med 2010;24(6):1358–68.

30. Porapakkham P, Porapakkham P, Zimmet H, et al. B-type natriuretic peptide-guided heart failure therapy: a meta-analysis. Arch Intern Med 2010;170(6):507–14.

31. Felker GM, Hasselblad V, Hernandez AF, et al. Biomarker-guided therapy in chronic heart failure: a meta-analysis of randomized controlled trials. Am Heart J 2009;158(3):422–30.

32. Wolf J, Gerlach N, Weber K, et al. Lowered N-terminal pro-B-type natriuretic peptide levels in response to treatment predict survival in dogs with symptomatic mitral valve disease. J Vet Cardiol 2012;14(3):399–408.

33. Herndon WE, Kittleson MD, Sanderson K, et al. Cardiac troponin I in feline hypertrophic cardiomyopathy. J Vet Intern Med 2002;16(5):558–64.

34. Connolly DJ, Cannata J, Boswood A, et al. Cardiac troponin I in cats with hypertrophic cardiomyopathy. J Feline Med Surg 2003;5(4):209–16.

35. Herndon WE, Rishniw M, Schrope D, et al. Assessment of plasma cardiac troponin I concentration as a means to differentiate cardiac and noncardiac causes of dyspnea in cats. J Am Vet Med Assoc 2008;233(8):1261–4.

36. Miyagawa Y, Tominaga Y, Toda N, et al. Relationship between glomerular filtration rate and plasma N-terminal pro B-type natriuretic peptide concentrations in dogs with chronic kidney disease. Vet J 2013, in press.

37. Lalor SM, Connolly DJ, Elliott J, et al. Plasma concentrations of natriuretic peptides in normal cats and normotensive and hypertensive cats with chronic kidney disease. J Vet Cardiol 2009;11(Suppl 1):S71–9.

38. Fine DM, Declue AE, Reinero CR. Evaluation of circulating amino-terminal-pro-B-type natriuretic peptide concentration in dogs with respiratory distress attributable to congestive heart failure or primary pulmonary disease. J Am Vet Med Assoc 2008;232(11):1674–9.

Practical Acid-Base in Veterinary Patients

Andrea A. Monnig, DVM, DACVECC

KEYWORDS

- Acid-base • Metabolic acidosis • Metabolic alkalosis • Respiratory acidosis
- Respiratory alkalosis • Base excess • Anion gap

KEY POINTS

- Acid-base assessment can be quickly and easily performed in veterinary patients.
- Rapid recognition of acid-base disorders can aid clinicians in developing a diagnostic and therapeutic plan, as well as monitor response to therapy.
- Four primary acid-base disturbances exist when using traditional means of acid-base interpretation: metabolic acidosis, metabolic alkalosis, respiratory acidosis, and respiratory alkalosis.
- Compensation for a primary acid-base disturbance is expected within a set time frame.
- Mixed disturbances may be present if Pco_2 and HCO_3^- are moving in opposite directions, pH is normal despite abnormalities in Pco_2 or HCO_3^-, the pH change is more significant than what is predicted for the primary disturbance, or the patient fails to mount the expected compensatory response.

Acid-base disturbances are commonly identified in critically ill veterinary patients. Disturbances should be expected in animals presenting for gastrointestinal, renal, respiratory, and neurologic diseases, as well as shock. Routine serum biochemical profile results may be suggestive of an acid-base disturbance when alterations of total carbon dioxide concentration, bicarbonate, electrolytes, and anion gap (AG) are present. Abnormalities in these variables should prompt clinicians to further investigate the patient's acid-base status through blood-gas analysis. Characterization of acid-base disturbances can provide insight into the underlying disease process, direct diagnostic resources, and help monitor response to therapy.

Multiple methods of acid-base interpretation have been developed. The traditional means of acid-base interpretation uses the Henderson-Hasselbalch method that utilizes partial pressure of carbon dioxide (Pco_2) and bicarbonate (HCO_3^-) to evaluate alterations in pH.[1] Base excess (BE) and AG have been incorporated into this

The author declares no conflicts of interest.
Department of Veterinary Clinical Sciences, College of Veterinary Medicine, The Ohio State University, 601 Vernon L. Tharp Street, Columbus, OH 43210, USA
E-mail address: andrea.monnig@cvm.osu.edu

Vet Clin Small Anim 43 (2013) 1273–1286
http://dx.doi.org/10.1016/j.cvsm.2013.07.009   vetsmall.theclinics.com
0195-5616/13/$ – see front matter © 2013 Elsevier Inc. All rights reserved.

methodology. The primary advantage of this approach is that it is both widely recognized and relatively simple to use and understand.[1] The greatest disadvantage of this method is its descriptive nature, rather than providing a mechanistic explanation for the changes observed in pH.[2,3] Another downside is that HCO_3^- is a dependent variable and can readily be influenced by variables in the system. The Stewart-Fencl approach to acid-base interpretation uses pH, Pco_2, electrolytes that make up strong ion difference, and quantity of weak acids, including albumin, globulins, and phosphorus, to provide a mechanistic explanation for the observed acid-base alterations.[1] This approach can be extremely helpful in cases of mixed acid-base disturbances or when alterations in weak acids exist. Similarly, the use of corrected serum chloride and predicated bicarbonate may help to identify acid-base abnormalities that are masked by changes in water balance or AG.[4] However, the formulas used in the Stewart-Fencl and the corrected chloride approaches can be somewhat cumbersome for routine clinical use. Therefore, this review focuses on the traditional means of acid-base analysis.

ACID-BASE HOMEOSTASIS

The body works to tightly regulate hydrogen ion (H^+) concentration. Alterations in $[H^+]$ can have profound physiologic effects, such as altered cardiac contractility, arrhythmias, hypotension, diminished responsiveness to catecholamines, insulin resistance, dysfunction of enzyme systems, and electrolyte disturbances.[5–8] Acid production in the body occurs in 2 forms: volatile acid (CO_2) and nonvolatile, or fixed, acid. Volatile acid production is the end product of aerobic metabolism. When CO_2 combines with water, the reaction is catalyzed by the enzyme carbonic anhydrase (CA) to form carbonic acid (H_2CO_3). Carbonic acid dissociates into H^+ and HCO_3^-.

$$CO_2 + H_2O \overset{CA}{\leftrightarrow} H_2CO_3 \leftrightarrow H^+ + HCO_3^-$$

Fixed acids are the end product of protein and phospholipid catabolism, such as sulfuric acid and phosphoric acid, respectively. Pathologic disease states such as diabetic ketoacidosis and tissue hypoxia can result in excessive production of fixed acids, including acetoacetate, β-hydroxybutyrate, and lactate. Fixed acids also can form as the result of ingestion of household items such as aspirin, ethylene glycol, or methanol-containing products.[9]

Body fluids contain several buffers that are the first line of defense against acute changes in pH. A buffer is simply a mixture of a weak acid and its conjugate base or a weak base and its conjugate acid. Buffered solutions resist changes in pH. Common body buffers include plasma HCO_3^-, proteins, and phosphates and intracellular proteins (eg, hemoglobin) and organic phosphates (eg, adenosine diphosphate, adenosine triphosphate, 2,3-diphosphoglycerate).[9] When alterations in H^+ exceed buffering capabilities, an acid-base disturbance will develop. Two primary organs, the lungs and kidneys, are responsible for maintenance of normal acid-base balance. The lungs alter CO_2 through change in alveolar ventilation. Peripheral and central chemoreceptors detect alterations in CO_2, O_2, and pH, and send afferent signals to the respiratory center located in the brainstem. Efferent signals are then sent to the muscles of respiration to modify respiratory rate and depth, affecting CO_2 gas exchange at the level of the alveolus.[10] The kidneys have the ability to excrete excess amounts of acid or base as needed to regulate systemic pH. Nearly all of the filtered HCO_3^- is reabsorbed in the proximal convoluted tubule and thick ascending limb of the loop of Henle. In addition, HCO_3^- lost in the buffering process is regenerated throughout the nephron, whereas excessive amounts of fixed acid are excreted into the urine with ammonium.[11]

EQUIPMENT AND SAMPLE COLLECTION

Point-of-care (POC) blood-gas analyzers in the form of hand-held devices and bench-top analyzers have added to the ease of acid-base assessment in general and specialty veterinary practice. However, several factors, including equipment, sample collection, and processing, must be considered. Not all variables reported by POC machines are measured directly; some are calculated from formulas and monograms programmed into the analyzer.[12] Calculated variables in those units designed and programmed for humans may not necessarily correlate to veterinary species.[12,13] Due diligence on the part of veterinary practitioners is necessary to ensure that the instrumentation being used has been validated for veterinary use.

Depending on the analyzer used, manufacturer-specific lyophilized lithium heparin syringes may be required for sample collection. Some syringes have a self-filling feature for arterial sample collection. These syringes cannot be used for direct sampling from a venous vessel. The sample is collected in a non-anticoagulated syringe and immediately transferred into a blood-gas–specific syringe. Alternatively, syringes can be heparinized with liquid sodium heparin, or samples can be placed into a heparinized green-top tube.[12] The use of liquid sodium heparin can introduce preanalytic error through dilution and binding of divalent cations, namely calcium.[14] One study in dogs demonstrated that dilution significantly changed measured values of P_{CO_2}, P_{O_2}, and base deficit, as well as concentrations of electrolytes and lactate.[15] Evacuation of sodium heparin by pushing air through the syringe 3 times, followed by collection of 1 mL of sample volume, can minimize this error.[15] If liquid sodium heparin green-top tubes are used, the manufacturer's guidelines for sample size should be used to ensure appropriate dilution.

Traditional assessment of acid-base can be performed on arterial or venous blood. Arterial samples are necessary only when one wishes to assess the patient's pulmonary function. Venous samples provide a more representative assessment of the acid-base status at the level of the tissues.[12] Location of sample collection will have subtle influences on results, as peripheral samples will reflect local tissue metabolism.[16] Ideally, samples should be obtained from a free-flowing venous site, minimizing venous stasis and muscle activity that can result in accumulation of acid metabolites (eg, lactate).[11,17] Despite these recommendations, one study found no statistical difference in lactate concentrations in cats noted to struggle during venipuncture.[18]

Syringe material and air bubbles have been demonstrated to affect the partial pressure of measured gases.[19,20] In addition, temperature and duration of sample storage before analysis can influence ongoing cellular metabolism within the sample.[19,21] Ultimately this can have an effect on gas tension and metabolites that directly contribute to acid-base assessment. To minimize artifact, it is recommended to remove air bubbles within 30 seconds, cork the sample to maintain anaerobic conditions, and analyze samples within minutes of collection. If this is not possible, the sample should be placed on ice until analysis.[19,22]

TRADITIONAL ACID-BASE INTERPRETATION

Traditional acid-base interpretation relies on the Henderson-Hasselbalch approach to calculate the pH using HCO_3^- and P_{CO_2}.

$$pH = 6.1 + \log[HCO_3^-]/(0.03 \times P_{CO_2})$$

Further analysis of pH, P_{CO_2}, and HCO_3^- will help determine the primary disturbance: metabolic acidosis, metabolic alkalosis, respiratory acidosis, or respiratory alkalosis. For each of these disturbances, compensation is expected in an effort to return the blood pH near normal. The body will never overcompensate for a single disorder. Timing and completeness of compensation will depend on the primary disturbance and species involved.[11] Acid-base disturbances can be described as simple if there is a primary disturbance with the expected compensatory response. Not uncommonly, multiple acid-base disturbances may be present concurrently. If 2 or 3 disturbances exist at once (ie, not the primary disturbance with its expected compensatory response), it is known as a mixed or triple disturbance.[11]

Developing a systematic approach to acid-base interpretation will aid the ease of disturbance identification, generation of a differential list, and subsequent diagnostic plan. A stepwise approach can be performed as follows[11]:

- Evaluate the pH. Is there an acidemia (decreased pH) or alkalemia (increased pH) present?
- Determine the primary disturbance. Is it metabolic or respiratory in origin?
- Establish whether there is compensation for the primary disturbance. If so, is the level of adaptation appropriate?
- Identify the underlying cause(s) of the acid-base disorder(s).

Evaluate the pH

Start by evaluating the pH. An increase in H^+ will result in acidemia, whereas a decrease in H^+ will result in an alkalemia. Note that mixed acid-base disorders can be present even if the pH is normal.

Determine the Primary Disturbance

Next, determine if the alteration in pH is the result of a metabolic (HCO_3^-) or respiratory (P_{CO_2}) abnormality. This step is important even if the pH is normal, because a mixed disturbance may be present. Once the primary disturbance has been identified, it will serve as the descriptor for the underlying process or "-osis" (eg, metabolic acidosis or alkalosis vs respiratory acidosis or alkalosis).

Establish if There is Compensation for the Primary Disturbance

Each primary acid-base disturbance has an expected compensatory response (**Table 1**). At quick glance, if the P_{CO_2} and HCO_3^- are moving in the same direction, the disorder is expected to be compensated. However, it is still important to make sure the response is adequate. Respiratory compensation occurs with primary metabolic disturbances, and the kidneys modulate metabolic compensation for primary respiratory disturbances. Evidence suggests that cats are not as effective as dogs at respiratory compensation for primary metabolic disorders, but they do exhibit expected metabolic responses to primary respiratory disorders.[23,24] The timing of respiratory compensation will start almost instantly and will take approximately 12 to 24 hours to complete. Evaluation of the adequacy of compensation for respiratory disturbances will depend on the chronicity of the disorder.

Identify the Underlying Cause(s) of the Acid-Base Disorder

Causes of the primary disturbances have been identified and are discussed later in greater detail. In addition to pH, P_{CO_2}, and HCO_3^-, BE, a calculated variable, can be helpful in determining the magnitude of nonrespiratory contribution to acid-base alterations because it is changed only by fixed acids. BE provides a truer

Table 1
Primary acid-base disturbances and expected compensatory response

Disorder	pH	Primary Change	Expected Compensatory Response
Metabolic acidosis	↓	↓ $[HCO_3^-]$	1.0-mm Hg decrement in P_{CO_2} for every 1-mEq/L decrement in $[HCO_3^-]$
Metabolic alkalosis	↑	↑ $[HCO_3^-]$	0.7-mm Hg increment in P_{CO_2} for every 1-mEq/L increment in $[HCO_3^-]$
Acute respiratory acidosis	↓	↑ P_{CO_2}	1.5-mEq/L increment in $[HCO_3^-]$ for every 10-mm Hg increment in P_{CO_2}
Chronic respiratory acidosis	↓	↑ P_{CO_2}	3.5-mEq/L increment in $[HCO_3^-]$ for every 10-mm Hg increment in P_{CO_2}
Acute respiratory alkalosis	↑	↓ P_{CO_2}	2.5-mEq/L decrement in $[HCO_3^-]$ for every 10-mm Hg decrement in P_{CO_2}
Chronic respiratory alkalosis	↑	↓ P_{CO_2}	5.5-mEq/L decrement in $[HCO_3^-]$ for every 10-mm Hg decrement in P_{CO_2}

Values from dogs.
Adapted from DiBartola SP. Metabolic acid-base disorders. In: DiBartola SP, ed. Fluid, electrolyte, and acid-base disorders in small animal practice. 4th ed. St. Louis: Elsevier; 2012. p. 239; with permission.

representation of metabolic disturbances then HCO_3^-. By definition, BE (or deficit) is the amount of strong acid or base that must be added to titrate 1 L of blood to a pH of 7.4 at 37°C while the P_{CO_2} is held constant at 40 mm Hg.[25] On some analyzers standard BE may be reported, which evaluates the amount of acid or base that is required to return the extracellular fluid space back to a pH of 7.4. A negative BE indicates a metabolic acidosis and a positive BE indicates a metabolic alkalosis.[11] In cases of metabolic acidosis, AG is also used to further characterize the disturbance and narrow the list of differentials.

METABOLIC ACIDOSIS

Metabolic acidosis is one of the most commonly identified acid-base disturbances in small animal practice. One recent retrospective review of 1805 blood gases performed in dogs and cats identified metabolic acidosis in 49% of the cases.[26] Metabolic acidosis is characterized by decreased pH, either from accumulation of fixed acids or loss of HCO_3^-, which exceeds the buffering systems in the body. The resultant compensatory mechanism is to decrease P_{CO_2} through hyperventilation. Metabolic acidosis can be further characterized as increased AG (normochloremic) metabolic acidosis or normal AG (hyperchloremic) metabolic acidosis. AG uses the concept of electroneutrality to balance measured and unmeasured cations (UC) and unmeasured anions (UA) in the body (**Fig. 1**).

$$Na^+ + K^+ + UC = Cl^- + HCO_3^- + UA$$

Rearranging this equation, one can calculate the AG:

$$UA - UC = (Na^+ + K^+) - (Cl^- + HCO_3^-) = AG$$

The AG is created from the presence of increased UA in comparison with UC. Serum proteins with a net negative charge (eg, albumin) are the predominant contributor to UA. In several disease states, accumulation of lactate, organic acids associated with uremia (eg, phosphates and sulfates), ketone bodies (eg, acetoacetate and

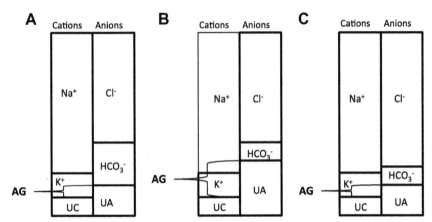

Fig. 1. Gamblegrams depicting the balance of cations and anions. (*A*) Normal plasma. (*B*) Increased anion gap (normochloremic) metabolic acidosis. (*C*) Normal anion gap (hyperchloremic) metabolic acidosis. AG, anion gap; UA, unmeasured anions; UC, unmeasured cations.

β-hydroxybutyrate), and toxins, such as ethylene glycol, salicylates, paraldehyde, and methanol, contribute to the AG. UC include calcium and magnesium.

Normal AG (hyperchloremic) metabolic acidosis is propagated by a loss of HCO_3^- through the gastrointestinal tract or kidneys, ineffective H^+ excretion in the kidneys, or via an increased concentration of Cl^- relative to Na^+ or loss of Na^+ relative to Cl^-.[9,27] A complete list of causes of metabolic acidosis are listed in **Box 1**.

The physiologic effects of acidemia include cardiovascular complications, dysfunction of enzyme systems and proteins, hyperkalemia, and ionized hypercalcemia.[5–8,27] Therapy is focused on treatment of the underlying cause. In cases of metabolic acidosis caused by hyperlactatemia, fluid therapy is crucial to optimizing tissue perfusion. In severe cases of metabolic acidosis (pH<7.2), alkalinizing agents, such as sodium bicarbonate ($NaHCO_3$), may be recommended. The goal of $NaHCO_3$ therapy is not to correct the pH to normal, but rather to raise it to a point at which cardiovascular complications are mitigated (eg, pH 7.2). The following formula can be used to estimate the HCO_3^- deficit[28,29]:

$$HCO_3^- \text{ (mEq)} = 0.3 \times \text{body weight (kg)} \times (HCO_3^- \text{ desired} - HCO_3^- \text{ of patient})$$

Consequences of overzealous $NaHCO_3$ administration may include hyperosmolality and fluid overload, hypokalemia, ionized hypocalcemia, overshoot alkalemia, and paradoxic central nervous system acidosis as CO_2 (product of carbonic acid dissociation) readily crosses the blood-brain barrier. In addition, the oxyhemoglobin dissociation curve shifts to the left, increasing the avidity of O_2 for the hemoglobin molecule.[27]

METABOLIC ALKALOSIS

Metabolic alkalosis characterized by increased pH, decreased H^+, increased HCO_3^-, and increased BE. The compensatory response is hypoventilation to increase P_{CO_2}. Metabolic alkalosis can result from loss of fixed acid via the kidneys and gastrointestinal tract, administration of alkaline-containing solutions, and volume contraction of the extracellular fluid (**Box 2**). Patients with metabolic alkalosis can be classified as having a chloride-responsive or chloride-nonresponsive metabolic alkalosis. Examples of chloride-responsive metabolic alkalosis include vomiting of stomach contents, diuretic

---

Box 1
Causes of metabolic acidosis

Increased Anion Gap (Normochloremic)

Ethylene glycol intoxication

Salicylate intoxication

Other rare intoxications (eg, paraldehyde, methanol)

Diabetic ketoacidosis[a]

Uremic acidosis[b]

Lactic acidosis

Normal Anion Gap (Hyperchloremic)

Diarrhea

Renal tubular acidosis

Carbonic anhydrase inhibitors (eg, acetazolamide)

Ammonium chloride

Cationic amino acids (eg, lysine, arginine, histidine)

Posthypocapneic metabolic acidosis

Dilutional acidosis (eg, rapid administration of 0.9% NaCl)

Hypoadrenocorticism[c]

[a] Patients with diabetic ketoacidosis may have some component of normal anion gap (hyperchloremic) metabolic acidosis in conjunction with increased anion gap (normochloremic) metabolic acidosis.[5,34]
[b] The metabolic acidosis early in renal failure may be hyperchloremic and later converted to typical increased anion gap acidosis.[35]
[c] Patients with hypoadrenocorticism typically have hypochloremia caused by impaired water excretion, absence of aldosterone, impaired renal function, and lactic acidosis. These factors prevent manifestation of hyperchloremia.
Adapted from DiBartola SP. Metabolic acid-base disorders. In: DiBartola SP, ed. Fluid, electrolyte, and acid-base disorders in small animal practice. 4th ed. St. Louis: Elsevier; 2012. p. 253–86; with permission.

---

therapy, and posthypercapnia. In the instance of vomiting, metabolic alkalosis develops from the loss of not only H^+ but also Cl^-. For each mole of H^+ lost, there is equimolar retention of HCO_3^-. In addition, Na^+, K^+, and fluid losses from the extracellular fluid compartment lead to volume contraction. Bicarbonate movement in the kidney is closely linked with Na^+. Volume depletion increases the kidney's avidity for Na^+. When Cl^- is present in adequate quantities, it is reabsorbed with Na^+. However, in states of Cl^- depletion, HCO_3^- is reabsorbed with Na^+, perpetuating metabolic alkalosis.[27,29] The resultant hypochloremic, hypokalemic metabolic alkalosis has been associated with proximal (gastric) obstruction. However, one study investigating acid-base and electrolyte abnormalities in dogs with foreign bodies concluded that hypochloremic metabolic alkalosis was associated with both proximal and distal foreign bodies.[30] Though rare in veterinary patients, chloride-nonresponsive metabolic alkalosis can develop from excessive quantities of mineralocorticoids, as observed in primary hyperaldosteronism and adrenal-dependent hyperadrenocorticism.[27]

Clinical signs associated with metabolic alkalosis are often related to the underlying cause or related electrolyte derangements. Treatment focuses on correction of the

---

Box 2
Causes of metabolic alkalosis

Chloride Responsive

Vomiting of stomach contents

Diuretic therapy

Posthypercapnia

Chloride Resistant

Primary hyperaldosteronism

Hyperadrenocorticism

Alkali Administration

Oral administration of sodium bicarbonate or other organic anions (eg, lactate, citrate, gluconate, acetate)

Oral administration of cation exchange resin with nonabsorbable alkali (eg, phosphorus binder)

Miscellaneous

Refeeding after fasting

High-dose penicillin

Severe potassium or magnesium deficiency

Adapted from DiBartola SP. Metabolic acid-base disorders. In: DiBartola SP, ed. Fluid, electrolyte, and acid-base disorders in small animal practice. 4th ed. St. Louis: Elsevier; 2012. p. 253–86; with permission.

---

underlying cause. In cases of chloride-responsive metabolic alkalosis, the chloride deficit must be addressed. Related electrolyte alterations such as hypokalemia will not completely resolve without sufficient quantities of chloride.

RESPIRATORY ACIDOSIS

Respiratory acidosis is characterized by decreased pH and increased P_{CO_2} with a compensatory increase in HCO_3^-. Respiratory acidosis can be classified as acute or chronic in nature, which will subsequently influence the degree of metabolic compensation expected. Metabolic compensation is recognized in both dogs and cats. Respiratory acidosis, or hypercapnia, is a complication of any disease process that can affect neuromuscular control of ventilation, loss of respiratory conduit, or alveolar gas exchange (**Box 3**). Common causes include large airway obstruction, respiratory center depression, increased CO_2 production with impaired alveolar ventilation, restrictive extrapulmonary disorders, parenchymal and small airway diseases, improper mechanical ventilation, and obesity.[10]

Clinical signs of respiratory acidosis may be more indicative of the underlying disease process than of the hypercapnia itself. Clinical signs are typically more severe in patients with acute disorders (eg, congestive heart failure, pneumonia) than in those with chronic, compensated respiratory disorders. Hypercapnia can result in cardiovascular changes such as tachycardia and vasodilation. Vasodilation can be of clinical significance in patients with intracranial disease. Altered mentation can occur when P_{CO_2} is significantly elevated.

Treatment of metabolic acidosis is aimed at the underlying cause. Oxygen therapy is indicated in the treatment of hypoxemia caused by hypoventilation. In cases of airway

| **Box 3** |
| **Causes of respiratory acidosis** |

Large Airway Obstruction

    Aspiration (eg, foreign body, vomitus)

    Mass (eg, neoplasia, abscess)

    Tracheal collapse

    Chronic obstructive pulmonary disease

    Asthma

    Obstructed endotracheal tube

    Brachycephalic syndrome

    Laryngeal paralysis/laryngospasm

Respiratory Center Depression

    Drug induced (eg, narcotics, barbiturates, inhalant anesthesia)

    Neurologic disease (eg, brainstem or high cervical cord lesion)

Increased CO_2 Production with Impaired Alveolar Ventilation

    Cardiopulmonary arrest

    Heatstroke

    Malignant hyperthermia

Neuromuscular Disease

    Myasthenia gravis

    Tetanus

    Botulism

    Polyradiculoneuritis

    Tick paralysis

    Electrolyte abnormalities (eg, hypokalemia)

    Drug induced (eg, neuromuscular blocking agents, organophosphates, aminoglycosides with anesthetics)

Restrictive Extrapulmonary Disorders

    Diaphragmatic hernia

    Pleural space disease (eg, pneumothorax, pleural effusion)

    Chest wall trauma/flail chest

Intrinsic Pulmonary and Small Airway Diseases

    Acute respiratory distress syndrome

    Chronic obstructive pulmonary disease

    Asthma

    Severe pulmonary edema

    Pulmonary thromboembolism

    Pneumonia

    Pulmonary fibrosis

Diffuse metastatic disease

Smoke Inhalation

Ineffective Mechanical Ventilation (eg, Inadequate Minute Ventilation, Improper CO_2 Removal)

Marked Obesity (Pickwickian Syndrome)

Adapted from DiBartola SP. Metabolic acid-base disorders. In: DiBartola SP, ed. Fluid, electrolyte, and acid-base disorders in small animal practice. 4th ed. St. Louis: Elsevier; 2012. p. 253–86; with permission.

obstruction, sedation, oxygen therapy, and airway management may be necessary to allow adequate ventilation. In some instances, mechanical ventilation may be required until the underlying disease process is corrected. Treatment with $NaHCO_3$ or other alkalizing agents is contraindicated because the CO_2 that is produced from the dissociation of H_2CO_3 will not be able to be effectively ventilated.

RESPIRATORY ALKALOSIS

Respiratory alkalosis is characterized by increased pH, decreased Pco_2, and compensatory decrease in HCO_3^-. Respiratory alkalosis, or hypocapnia, occurs when alveolar ventilation exceeds what is necessary to expire the CO_2 produced through normal metabolic processes. Common causes include hypoxemia, pulmonary parenchymal disease independent of hypoxemia, centrally mediated hyperventilation, muscle metaboreceptor overactivity, overzealous mechanical ventilation, or situations that induce pain, fear, or anxiety (**Box 4**).[10]

Clinical signs of metabolic alkalosis can be attributed to the underlying disease process. Physiologic consequences of hypocapnia include vasoconstriction that may decrease myocardial and cerebral perfusion, arrhythmias, and electrolyte disturbances. Treatment is aimed at addressing the underlying cause, and may include sedation, pain medications, and diuretics. Oxygen should be provided when hypoxemia contributes to respiratory alkalosis.

MIXED DISTURBANCES

Mixed disturbances result when 2 or more acid-base disturbances occur simultaneously. A mixed disturbance should be suspected if the following criteria are present[29,31]:

- Pco_2 and HCO_3^- are moving in opposite directions
- pH is normal despite an abnormal Pco_2 and/or HCO_3^-
- pH change is more significant that what is predicted for a known primary disorder
- Failure to mount the expected compensatory response

To gain more insight into whether a mixed disturbance is present, clinicians can review historical, physical examination, and laboratory data to determine if multiple disease processes exist that could result in the blood-gas findings consistent with a mixed disorder. Particular attention must be paid to alterations in Na^+, Cl^-, phosphorus, and serum proteins, particularly albumin. Abnormalities of these variables may be better investigated through the Stewart-Fencl approach, besides which the reader is referred to additional resources.[32,33] Other spurious reasons why a blood-gas result may be interpreted as mixed include inadequate time for compensation, use of venous samples in which local tissue metabolism may be altered, liquid sodium

Box 4
Causes of respiratory alkalosis

Hypoxemia (Stimulation of Peripheral Chemoreceptors by Decreased Oxygen Delivery)

　Right-to-left shunting

　Decreased Pio_2 (partial pressure of inspired oxygen, eg, high altitude)

　Congestive heart failure

　Severe anemia

　Severe hypotension

　Decreased cardiac output

　Pulmonary diseases with ventilation-perfusion mismatch

　　• Pneumonia

　　• Pulmonary thromboembolism

　　• Pulmonary fibrosis

　　• Pulmonary edema

　　• Acute respiratory distress syndrome

Pulmonary Disease (Simulation of Stretch/Nocioceptors Independent of Hypoxemia)

　Pneumonia

　Pulmonary thromboembolism

　Interstitial lung disease

　Pulmonary edema

　Acute respiratory distress syndrome

Centrally Mediated Hyperventilation

　Liver disease

　Hyperadrenocorticism

　Gram-negative sepsis

　Drugs

　　• Salicylates

　　• Corticosteroids

　　• Progesterone (pregnancy)

　　• Xanthines (eg, aminophylline)

　Recovery from metabolic acidosis

　Central neurologic disease

　　• Trauma

　　• Neoplasia

　　• Infection

　　• Inflammation

　　• Cerebrovascular accident

　Exercise

　Heatstroke

Muscle Metaboreceptor Overactivity

   Heart Failure

Overzealous Mechanical Ventilation

Situations Causing Pain, Fear, or Anxiety

Adapted from DiBartola SP. Metabolic acid-base disorders. In: DiBartola SP, ed. Fluid, electrolyte, and acid-base disorders in small animal practice. 4th ed. St. Louis: Elsevier; 2012. p. 253–86; with permission.

heparin dilution of sample, sample storage time, or machine errors in the calculation of HCO_3^-.[31] Every effort must be made to tease out the underlying conditions so that they can be appropriately addressed. Treatment should first be aimed at the most life-threatening disorder, followed by the most treatable disorder.[31]

SUMMARY

Incorporating acid-base assessment into routine clinical use will provide the veterinary practitioner with valuable insight into the patient's underlying disease process. It is important to take a stepwise approach toward identifying the primary disturbance and assessing for compensation. Routine use will make this tool quick and easy to use in patient assessment.

REFERENCES

1. Constable PD. Clinical assessment of acid-base status: comparison of the Henderson-Hasselbalch and strong ion approaches. Vet Clin Pathol 2000;29: 115–28.
2. Stewart P. Strong ions, plus carbon dioxide, plus weak acid, isolated blood plasma and isolated intracellular fluid. How to understand acid-base. New York: Elsevier; 1981. p. 110–44.
3. Constable PD. A simplified strong ion model for acid-base equilibria: application to horse plasma. J Appl Physiol 1997;83:297–311.
4. Meltesen HS, Bohn AA. Using corrected serum chloride and predicted bicarbonate concentrations to interpret acid-base status in dogs. Vet Clin Pathol 2012;41: 509–17.
5. Adrogue HJ, Madias NE. Management of life-threatening acid-base disorders. First of two parts. N Engl J Med 1998;338:26–34.
6. Adrogue HJ, Brensilver J, Madias NE. Changes in the plasma anion gap during chronic metabolic acid-base disturbances. Am J Physiol 1978;235:F291–7.
7. Mitchell JH, Wildenthal K, Johnson RL Jr. The effects of acid-base disturbances on cardiovascular and pulmonary function. Kidney Int 1972;1:375–89.
8. Orchard CH, Kentish JC. Effects of changes of pH on the contractile function of cardiac muscle. Am J Physiol 1990;258:C967–81.
9. Costanzo LS. Acid-base physiology. In: Costanzo LS, editor. Physiology. 4th edition. Philadelphia: Saunders/Elsevier; 2010. p. 299–325.
10. Johnson RA, de Morais HA. Respiratory acid-base disorders. In: DiBartola SP, editor. Fluid, electrolyte, and acid-base disorders in small animal practice. 4th edition. St Louis (MO): Saunders; 2012. p. 287–301.
11. DiBartola SP. Introduction to acid-base disorders. In: DiBartola SP, editor. Fluid, electrolytes, and acid-base disorders in small animal practice. 4th edition. St Louis (MO): Saunders; 2012. p. 231–52.

12. Bateman SW. Making sense of blood gas results. Vet Clin North Am Small Anim Pract 2008;38:543–57, x.
13. Raffe MR. Point-of-care laboratory testing in the intensive care unit. In: Bonagura J, editor. Kirk's current veterinary therapy. 13th edition. Philadelphia: WB Saunders; 2000. p. 110–2.
14. Landt M, Hortin GL, Smith CH, et al. Interference in ionized calcium measurements by heparin salts. Clin Chem 1994;40:565–70.
15. Hopper K, Rezende ML, Haskins SC. Assessment of the effect of dilution of blood samples with sodium heparin on blood gas, electrolyte, and lactate measurements in dogs. Am J Vet Res 2005;66:656–60.
16. Ilkiw JE, Rose RJ, Martin IC. A comparison of simultaneously collected arterial, mixed venous, jugular venous and cephalic venous blood samples in the assessment of blood-gas and acid-base status in the dog. J Vet Intern Med 1991;5: 294–8.
17. Rand JS, Kinnaird E, Baglioni A, et al. Acute stress hyperglycemia in cats is associated with struggling and increased concentrations of lactate and norepinephrine. J Vet Intern Med 2002;16:123–32.
18. Redavid LA, Sharp CR, Mitchell MA, et al. Plasma lactate measurements in healthy cats. J Vet Emerg Crit Care (San Antonio) 2012;22:580–7.
19. Haskins SC. Sampling and storage of blood for pH and blood gas analysis. J Am Vet Med Assoc 1977;170:429–33.
20. Kennedy SA, Constable PD, Sen I, et al. Effects of syringe type and storage conditions on results of equine blood gas and acid-base analysis. Am J Vet Res 2012;73:979–87.
21. Reeves RB. Temperature-induced changes in blood acid-base status: pH and PCO2 in a binary buffer. J Appl Physiol 1976;40:752–61.
22. Madiedo G, Sciacca R, Hause L. Air bubbles and temperature effect on blood gas analysis. J Clin Pathol 1980;33:864–7.
23. Watson AD, Culvenor JA, Middleton DJ, et al. Distal renal tubular acidosis in a cat with pyelonephritis. Vet Rec 1986;119:65–8.
24. Lemieux G, Lemieux C, Duplessis S, et al. Metabolic characteristics of cat kidney: failure to adapt to metabolic acidosis. Am J Physiol 1990;259:R277–81.
25. Siggaard-Andersen O, Astrup P, Campbell E. Report of ad hoc committee on acid-base terminology. Ann N Y Acad Sci 1966;133(1):59–65.
26. Hopper K, Epstein SE. Incidence, nature, and etiology of metabolic acidosis in dogs and cats. J Vet Intern Med 2012;26:1107–14.
27. DiBartola SP. Metabolic acid-base disorders. In: DiBartola SP, editor. Fluid, electrolyte and acid-base disorders in small animal practice. 4th edition. St Louis (MO): Saunders; 2012. p. 253–86.
28. Robertson SA. Simple acid-base disorders. Vet Clin North Am Small Anim Pract 1989;19:289–306.
29. Day TK. Blood gas analysis. Vet Clin North Am Small Anim Pract 2002;32: 1031–48.
30. Boag AK, Coe RJ, Martinez TA, et al. Acid-base and electrolyte abnormalities in dogs with gastrointestinal foreign bodies. J Vet Intern Med 2005;19:816–21.
31. de Morais HA, Leisewitz AL. Mixed acid-base disturbances. In: DiBartola SP, editor. Fluid, electrolytes, and acid-base disorders in small animal practice. 4th edition. St Louis (MO): Saunders; 2012. p. 302–15.
32. Russell KE, Hansen BD, Stevens JB. Strong ion difference approach to acid-base imbalances with clinical applications to dogs and cats. Vet Clin North Am Small Anim Pract 1996;26:1185–201.

33. Hopper K, Haskins SC. A case-based review of a simplified quantitative approach to acid-base analysis. J Vet Emerg Crit Care 2008;18:467–76.
34. Adrogue HJ, Wilson H, Boyd AE 3rd, et al. Plasma acid-base patterns in diabetic ketoacidosis. N Engl J Med 1982;307:1603–10.
35. Widmer B, Gerhardt RE, Harrington JT, et al. Serum electrolyte and acid base composition. The influence of graded degrees of chronic renal failure. Arch Intern Med 1979;139:1099–102.

Use of Lactate in Small Animal Clinical Practice

Leslie C. Sharkey, DVM, PhD[a],*, Maxey L. Wellman, DVM, MS, PhD[b]

KEYWORDS

- Lactate • L-Lactate • D-Lactate • Lactic acidosis • Hypoxia • Hypoperfusion
- Metabolic acidosis

KEY POINTS

- Lactate concentration is used as an indicator of tissue hypoperfusion and hypoxia, particularly in critical care or perioperative settings.
- Lactate concentration is used to determine the severity of an underlying disorder, assess response to therapy, and predict outcome, especially if serial lactate levels are measured.
- Decreasing levels of lactate suggest improvement, whereas prolonged increases in lactate concentration imply deterioration with a poor prognosis.
- Repeated lactate concentrations should be determined on the same instrument with close attention to sample collection and processing and adherence to recommendations for instrument quality control.

INTRODUCTION

Lactate is formed primarily as the end product of anaerobic glycolysis, although small amounts are produced during aerobic metabolism. Hyperlactatemia refers to mildly increased lactate concentration without concurrent metabolic acidosis. Lactic acidosis occurs when hyperlactatemia is more severe and is accompanied by a decrease in blood pH.[1–3] Lactic acidosis occurs most commonly with tissue hypoperfusion and hypoxia, often as a consequence of systemic or regional hypoperfusion, severe anemia, or hypermetabolic states. Liver disease, kidney disease, diabetes mellitus, sepsis, drugs and toxins, and uncommon mitochondrial defects can cause lactic acidosis from various mechanisms including decreased aerobic metabolism and lactate consumption.[4]

In healthy adult dogs, serum lactate measures 0.3 to 2.5 mmol/L.[5] Puppies have higher lactate concentrations that decrease to adult values by 2 to 3 months of age.[6]

Disclosures: Dr M.L. Wellman is a paid consultant for IDEXX Laboratories and Marshfield Labs.
[a] Veterinary Clinical Sciences Department, University of Minnesota College of Veterinary Medicine, 1352 Boyd Avenue, St Paul, MN 55108, USA; [b] Department of Veterinary Biosciences, The Ohio State University, 1925 Coffey Road, Columbus, OH 43210, USA
* Corresponding author.
E-mail address: Shark009@umn.edu

Serum lactate in healthy adult cats is 0.5 to 2.0 mmol/L.[7] Indications for measuring serum lactate include assessment of tissue perfusion and oxygenation, predicting outcome or response to therapy in critically ill patients, and evaluation of metabolic acidosis. In people, serum lactate concentration has been used as a risk stratification biomarker.[8] Several studies in veterinary medicine indicate that lactate concentration may have similar implications for prognosis.[4,9–11] In dogs, 3 to 5 mmol/L is considered a mild increase; 5 to 8 mmol/L is considered a moderate increase, and greater than 8 mmol/L is considered a marked increase in blood lactate concentration.[12]

LACTATE PHYSIOLOGY AND METABOLISM

Under aerobic conditions, glucose is metabolized to pyruvic acid, which diffuses into mitochondria to enter the Krebs cycle and undergo oxidative phosphorylation for energy production or transformation in glucose via gluconeogenesis (**Fig. 1**). However, in red blood cells (RBC) and other cells that lack mitochondria, and in other tissues during periods of hypoxia, glucose is metabolized to pyruvic acid by anaerobic glycolysis. In the final step of anaerobic glycolysis, lactic acid dehydrogenase catalyzes the conversion of pyruvic acid to lactic acid, a reaction that favors lactic acid formation by a ratio of 10:1 during normal metabolism (**Fig. 2**).[8]

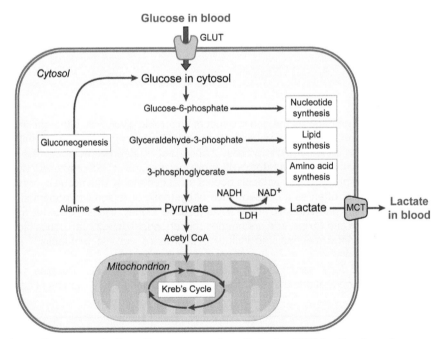

Fig. 1. Glucose metabolism. Glucose enters the cell via the GLUT family of membrane proteins. Glucose is metabolized through several steps (only some of which are shown in the diagram) to pyruvate. Pyruvate can be oxidized via the Kreb's cycle in the mitochondrion or transformed to glucose via the gluconeogenesis pathway. Pyruvate also can be converted to lactate via the enzyme lactate dehydrogenase (LDH), which generates nicotine adenine dinucleotide (NAD). This reaction occurs more readily when there is tissue hypoxia. Lactate in the cytoplasm crosses the cell membrane into the blood via a monocarboxylate-proton cotransporter (MCT), an anion exchange system, and simple diffusion.

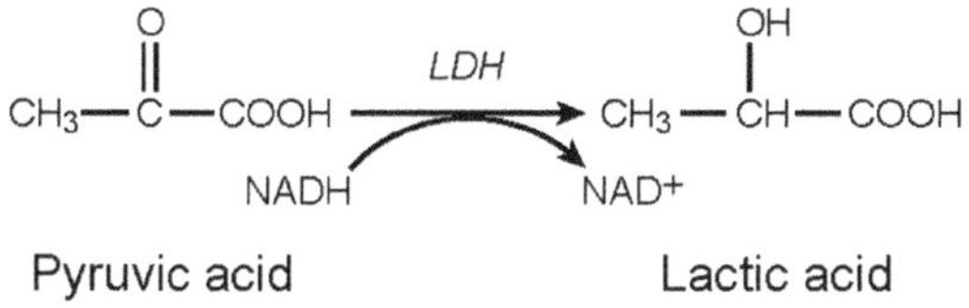

Fig. 2. The final step of anaerobic glycolysis.

Lactic acid ($C_3H_6O_3$) is a nonvolatile (fixed) acid that readily dissociates into a lactate ion [$C_3CH(OH)COO^-$] and a hydrogen ion (H^+) in body fluids at physiologic pH. Lactate ion most often is referred to simply as lactate. A monocarboxylate-proton cotransporter, an anion exchange system, and simple diffusion allow lactate to cross the cell membrane into the blood. The H^+ ions are titrated by various body buffers, but when lactate production is increased, the buffers are depleted and acidemia develops. Lactate and H^+ are metabolized to glucose or oxidized to H_2O and CO_2 when aerobic conditions are restored.[4]

The concentration of lactate in blood depends on the balance between formation and clearance. Daily lactate production is generated primarily by skeletal muscle, skin, brain, heart, intestine, renal medulla, and RBC, but lactate production occurs in many other tissues during illness.[1,4,8] For example, large amounts of lactate are produced by the lungs during acute lung injury and by leukocytes during phagocytosis or from leukocyte activation associated with sepsis. Lactate is metabolized primarily by the liver (60%–70%) and kidney (20%–30%) via the Cori cycle, in which lactate produced in other tissues is converted back to pyruvate and then to glucose through gluconeogenesis.[8,13] Lactate is freely filtered by the glomerulus and most is reabsorbed in the proximal tubules, with only minimal amounts being excreted in urine.[1,8,14] In chronic liver disease like cirrhosis, lactate clearance is maintained, but in acute liver disease and impaired renal function can contribute to increased blood levels of lactate due to decreased clearance. Acidosis decreases hepatic clearance and may cause increased hepatic lactate production, whereas renal clearance is increased with acidosis.[4,15] In marked hypoperfusion associated with shock, the liver and kidney may switch from lactate consumption to lactate production, emphasizing the importance of reinstating adequate perfusion and oxygen delivery.[1]

Lactate has 2 optical isomers, L-lactate, and its mirror image, D-lactate. L-Lactate is produced almost exclusively in healthy monogastric animals. D-Lactate can come from bacterial fermentation of carbohydrates in the intestinal tract or from alternate metabolic pathways that occur with some toxins or in certain diseases. Increases in D-lactate have been reported in diabetes mellitus and propylene glycol toxicity, or from intestinal bacterial overgrowth (small intestinal dysbiosis).[4,16,17] Routine testing measures only L-lactate concentration. D-Lactic acidosis is sometimes suspected when there is unexplained metabolic acidosis with an increased anion gap and normal L-lactate concentration. D-Lactate can be measured by high-pressure liquid chromatography or mass spectrometry in select laboratories.[17]

CLASSIFICATION OF LACTIC ACIDOSIS

There are 3 types of lactic acidosis. Type A lactic acidosis is more common and occurs when there is tissue hypoperfusion and hypoxia from either decreased oxygen delivery or increased oxygen demand. Shock is an example of hypoperfusion; anemia is an example of decreased oxygen delivery, and seizures are an example of increased oxygen demand (**Box 1**). Type B lactic acidosis occurs when oxygen delivery

Box 1
Causes of lactic acidosis

Type A lactic acidosis

Decreased oxygen delivery

  Hypovolemic, cardiogenic, or septic shock

  Severe anemia (PCV <10%) or severe hypoxemia (Po_2 <30 mm Hg)

  Global or regional hypoperfusion

  Carbon monoxide toxicity

Increased oxygen demand

  Exercise, seizures, uncontrolled shivering

Type B lactic acidosis

Type B_1 (underlying disease)

  Acute liver disease

  Chronic kidney disease (renal failure)

  Hyperthyroidism

  Diabetes mellitus

  Neoplasia

  Sepsis

  Systemic inflammatory response syndrome

  Alkalosis

Type B_2 (drugs or toxins)

  Aceteminophen, salicylates

  Ethylene glycol, propylene glycol

  Catecholamines

  Carbon monoxide

  Bicarbonate

  Others: cyanide, strychnine, nitroprusside, halothane, terbutaline, activated charcoal

Type B_3 (mitochondrial diseases)

  Mitochondrial myopathies

  Mitochondrial encephalomyopathy with lactic acidosis and stroke syndrome (MELAS)

D-Lactic acidosis

Diabetes mellitus

Intestinal bacterial overgrowth (small intestinal dysbiosis)

Exocrine pancreatic insufficiency

Propylene glycol toxicity

Data from Pang DS, Boysen S. Lactate in veterinary critical care: pathophysiology and management. J Am Anim Hosp Assoc 2007;43:273–4; and Allen SE, Holm JL. Lactate: physiology and clinical utility. J Vet Emerg Crit Care 2008;18:125.

is adequate but there is altered carbohydrate metabolism or mitochondrial function. Type B_1 lactic acidosis occurs in acute hepatitis, chronic kidney disease (see **Box 1**), and other diseases associated with decreased lactate clearance. Type B_2 lactic acidosis occurs with some toxins or medications that inhibit oxidative phosphorylation. Type B_3 is the least common form of lactic acidosis and occurs when there are inborn errors of mitochondrial metabolism.[4,8,18-20] As mentioned above, type D-lactic acidosis has been reported in diabetes mellitus, intestinal bacterial overgrowth (small intestinal dysbiosis), exocrine pancreatic insufficiency, and propylene glycol toxicity.[4,16,17]

During classic type A lactic acidosis, there is increased anaerobic glycolysis and accumulation of pyruvate, which cannot enter the mitochondrion for oxidative phosphorylation because of low levels of oxygen. Hypoxia also inhibits the enzyme that converts pyruvate to acetyl coenzyme A for entry into the Krebs cycle and the enzyme that converts pyruvate into oxaloacetate, both of which contribute to an accumulation of pyruvate and the shift of pyruvate metabolism to form lactate. Intracellular lactate concentration increases and is shuttled to the bloodstream via the monocarboxylate transporter.[8,21] There may be features of both type A and type B lactic acidosis in critically ill patients. For example, in sepsis, there may be tissue hypoperfusion, increased metabolism associated with inflammation, diminished lactate clearance, decreased entry of pyruvate into the Krebs cycle, and abnormal mitochondrial function.[1,4]

SAMPLE COLLECTION AND LACTATE ANALYSIS

Lactate is measured in plasma by automated chemistry analyzers or in whole blood by point-of-care (POC) instruments. Although sampling site affects lactate concentration, differences are not clinically relevant.[5] For plasma samples, anti-coagulated blood should be centrifuged and the plasma removed from the RBCs to avoid false increases in lactate concentration because of in vitro metabolism. Plasma samples should be kept at $4°C$ if analysis is delayed for more than 30 minutes for samples collected in heparin.[22] Plasma can be stored longer at $-20°C$, although immediate analysis is useful for most clinical patients. For POC instruments using whole blood, 0.5 to 1.0 mL of venous or arterial blood should be collected in lithium heparin (preferred) or sodium fluoride and samples should be processed immediately.[1,12,23] Recent exercise, seizures, stress, excitement, food intake, and prolonged venous stasis during sample collection can increase lactate concentration 2.5 to 10.0 mmol/L.[1,22] One study showed a transient 10-fold increase in lactate in healthy cats that were stressed before sample collection.[24] However, a more recent study found that struggling during venipuncture caused no statistical differences in lactate concentrations in cats.[25] Increases from exercise, restraint, and seizures typically return to normal within 2 hours.

Lactate can be measured by enzymatic colorimetry or enzymatic amperometry.[1,4] In automated chemistry analyzers, which use enzymatic colorimetry, oxidation of L-lactate is catalyzed by lactic acid dehydrogenase to produce the reduced form of nicotinamide adenine dinucleotide, which is detected by spectrophotometry and is proportional to the sample lactate concentration. Enzymatic amperometry is used in POC instruments because results are available in minutes. The enzymatic activity of lactate oxidase on lactate generates H_2O_2, an electroactive analyte that is oxidized by an electrical potential to generate an electrical current on a platinum electrode that is proportional to the sample lactate concentration.[1,4] POC instruments are useful in critical care and intraoperative settings during which serial lactate measurements guide patient management. Recent studies in people have shown that more rapid turnaround time for lactate results in improved clinical outcomes for critically ill patients.[23] Comparison of lactate values obtained from POC instruments with those determined by automated chemistry analyzers indicate that POC performance is acceptable as long as there is close attention to sample collection and processing and adherence to recommendations for quality control of the instrument.[26,27] However, using the same instrument for repeated measurements is recommended because of differences in methodology and sample requirements.

ANALYTICAL INTERFERENCES

Ethylene glycol exposure may falsely increase plasma lactate concentration measured by some instruments that use enzymatic amperometry, likely because glycolate, a major metabolite of ethylene glycol, is chemically similar to lactate,[28] which is different from propylene glycol intoxication, in which L-lactate and D-lactate are metabolites of propylene glycol.[16] Lactate is one of the main components of lactated Ringer's solution (LRS). The lactate in LRS is metabolized to glucose or is oxidized to water and CO_2, both of which consume H^+ ions and contribute to an overall alkalinizing effect. Administration of LRS does not typically cause an increase in lactate.[1,29–31] Although increased lactate associated with LRS administration has been described in dogs with lymphoma, recent studies are less convincing.[32,33] However, small amounts of LRS in catheters that are not appropriately flushed before sample collection can cause a falsely increased lactate concentration.[4,34] Solutions that do not contain lactate can cause a dilutional effect if the sample is collected from a catheter that is inadequately cleared.

DIAGNOSTIC APPLICATION OF LACTATE CONCENTRATION

Metabolic acidosis is a common disorder in small animal patients, particularly in dogs, and increased lactate concentration causes a significant proportion of high anion gap metabolic acidoses in dogs and cats.[35,36] A study of serial lactate concentrations in systemically ill dogs found that although increases in initial lactate concentrations were not related to outcome, failure of lactate concentration to improve by $\geq$50% was associated with increased mortality.[11] More targeted studies have evaluated lactate concentrations in specific conditions that cause type A, type B, or D-lactic acidosis in dogs and cats.

Type A Lactic Acidosis

Although tissue hypoperfusion from hypovolemic or cardiogenic shock likely is a common cause of lactic acidosis in dogs and cats, there are few studies in specific subpopulations of animals that show the consistent occurrence of hyperlactatemia and lactic acidosis that has been shown in human patients with shock.[1,10] Lactate levels have been used as a prognostic indicator in people, but prognostic implications may vary with the cause of lactic acidosis. Human patients with hemorrhagic shock and high lactate levels may have a better prognosis than patients with cardiogenic shock and similar lactate levels.[1,37] Lactic acidosis has been used as a prognostic indicator in critically ill human patients with septic shock, and lactate concentration has been used to determine efficacy of interventions in canine models of septic shock.[38] However, evaluation of blood lactate in a cohort of dogs with pyometra failed to demonstrate differences in plasma lactate between affected and control dogs, or between dogs with pyometra with or without evidence of systemic inflammatory response syndrome.[39]

Several studies have evaluated the prognostic value of lactate in dogs with gastric dilatation volvulus, which could cause lactic acidosis because of either regional or systemic hypoperfusion.[40,41] One study found that survival was significantly higher in dogs with an initial lactate concentration $\leq$9.0 mmol/L. In dogs with a lactate concentration greater than 9.0 mmol/L, there was no difference in mean lactate values between survivors and nonsurvivors, although posttreatment lactate of greater than 6.4 mmol/L or a reduction of $\leq$4 mmol/L or $\leq$42.5% was a negative prognostic indicator.[41] In another study, an initial plasma lactate of greater than 6.0 mmol/L failed to predict macroscopic gastric wall necrosis or a negative outcome consistently. However, a greater than 50% reduction in plasma lactate was a positive prognostic indicator.[40] Similarly, a more recent study found that an initial plasma lactate concentration of 7.4 mmol/L was a strong prognostic indicator of gastric necrosis and outcome.[42]

Hypoxemia associated with severe anemia causes type A lactic acidosis. A large retrospective study of dogs with immune-mediated hemolytic anemia found that blood lactate was inversely correlated with PCV and nonsurvivors had higher median blood lactate concentrations at presentation than survivors (4.8 mmol/L vs 2.9). All dogs in which blood lactate normalized by 6 hours survived, whereas 71% of dogs with persistent hyperlactatemia survived, implying that serial monitoring may improve the predictive value of lactate evaluation.[43] Canine babesiosis is another cause of anemia associated with hyperlactatemia. However, the pathophysiology is complex and includes neurologic and respiratory abnormalities as other potential causes of increased lactate. In one cohort of 90 dogs with babesiosis, 50% had increased blood lactate and persistent hyperlactatemia despite therapy as a negative prognostic indicator.[11]

Hypoxemia due to exercise-induced increases in oxygen demand can cause increased blood lactate, and this is a potential source of preanalytical error. However, in a study of healthy Labrador retrievers exercised to exhaustion, there was no significant increase in blood lactate.[44] In another study, lactate levels in agility dogs evaluated immediately, within 2 minutes after, and 4 hours after completing an agility course increased incrementally more in dogs with higher agility immediately after course completion, were close to baseline at the final time point, and all values remained within the reference interval.[45]

Type B Lactic Acidosis

The most common type B lactic acidosis in veterinary species is type B_1 associated with underlying disease. Proposed mechanisms for lactic acidosis in the presence of other diseases include decreased clearance, as in acute hepatic failure or chronic kidney disease, or dysfunctional carbohydrate metabolism, as in hyperthyroidism and sepsis, but multiple mechanisms likely occur, including combinations of type B and type A lactic acidosis. Serum lactate concentrations were higher in hyperthyroid cats compared with diabetic or control cats, possibly related to increased rates of glucose use.[46] Neoplasia has been implicated as a cause of hyperlactatemia, but the veterinary medical literature does not support a strong association. In a retrospective study of dogs with intracranial disease or intervertebral disc disease anesthetized for advanced imaging or surgery revealed that dogs with meningioma or hydrocephalus had higher lactate concentrations than dogs with intervertebral disc disease. However, only one dog with meningioma had clinically significant hyperlactatemia.[47] One prospective study of 37 dogs with various hematopoietic or solid tumors failed to identify increased lactate concentrations and concluded that neoplasia is associated with an increase in lactate only in rare or complicated cases.[48] A more focused retrospective study of 55 dogs with lymphoma observed hyperlactatemia in 40%, but the authors concluded that only 5 had cancer-related increases, and the authors reported that the mean blood lactate concentration in dogs with lymphoma was not statistically different from their normal value of 2.5 mmol/L.[49]

As discussed previously, exposure to exogenous compounds such as ethylene and propylene glycol may be associated with type B_2 hyperlactatemia. A prospective cross-over study of healthy adult Beagles demonstrated significantly increased blood lactate levels 4 and 14 days after receiving daily anti-inflammatory (1 mg/kg) and immunosuppressive (4 mg/kg) oral prednisone.[49] Although not directly evaluated, corticosteroid-mediated increases in gluconeogenesis from protein and enhanced use of glucose were implicated as mechanisms for the modest but significant increase greater than 2.5 mmol/L. Type B_3 hyperlactatemia seems to be rare in dogs and cats.[50] However, increased lactate was reported in a Sussex spaniel with pyruvate dehydrogenase deficiency.[51]

D-Lactic Acidosis

Marked increases in blood and urine D-lactic acid with normal blood L-lactate were reported in a cat with exocrine pancreatic insufficiency.[7] Cats with gastrointestinal disease have increased blood D-lactate compared with healthy control cats, whereas L-lactate levels were not significantly different in sick cats.[17] In cats with gastrointestinal disease, D-lactate concentrations were not correlated with the presence of neurologic abnormalities or the results of other gastrointestinal function tests, such as pancreatic lipase immunoreactivity, trypsin-like immunoreactivity, or serum cobalamin and folate levels.[17] In propylene glycol intoxication, the L-lactate metabolite is metabolized much faster than the D-lactate metabolite, which may result in persistent metabolic acidosis from D-lactate, which typically is not measured.[16]

LACTATE CONCENTRATION IN OTHER BODY FLUIDS

Lactate concentration has been evaluated in other body fluids as an indication of sepsis or neoplasia. Lactate concentrations are higher in abdominal fluid in dogs and cats with septic peritonitis than in those with nonseptic or nonneoplastic effusions.[52–54] In dogs, fluid lactate levels of greater than 5.5 mmol/L or a difference of greater than 2 mmol/L between fluid and peripheral blood lactate are suggestive of bacterial peritonitis.[52] Dogs with neoplastic effusions have higher abdominal fluid lactate concentrations than dogs with nonneoplastic effusions but lactate levels in pericardial fluid are not as helpful in differentiating neoplastic from nonneoplastic effusions.[55,56]

SUMMARY

Lactate forms primarily during anaerobic glycolysis. Lactate concentration is used clinically as an indicator of tissue hypoperfusion and hypoxia, particularly in critical care or perioperative settings, to determine the severity of an underlying disorder, assess response to therapy, and predict outcome. Serial determination of lactate levels may be more helpful than a single lactate concentration. Decreasing levels of lactate suggest improvement, whereas prolonged increases in lactate concentration imply deterioration with a poor prognosis. Repeated lactate concentrations should be determined on the same instrument with close attention to sample collection and processing and adherence to recommendations for instrument quality control.

REFERENCES

1. Pang DS, Boysen S. Lactate in veterinary critical care: pathophysiology and management. J Am Anim Hosp Assoc 2007;43:270–9.

2. Shapiro BA, Peruzzi WT. Interpretation of blood gases. In: Ayres SM, Grenvik A, Holbrook PR, et al, editors. Textbook of critical care. 3rd edition. Philadelphia: WB Saunders; 1995. p. 278–94.
3. Tonnessen TI. Intracellular pH and electrolyte regulation. In: Ayres SM, Grenvik A, Holbrook PR, et al, editors. Textbook of critical care. 3rd edition. Philadelphia: WB Saunders; 1995. p. 172–87.
4. Allen SE, Holm JL. Lactate: physiology and clinical utility. J Vet Emerg Crit Care 2008;18:123–32.
5. Hughes D, Rozanski ER, Shofer FS, et al. Effect of sampling site, repeated sampling, pH, and PCO_2 on plasma lactate concentrations in healthy dogs. Am J Vet Res 1999;60:521–4.
6. McMichael MA, Lees GE, Hennessey J, et al. Serial plasma lactate concentrations in 68 puppies aged 4 to 80 days. J Vet Emerg Crit Care 2005;15: 17–21.
7. Packer RA, Cohn LA, Wohlstadter DR, et al. D-Lactic acidosis secondary to exocrine pancreatic insufficiency in a cat. J Vet Intern Med 2005;19:106–10.
8. Vernon C, LeTourneau JL. Lactic acidosis: recognition, kinetics, and associated prognosis. Crit Care Clin 2010;26:255–83.
9. dePapp E, Drobatz KJ, Hughes D. Plasma lactate concentration as a predictor of gastric necrosis and survival among dogs with gastric dilatation-volvulus: 102 cases (1995–1998). J Am Vet Med Assoc 1999;215(1):49–52.
10. Lagutchik MS, Ogilvie GK, Hackett TB, et al. Increased lactate concentrations in ill and injured dogs. J Vet Emerg Crit Care 1998;8:117–27.
11. Nel M, Lobetti RG, Keller N, et al. Prognostic value of blood lactate, blood glucose, and hematocrit in canine babesiosis. J Vet Intern Med 2004;18: 471–6.
12. Mathews KA. Monitoring fluid therapy and complications of fluid therapy. In: DiBartola SP, editor. Fluid, electrolyte, and acid-base disorders in small animal practice. 4th edition. St Louis (MO): Elsevier Saunders; 2012. p. 386–404.
13. Madias NE. Lactic acidosis. Kidney Int 1986;29:752–74.
14. Yudkin J, Cohen RD. The contribution of the kidney to the removal of a lactic acid load under normal and acidotic conditions in the conscious rat. Clin Sci Mol Med 1975;48:121–31.
15. Record CO, Iles RA, Cohen RD, et al. Acid-base and metabolic disturbances in fulminant hepatic failure. Gut 1975;16(2):144–9.
16. Claus MA, Jandrey KE, Poppenga RH. Propylene glycol intoxication in a dog. J Vet Emerg Crit Care 2011;21:679–83.
17. Packer RA, Moore GE, Chang CY, et al. Serum D-lactate concentrations in cats with gastrointestinal disease. J Vet Intern Med 2012;26:905–10.
18. Kruse JA, Carlson RW. Lactate metabolism. Crit Care Clin 1987;5(4):725–46.
19. Luft FC. Lactic acidosis update for critical care clinicians. J Am Soc Nephrol 2001;12:S15–9.
20. Mizock BA, Falk JL. Lactic acidosis in critical illness. Crit Care Med 1992;20(1): 80–93.
21. Stryer L. Oxidative phosphorylation. In: Stryer L, editor. Biochemistry. 4th edition. New York: WH Freeman and Company; 1995. p. 529–58.
22. Lagutchik MS. Lactate. In: Vade SL, Knoll JS, Smith FW, et al, editors. Blackwell's five-minute veterinary consult: laboratory tests and diagnostic procedures. Ames (IA): Wiley-Blackwell Publishing; 2009. p. 388–9.
23. Karon BS, Scott R, Burritt MF, et al. Comparison of lactate values between point-of-care and central laboratory analyzers. Am J Clin Pathol 2007;128:168–71.

24. Rand JS, Kinnaird E, Baglioni A, et al. Acute stress hyperglycemia in cats is associated with struggling and increased concentrations of lactate and norepinephrine. J Vet Intern Med 2002;16:123–32.
25. Redavid LA, Sharp CR, Mitchell MA, et al. Plasma lactate measurement in healthy cats. J Vet Emerg Crit Care 2012;22:580–7.
26. Karagiannis MH, Mann FA, Madsen RW, et al. Comparison of two portable lactate meters in dogs. J Am Anim Hosp Assoc 2013;49:8–15.
27. Thorneloe C, Bedard C, Boysen S. Evaluation of a hand held lactate analyzer in dogs. Can Vet J 2007;48:283–7.
28. Hopper K. Falsely increased plasma lactate concentration due to ethylene glycol poisoning in 2 dogs. J Vet Emerg Crit Care 2013;23:63–7.
29. Didwania A, Miller J, Kassel D, et al. Effect of intravenous lactated ringer's solution infusion on the circulating lactate concentration: part 3. Results of a prospective, randomized, double-blind, placebo-controlled trial. Crit Care Med 1997;25(11):1851–4.
30. Pascoe PJ. Perioperative management of fluid therapy. In: DiBartola SP, editor. Fluid, electrolyte, and acid-base disorders in small animal practice. 3rd edition. St Louis (MO): Elsevier; 2006. p. 391–419.
31. Us MH, Ozcan S, Oral L, et al. Comparison of the effects of hypertonic saline and crystalloid infusions on haemodynamic parameters during haemorrhagic shock in dogs. J Int Med Res 2001;29:508–15.
32. Vail DM, Ogilvie GK, Fettman MJ, et al. Exacerbation of hyperlactemia by infusion of lactated ringer's solution in dogs with lymphoma. J Vet Intern Med 1990; 4(5):228–32.
33. Touret M, Boysen SR, Nadeau ME. Retrospective evaluation of potential causes associated with clinically relevant hyperlactatemia in dogs with lymphoma. Can Vet J 2012;53:511–7.
34. Jackson EV, Wiese J, Sigal B, et al. Effects of crystalloid solutions on circulating lactate concentrations: part I. Implications for the proper handling of blood specimens obtained from critically ill patients. Crit Care Med 1997;25(11): 1840–6.
35. Hopper K, Epstein SE. Incidence, nature, and etiology of metabolic acidosis in dogs and cats. J Vet Intern Med 2012;26:1107–14.
36. Stevenson CK, Kidney BA, Duke T, et al. Serial blood lactate concentrations in systemically ill dogs. Vet Clin Pathol 2007;36:234–9.
37. Vitek V, Cowle RA. Blood lactate in the prognosis of various forms of shock. Ann Surg 1971;173:308–13.
38. Hicks CW, Sweeney DA, Danner RL, et al. Efficacy of selective mineralocorticoid and glucocorticoid agonists in canine septic shock. Crit Care Med 2012;40: 199–207.
39. Hagman R, Reezigt BJ, Ledin HB, et al. Blood lactate levels in 31 female dogs with pyometra. Acta Vet Scand 2009;51:2–9.
40. Green TI, Tonozzi CC, Kirby R, et al. Evaluation of initial plasma lactate values as a predictor of gastric necrosis and initial and subsequent plasma lactate values as a predictor of survival in dogs with gastric dilatation-volvulus: 84 dogs (2003-2007). J Vet Emerg Crit Care 2011;21:36–44.
41. Zacher LA, Berg J, Shaw SP, et al. Association between outcome and changes in plasma lactate concentration during presurgical treatment in dogs with gastric dilatation-volvulus; 64 cases. J Am Vet Med Assoc 2010;236:892–7.
42. Beer KA, Syring RS, Drobatz KJ. Evaluation of plasma lactate concentration and base excess at the time of hospital admission as predictors of gastric necrosis

and outcome and correlation between those variables in dogs with gastric dilatation-volvulus: 78 cases (2004-2009). J Am Vet Med Assoc 2013;242:54–8.

43. Holahan ML, Brown AJ, Drobatz KJ. The association of blood lactate concentration with outcome in dogs with idiopathic immune-mediated hemolytic anemia: 173 cases. J Vet Emerg Crit Care 2010;20:413–20.

44. Ferasin L, Marcora S. Reliability of an incremental exercise test to evaluate acute blood lactate, heart rate, and body temperature responses in Labrador Retrievers. J Comp Physiol B 2009;179:839–45.

45. Baltzer WI, Firshman AM, Stang B, et al. The effect of agility exercise on eicosanoid excretion, oxidant status, and plasma lactate in dogs. BMC Vet Res 2012; 8:249–59.

46. Christopher MM, O'Neill S. Effect of specimen collection and storage on blood glucose and lactate concentrations in healthy, hyperthyroid and diabetic cats. Vet Clin Pathol 2000;29:22–8.

47. Sullivan LA, Campbell VL, Klopp LS, et al. Blood lactate concentrations in anesthetized dogs with intracranial disease. J Vet Intern Med 2009;23:488–92.

48. Touret M, Boysen SR, Nadeau ME. Prospective evaluation of clinically relevant type B hyperlactatemia in dogs with cancer. J Vet Intern Med 2010;24:1458–61.

49. Boysen SR, Bozzetti M, Rose L, et al. Effects of prednisone on blood lactate concentrations in healthy dogs. J Vet Intern Med 2009;23:1123–5.

50. Shelton GD. Routine and specialized laboratory testing for the diagnosis of neuromuscular diseases in dogs and cats. Vet Clin Pathol 2010;39:278–95.

51. Abramson CJ, Platt SR, Shelton GD. Pyruvate dehydrogenase deficiency in a Sussex spaniel. J Small Anim Pract 2004;45:162–5.

52. Bonczynski JJ, Ludwig LL, Tarton LF, et al. Comparison of peritoneal fluid and peripheral blood pH, bicarbonate, glucose and lactate concentrations a diagnostic tool for septic peritonitis in dogs and cats. Vet Surg 2003;32:161–6.

53. Levin GM, Bonczynski JJ, Ludwig LL, et al. Lactate as a diagnostic test for septic peritoneal effusions in dogs and cats. J Am Anim Hosp Assoc 2004; 40:364–71.

54. Swann H, Hughes D. Use of abdominal fluid pH, pO2, [glucose], and [lactate] to differentiate bacterial peritonitis from non-bacterial causes of abdominal effusion in dogs and cats. Proceed International Veterinary Emergency and Critical Care Society Meeting. San Antonio (TX): 1996. p. 884.

55. Nestor DD, McCullough SM, Schaeffer DJ. Biochemical analysis of neoplastic versus nonneoplastic abdominal effusions in dogs. J Am Anim Hosp Assoc 2004;40:372–5.

56. de Laforcade AM, Freeman LM, Rozanski EA, et al. Biochemical analysis of pericardial fluid and whole blood in dogs with pericardial effusion. J Vet Intern Med 2005;19:833–6.

Hypocalcemia of Critical Illness in Dogs and Cats

Marie K. Holowaychuk, DVM

KEYWORDS

- Ionized calcium • Parathyroid hormone • Vitamin D • Calcitriol • Magnesium

KEY POINTS

- Hypocalcemia is an important electrolyte disturbance in critically ill dogs and cats best detected by measuring ionized calcium, the biologically active form, rather than total or adjusted calcium.
- Hypocalcemia is associated with certain medications and treatments commonly administered to critically ill patients, as well as with various underlying diseases such as acute kidney disease, pancreatitis, parathyroid disease, sepsis, and trauma.
- Suggested underlying mechanisms include hypovitaminosis D, acquired or relative hypoparathyroidism, or hypomagnesemia, as well as alterations in the ionized fraction of calcium caused by changes in chelated or protein-bound calcium.
- If severe or acute, hypocalcemia can cause obvious clinical signs of hyperexcitability, including tremors, twitching, spasms, or seizures, or more subtle signs related to cardiovascular collapse.
- Emergency treatment with calcium gluconate is recommended when clinical signs are present or if there is moderate to severe ionized hypocalcemia.

INTRODUCTION

Relevance

Hypocalcemia is an increasingly recognized and important electrolyte disturbance in critically ill dogs and cats. It occurs in approximately 16% of dogs admitted to the intensive care unit (ICU) and is associated with prolonged hospitalization.[1] In many small animals, detection of hypocalcemia can give insight to the underlying condition and can even be used to predict outcome with certain diseases. If unrecognized or unmanaged, hypocalcemia can result in serious clinical signs, necessitating emergency treatment. Therefore, the routine measurement of ionized calcium (iCa) concentration is recommended in all critically ill dogs and cats.

Disclosures: The author has nothing to disclose.
Department of Clinical Studies, Ontario Veterinary College, University of Guelph, 50 Stone Road East, Guelph, Ontario N1G 2W1, Canada
E-mail address: mholoway@uoguelph.ca

Vet Clin Small Anim 43 (2013) 1299–1317
http://dx.doi.org/10.1016/j.cvsm.2013.07.008

Physiologic Role of Calcium

In addition to providing skeletal support, calcium is required for a multitude of important intracellular and extracellular processes throughout the body (**Box 1**). Because calcium is often necessary for receptor activation, it is a major regulator of intracellular metabolic processes and plays an important role in maintaining cellular and organ integrity.[2]

Distribution of Calcium in the Body

Most calcium is stored in bone as hydroxyapatite, with only 1% of bone stores considered readily available.[3] Almost all nonskeletal calcium is located extracellularly in plasma or serum, with a small but biologically important quantity located intracellularly. Extracellular calcium exists in 3 fractions: ionized (free), complexed (with bicarbonate, citrate, free fatty acids, lactate, phosphate, or sulfate), and protein bound, most (80%–90%) of which is bound to albumin.[4] In healthy dogs, approximately 56% of total calcium (tCa) exists in the ionized form, which is considered the most biologically activate and tightly regulated form.[4] The protein-bound form constitutes 34% of the total, whereas 10% is complexed and might have a lesser biologically active role.[4] In healthy cats, the ionized, protein-bound, and chelated fractions of calcium are 52%, 40%, and 8%, respectively.[5]

Alterations in the Fraction of Extracellular Calcium

Many disturbances that occur commonly in critically ill small animals can change the percentage of calcium in the ionized, complexed, and protein-bound forms (**Box 2**). Specifically, increases in the amount of complexed or protein-bound calcium decrease the biologically active iCa concentration. Lactic acidosis occurs commonly in critically ill dogs and cats and results in increased calcium complexed with lactate. Likewise, sodium bicarbonate, citrate (anticoagulant), phosphate, or sulfate administration also has the potential to increase complexed calcium. Similarly, alkalosis increases the anion groups available for protein binding, thereby increasing the amount of protein-bound calcium and resulting in ionized hypocalcemia (iHCa).

Box 1
Physiologic processes requiring calcium

- Blood coagulation
- Bone metabolism
- Cardiac contractility
- Enzyme reactions
- Hormone secretion
- Intestinal motility
- Mitotic division
- Muscle contraction
- Neurotransmitter secretion
- Nerve conduction
- Vasomotor tone

Box 2
Situations altering the fractions of extracellular calcium

- Acid-base disturbances
- Bicarbonate administration
- Citrate (anticoagulant) administration
- Increased free fatty acids
- Lactic acidosis
- Phosphate administration
- Protein loss or gain
- Sulfate administration

MAINTENANCE OF CALCIUM HOMEOSTASIS
Regulation of Intracellular Calcium Concentrations

Intracellular iCa is maintained at a very low concentration, approximately 10,000-fold less than the extracellular concentration, to enable rapid diffusion into the cell from the extracellular fluid or endoplasmic reticulum in response to chemical signals.[3] Uncontrolled increases in intracellular calcium can activate harmful enzymes, including lipases, proteases, or nucleases, and result in free radical generation and cell destruction.[2] Intracellular calcium is often bound to specific proteins in the cytosol or membrane (eg, calbindin, calmodulin, troponin C) to provide intracellular buffering.[6] This characteristic maintains cellular calcium concentrations within narrow limits to prevent cell damage but achieve cellular processes when needed.

Regulation of Extracellular Calcium Concentrations

Concentrations of extracellular iCa are tightly regulated by the actions of parathyroid hormone (PTH), vitamin D metabolites, and calcitonin. PTH and calcitriol (1,25-dihydroxyvitamin D_3) are the primary regulators of iCa, the main targets of which include the intestines, kidneys, and bone. PTH is mainly responsible for the minute-to-minute control of iCa concentration, whereas calcitriol achieves the day-to-day control.[7] During growth, lactation, or disease, other hormones, including corticosteroids, estrogen, glucagon, growth hormone, prolactin, and thyroxine, can also affect iCa concentrations.[7]

Response to iHCa

Within seconds of a mild decrease in iCa concentration, PTH secretion occurs to directly affect calcium mobilization and retention from the bone and kidneys. This situation happens because of the interaction between extracellular iCa with specific calcium-sensing receptors expressed on the surface of parathyroid cells.[8] Once secreted, PTH increases osteoclast number and function to increase bone resorption and the subsequent release of iCa from bone.[7] In addition, PTH increases tubular reabsorption of calcium and decreases tubular reabsorption of phosphorus from the glomerular filtrate, thus decreasing calcium excretion.[7] Within 1 to 2 hours of iHCa, PTH indirectly increases iCa concentrations by activating renal mitochondrial hydroxylation of 25-hydroxycholecalciferol to synthesize calcitriol.[7] Subsequently, calcitriol increases calcium transport across the enterocytes into the bloodstream[9] and also stimulates osteoclastic bone resorption by enabling differentiation of osteo-clasts from precursor mononuclear cells.[7] After days or weeks of iHCa, further increases in PTH secretion are achieved by hypertrophy and hyperplasia of the chief cells of the parathyroid gland, with a larger proportion of chief cells synthesizing and secreting PTH.[7]

MEASUREMENT OF TCA AND ICA CONCENTRATIONS
Measurement of tCa

Traditionally, serum total calcium (tCa) has been used to assess calcium status in small animals, even although iCa is the biologically active and tightly regulated form. Fasted serum or heparinized plasma samples can be used to measure tCa; however, other anticoagulants including citrate or ethylenediaminetetraacetic acid (EDTA) complex with calcium and should be avoided.

Normal tCa Concentrations

Normal serum tCa concentrations in healthy dogs and cats are included in **Table 1**. Dogs younger than 3 months old have slightly higher serum tCa concentrations than dogs older than 1 year, with some young growing dogs having serum tCa concentrations as high as 12 to 15 mg/dL (3.0–5.0 mmol/L).

Usefulness of tCa to Predict iCa

It is important that tCa is not considered directly proportional to or representative of iCa, especially during critical illness. Several studies in critically ill people, dogs, and cats reveal that tCa and iCa disagree at least 30% to 40% of the time.[10–14] When tCa and iCa are compared using more than 1600 canine serum samples, the diagnostic disagreement is 27% overall, and increases to 36% in dogs with chronic kidney disease.[12] Likewise, assessment of more than 400 feline serum samples reveals a 40% diagnostic disagreement.[10] In healthy and critically ill dogs, tCa tends to overestimate normocalcemia and underestimate iHCa,[11,12] whereas in healthy cats, tCa overestimates iHCa.[10]

Usefulness of Adjusted Calcium to Predict iCa

Formulas to adjust tCa according to total protein or albumin concentrations were derived decades ago to assist clinicians in assessing calcium status. These formulas were derived using tCa concentrations measured by outdated technology and were not verified by iCa concentrations. Since then, comparisons of adjusted tCa and iCa show its inaccuracy in healthy and critically ill patients. The use of an adjustment formula in dogs results in a diagnostic discordance of 37% to 38%, which is higher than using an unadjusted tCa measurement to estimate iCa.[12] This diagnostic discordance increases to 53% in dogs with chronic kidney disease.[12] In healthy and critically ill

Table 1					
Normal tCa and iCa concentrations in dogs and cats					
	tCa			iCa	
	mmol/L	mg/dL		mmol/L	mg/dL
Dogs <3 mo old	2.5–2.9	10.0–11.5		1.30–1.55	5.1–6.2
Dogs >1 y old	2.2–2.5	9.0–10.0		1.25–1.45	5.0–5.8
Adult cats	2.0–2.6	8.0–10.5		1.15–1.40	4.6–5.6

dogs, the adjustment formulas tend to overestimate ionized hypercalcemia and underestimate iHCa.[11,12] Given the consistently high diagnostic discordance of adjusted tCa formulas, adjustment formulas are no longer recommended for estimation of iCa.

Measurement of iCa

iCa should always be measured to accurately assess calcium status, especially in patients with critical illness, acid-base disturbances, alterations in protein concentrations, or kidney or parathyroid disease.[10–14] Given the increase in bench-top analyzers with ion-selective electrodes, the measurement of iCa has become more readily available in veterinary practice. Serum can be used to measure iCa concentrations, but should ideally be collected anaerobically. Aerobic collection allows the mixing of air and a decrease in CO_2, which increases the pH in the sample and decreases protein binding, thereby decreasing iCa concentrations.[15] Exposure to air in partially filled serum tubes results in a decrease of up to 0.07 mmol/L in iCa concentration compared with filling the tubes completely.[16] It is also important to use regular serum vacutainer tubes rather than serum separator (silicone) tubes, because the iCa concentration might increase because of release of iCa from the silicone gel.[17] Once blood is collected in a regular serum tube, it should be allowed to clot, and then separated by centrifugation. Thereafter, the serum can be removed using a long needle attached to a non–air-containing syringe that punctures the red-top stopper without exposing the sample to air.[15]

Heparinized blood samples

Many cage side analyzers perform iCa measurements on heparinized plasma or whole blood. iCa is less stable in whole or heparinized blood compared with plasma and must therefore be analyzed immediately. In dogs, iCa concentrations are approximately 0.05 mmol/L lower in heparinized plasma compared with serum.[16] Liquid heparin also can result in dilution of the sample and false decrease of iCa concentration.[18] Ideally, commercially available syringes containing a premeasured quantity of dry heparin are preferable to manually coating a syringe with an unknown or variable quantity of liquid heparin. However, it is still important to ensure that these syringes are filled according to the manufacturer's recommendations, to avoid underfilling and subsequent underestimation of iCa concentration.

Portable electrolyte analyzers

Portable analyzers are conveniently available for cage side analysis of iCa concentration. They require a heparinized whole blood sample and use a disposable cartridge with an impregnated biosensor for iCa and other analytes. However, iCa concentrations are typically 0.05 to 0.26 mmol/L lower in dogs and 0.05 to 0.14 mmol/L lower in cats when measured using this method compared with serum iCa measurements.[19] Given the effect of heparin on iCa measurements, it is important that reference ranges using standardized blood collection and heparinization protocols are established using these analyzers and that results are not directly compared with measurements obtained using ion-selective methods.

Normal iCa Concentrations

Normal serum iCa concentrations in healthy dogs and cats are included in **Table 1**. Young dogs and cats have serum iCa concentrations approximately 0.1 to 0.4 mg/dL (0.03–0.1 mmol/L) higher than those reported in older animals.[7]

HYPOCALCEMIA OF CRITICAL ILLNESS
Incidence in Critically Ill People

Mild iHCa (iCa ≤1.15 mmol/L) measured at admission or during hospitalization occurs in 58% to 88% of adult human patients admitted to medical-surgical ICUs.[20–22] Conversely, episodes of severe iHCa (iCa <0.80 mmol/L) occur in approximately 3% of critically ill adults during hospitalization in the ICU.[22] The few investigations of hypocalcemia in pediatric ICU populations reveal an overall incidence of iHCa of 12% to 18%, which increases to 37% in children with total hypocalcemia.[23,24] iHCa (iCa <1.10 mmol/L) occurs more commonly in critically ill people with sepsis compared to those without, with an incidence of approximately 77%.[25]

Incidence in Critically Ill Small Animals

Although the incidence of iHCa has been studied in certain diseases in dogs and cats, there are limited published studies investigating the incidence of iHCa in general populations of critically ill animals. Of 141 adult dogs admitted to a veterinary teaching hospital ICU, 16% showed iHCa (iCa <1.11 mmol/L) at ICU admission.[1] The median iCa was 1.03 mmol/L for the dogs with iHCa and ranged from 0.64 to 1.10 mmol/L.[1] Dogs diagnosed with sepsis as defined by meeting at least 2 criteria for systemic inflammatory response syndrome (SIRS) and having a positive culture were more likely to have iHCa.[1]

Prognostic Value of Hypocalcemia in Critically Ill Patients

Although there is no association between admission iHCa and outcome in critically ill dogs hospitalized in an ICU,[1] many human studies reveal that iHCa is associated with increased mortality during critical illness. However, concurrent associations with increased severity of illness make it unclear whether lower iCa concentrations are a marker of severe disease or are attributable to the poorer outcome.[20–24] However, a recent investigation of iCa measurements in more than 7000 critically ill adults shows that an iCa level less than 0.80 mmol/L predicts a 150% increase in mortality and is independently associated with outcome regardless of illness severity.[22]

MECHANISMS UNDERLYING HYPOCALCEMIA OF CRITICAL ILLNESS

Many underlying conditions are associated with hypocalcemia in critically ill dogs and cats, most of which have an obvious pathophysiologic mechanism for the hypocalcemia (Box 3). In addition, several treatments and medications are consistently associated with hypocalcemia in critically ill people and animals (Table 2). Examples include drugs that decrease bone turnover (eg, bisphosphonates) or blood products that contain citrate anticoagulant, which complexes with calcium. In addition, aggressive intravenous fluid therapy can result in calciuresis or a dilutional hypocalcemia, which might be exacerbated in patients with dysfunctional renal calcium reabsorption or those receiving loop diuretics. Nevertheless, many patients with hypocalcemia of critical illness do not have an obvious reason for the hypocalcemia. Several proposed mechanisms might account for the hypocalcemia in these patients, including vitamin D deficiency or resistance, acquired or relative hypoparathyroidism, and hypomagnesemia.

Vitamin D Deficiency or Resistance

Vitamin D deficiency is the most recently investigated and heavily supported mechanism for hypocalcemia of critical illness. Numerous studies investigating vitamin D status in critically ill adults and children admitted to medical and surgical ICUs show

Box 3
Diseases associated with hypocalcemia in critically ill dogs and cats

- Acute kidney failure
- Acute pancreatitis
- Diabetic ketoacidosis
- Eclampsia
- Ethylene glycol intoxication
- Parathyroid disease
- Protein-losing enteropathies
- Renal transplant
- Sepsis
- Trauma
- Tumor lysis syndrome
- Urethral obstruction

hypovitaminosis D defined as serum 25-hydroxyvitamin D less than 15 to 30 ng/mL (37–75 nmol/L) in 26% to 82% of patients.[26–29] These studies also reveal an association between 25-hydroxyvitamin D deficiency and increased length of hospital or ICU stay, severity of illness, organ dysfunction, infection, and mortality.[26–29] Although

Table 2
Drugs or therapies associated with hypocalcemia and the proposed mechanism

Drug or Therapy	Mechanism
Albumin	Increased protein binding
Aminoglycosides	Renal magnesium wasting
Amphotericin B	Decreased bone resorption
Bisphosphonates	Decreased bone resorption
Calcitonin	Decreased bone resorption, decreased PTH secretion/action
Cimetidine	Decreased bone resorption
Cisplatin, carboplatin	Decreased bone resorption
Citrated blood products	Calcium chelation
Cyclophosphamide	Decreased bone resorption
Diuretics (eg, furosemide)	Renal calcium and magnesium wasting, decreased PTH secretion/action
Ethanol	Decreased bone resorption
Heparin	Calcium chelation
Lipid emulsion solutions	Calcium chelation
Magnesium sulfate	Decreased PTH secretion/action
Phosphate preparations (oral, parenteral, enema)	Calcium chelation
Radiographic contrast dyes (eg, gadolinium)	Calcium chelation
Sodium bicarbonate	Calcium chelation

Data from Refs.[2,38–40,88–90]

vitamin D is traditionally thought of as playing an important role in calcium homeostasis, during the past decade, there has been increasing evidence that vitamin D is also required for antimicrobial activity, antiinflammation, cardioprotection, immunomodulation, and metabolic regulation.[30,31] It is not surprising that hypovitaminosis D is associated with comorbidities in critically ill patients, including SIRS, sepsis, and kidney injury.[26,27,29]

Suggested mechanisms by which critically ill patients become deficient in vitamin D include reduced intake during malnutrition, decreased synthesis because of insufficient 1α-hydroxylase, increased tissue demand during critical illness, and renal wasting as a result of loss of vitamin D–binding protein.[30,31] PTH resistance also contributes to hypovitaminosis D and can occur in patients with hypomagnesemia, kidney failure, or hypoparathyroidism.[31] It remains to be determined whether hypovitaminosis D occurs because of critical illness or is implicated in the pathogenesis of comorbidities in critically ill patients, and if vitamin D supplementation improves outcome. The incidence and impact of hypovitaminosis D in critically ill small animals have not been investigated.

Acquired or Relative Hypoparathyroidism

Hypocalcemia can occur in patients with critical illness caused by acquired or relative hypoparathyroidism, which results in impaired synthesis or secretion of PTH. Studies investigating PTH as a contributor to hypocalcemia in critically ill people reveal that PTH concentrations can be low, appropriately high, or inappropriately normal in the face of a concurrent iHCa; the last situation is referred to as relative hypoparathyroidism.[25,32] The most compelling mechanism for low or inappropriately normal PTH concentrations in critically ill patients is cytokine-mediated suppression of PTH secretion. Studies show an association between inflammatory cytokines (eg, tumor necrosis factor α, interleukin 1 (IL-1), IL-6) and decreased PTH secretion.[25] IL-1 and IL-6 in particular are associated with upregulation of calcium-sensing receptors in the kidney and parathyroid, which leads to decreased stimulation for release of PTH.[33]

Hypomagnesemia

Because of the role of magnesium in PTH secretion and activity, hypomagnesemia is implicated as a cause of hypocalcemia of critical illness. Decades-old studies show that magnesium deficiency results in hypoparathyroidism and end-organ (ie, bone, kidney) PTH resistance.[34] Magnesium is a cofactor in many pathways, including the activation of adenylate cyclase, which likely contributes to the deranged release of and resistance to PTH in hypomagnesemic patients.[35] Because of the role of PTH in vitamin D activation, hypomagnesemia likely also contributes to hypovitaminosis D.

Hypomagnesemia occurs in 20% to 65% of critically ill human patients,[35] 54% of critically ill dogs,[36] and 23% of critically ill cats.[37] Inability to measure ionized magnesium (biologically active form) or interpret the meaning of total serum magnesium makes the diagnosis of hypomagnesemia difficult. Many syndromes that affect critically ill patients can lead to hypomagnesemia, including gastrointestinal disorders (eg, malnutrition, malabsorption, pancreatitis, diarrhea, vomiting), renal loss (eg, fluid therapy, osmotic diuresis, metabolic acidosis, kidney disease), and drug administration (see **Table 2**).[2,35,38]

THERAPIES ASSOCIATED WITH HYPOCALCEMIA IN SMALL ANIMALS DURING CRITICAL ILLNESS

In addition to many routinely administered medications (see **Table 2**), several therapies performed in critically ill small animals are also associated with hypocalcemia.

Sodium bicarbonate administration is associated with transient total and iHCa in dogs and cats.[39,40] Administration of citrated blood products in large volumes can also lead to iHCa. Dogs requiring massive transfusions defined as transfusion of a volume of blood products in excess of the estimated blood volume (90 mL/kg) in a 24-hour period or in excess of half of the estimated blood volume in a 3-hour period all develop iHCa (mean iCa 0.89 mmol/L).[41] The iHCa that occurs due to chelation of calcium with citrate is likely exacerbated by the ionized hypomagnesemia that occurs concurrently in these dogs.[41]

Prolonged cardiopulmonary resuscitation (CPR) is also associated with iHCa in dogs. After 7.5 minutes of induced ventricular fibrillation followed by performing CPR in dogs, iCa decreases from 1.24 to 0.86 mmol/L after 10 minutes of CPR and from 1.27 to 0.80 mmol/L after 20 minutes of CPR.[42,43] Proposed mechanisms include chelation with lactate or transcellular diffusion of calcium caused by ischemia-induced phosphate depletion or increased membrane permeability.[42,43]

CONDITIONS ASSOCIATED WITH HYPOCALCEMIA IN CRITICALLY ILL SMALL ANIMALS

Several conditions are commonly associated with hypocalcemia in critically ill dogs and cats (see **Box 3**). Some conditions have proposed mechanisms unique to the underlying disease that explain the development of the hypocalcemia. However, it is likely that some of the mechanisms attributed to hypocalcemia of critical illness already discussed also contribute.

Acute Kidney Disease

Acute kidney disease occurs in critically ill dogs and cats and is associated with total and iHCa. iHCa (median nadir iCa <0.7 mmol/L) occurs in 100% of cats and dogs undergoing continuous renal replacement therapy (CRRT) for acute or acute-on-chronic kidney disease, likely because of citrate anticoagulant administration.[44] Dogs with acute kidney disease and tCa concentrations less than 8.6 mg/dL (<2.15 mmol/L) are more than 4 times less likely to survive to hospital discharge compared with dogs with normal tCa concentrations.[45] Hypocalcemia in patients with acute kidney disease is attributed to an abrupt decrease in glomerular filtration rate, causing a rapid increase in serum phosphorus concentration, which results in a reciprocal secondary hypocalcemia.[45] In addition, ethylene glycol ingestion, pancreatitis, and sepsis often cause acute kidney injury and cannot be excluded as other causes of the hypocalcemia in these patients.[45]

Diabetic Ketoacidosis

Total and iHCa occur in dogs and cats with diabetic ketoacidosis (DKA) and is mild in most cases. Of cats with DKA, 76% show total hypocalcemia, and of those cats with iCa measurements, 21% have iHCa.[46] Conversely, approximately 86% of dogs with DKA have total hypocalcemia, and 52% have iHCa ranging from 0.55 to 1.12 mmol/L.[47] tCa and iCa concentrations are significantly higher in dogs that survive DKA compared with dogs that do not survive.[47] Cats and dogs with DKA and concurrent hypocalcemia do not tend to show signs of hypocalcemia or receive treatment with calcium supplementation.[46,47] Possible causes of the hypocalcemia in dogs and cats with DKA include osmotic diuresis, administration of corticosteroids, bicarbonate, or potassium phosphate supplementation, or concurrent pancreatitis or acute kidney disease.[46,47] Concurrent conditions are diagnosed in 70% of dogs with DKA, and approximately 40% of those dogs have acute pancreatitis.[47]

Eclampsia

Eclampsia or puerperal tetany is postpartum hypocalcemia that occurs during the first 4 weeks of lactation.[48,49] It is more likely to occur in small-breed dogs and is possibly more common with large litter sizes.[48] The cause is not understood, but it might be caused by increase calcium drain during fetal skeletal ossification, massive calcium loss during lactation, parathyroid gland atrophy, or poor dietary calcium sources.[48] iCa concentrations range from 0.42 to 0.81 mmol/L.[48,49] Treatment is typically required in all dogs presenting with eclampsia, and relapses occur in 10% of dogs, despite at-home calcium supplementation.[48]

Ethylene Glycol Intoxication

Intoxication occurs with ingestion of antifreeze products that contain ethylene glycol, which is metabolized in the liver to form the toxic metabolites glycoaldehyde, glycolate, and oxalate. Oxalate combines with calcium to form calcium oxalate crystals, which precipitate in the renal tubules, causing acute kidney injury. Total hypocalcemia occurs in 44% of dogs and 50% of cats after ethylene glycol intoxication.[50] iHCa is more recently reported in dogs and cats with ethylene glycol intoxication.[51,52]

Kidney Transplant

iHCa occurs in 100% of feline kidney transplant recipients.[53] iHCa is commonly accompanied by total hypomagnesemia, which might account for the iHCa.[53] Other proposed mechanisms include renal loss or a reciprocal decrease in iCa in response to a decreased glomerular filtration rate and subsequent hyperphosphatemia.

Pancreatitis

iHCa occurs in 43% to 61% of cats with acute pancreatitis.[54,55] Cats with acute pancreatitis that do not survive have significantly lower iCa concentrations compared with cats that survive; 77% of cats with acute pancreatitis and iCa 1.00 mmol/L or less die or are euthanized.[54] Hypocalcemia occurs infrequently in dogs with acute pancreatitis,[56,57] but approximately 40% of dogs with chronic pancreatitis have total hypocalcemia.[58] Proposed mechanisms for hypocalcemia in patients with pancreatitis include increased free fatty acids, which chelate with calcium, or sequestration of calcium in the soft tissues or peripancreatic fat as a result of saponification.[54]

Parathyroid Disease

Primary hypoparathyroidism is a common cause of severe hypocalcemia in dogs.[59,60] Severe total hypocalcemia is also seen in dogs with infarction of parathyroid gland adenomas.[61] Likewise, iHCa (iCa 0.75–1.1 mmol/L) occurs commonly in 36% to 71% of dogs 2 to 3 days after parathyroidectomy for primary hyperparathyroidism or parathyroid carcinoma excision.[62–64] Risk factors for the development of postoperative hypocalcemia remain unclear, but the degree of preoperative hypercalcemia is an inconsistent predictor.[62,63]

Protein-Losing Enteropathies

tCa and iHCa (iCa 0.50–0.88 mmol/L) occur in dogs with protein-losing enteropathies.[65,66] PTH is appropriately increased in these dogs; however, 25-hydroxyvitamin D, 1,25-dihydroxyvitamin D, and serum total magnesium concentrations are consistently decreased.[65,66] Therefore, it is likely that the hypocalcemia is caused by intestinal loss of magnesium and malabsorption of magnesium and vitamin D, with subsequent impaired intestinal absorption of calcium and an abnormal homeostatic response to iHCa.[65,66]

Sepsis

Sepsis is a common cause of hypocalcemia in critically ill small animals. Approximately 90% of cats with septic peritonitis have iHCa at the time of sepsis diagnosis.[67] Clinical signs of hypocalcemia were not documented in any of those cats, but intravenous calcium supplementation was administered to 20% of cats with an iCa ranging from 0.73 to 0.89 mmol/L.[67] Cats with iHCa that did not normalize during hospitalization were less likely to survive.[67] Conversely, 24% of dogs with sepsis have iHCa, including 67% of dogs that experience cardiopulmonary arrest and die during hospitalization.[68] Proposed mechanisms include accumulation of calcium in tissues or cells, acquired or relative hypoparathyroidism, chelation of calcium with lactate or free fatty acids, hypomagnesemia, hypovitaminosis D or vitamin D resistance, as well as alkalosis and subsequent increased protein binding of calcium.[69] In dogs with experimentally induced endotoxemia, iHCa is associated with hypovitaminosis D, but not hypomagnesemia, hypoparathyroidism, alkalosis, or increased calciuresis.[70]

Trauma

iHCa occurs in 16% of dogs admitted to a veterinary teaching hospital after trauma.[71] It is more likely to occur in dogs with abdominal injuries and is associated with an increased requirement for synthetic colloids, vasopressors, and blood transfusions.[71] Dogs with iHCa after trauma are more severely injured, have decreased systolic blood pressure, have a longer duration of hospitalization, and are less likely to survive, compared with dogs with normal iCa concentrations.[71] Proposed mechanisms include acquired or relative hypoparathyroidism, hypovitaminosis D, chelation with lactate, or increased calcium deposition intracellularly or extracellularly.[72]

Tumor Lysis Syndrome

Acute tumor lysis syndrome occurs rarely in small animals and occurs most commonly in human patients with aggressive hematopoietic malignancies and less commonly with solid tumors, including lymphoma.[73–77] Risk factors include rapid cytoreduction of a large tumor burden and pretreatment kidney insufficiency.[76,77] Acute tumor lysis results in the release of large amounts of intracellular purines, phosphorus, uric acid, potassium, and lactate from neoplastic cells, which results in metabolic derangements, including hyperphosphatemia, hyperkalemia, hyperuricemia, and acidosis.[76,77] tCa and iHCa likely occur secondary to the hyperphosphatemia and are documented in dogs and cats with tumor lysis syndrome after treatment of lymphoma.[73–75]

Urethral Obstruction

iHCa occurs in 75% of cats presented for urethral obstruction, with values ranging from 0.55 to 1.19 mmol/L.[78] iCa concentrations are negatively correlated with potassium, phosphorus, creatinine, and urea, and positively correlated with heart rate and pH.[78] Likewise, iCa is inversely correlated with PTH, suggesting an appropriate response to iHCa in these cats.[79] 25-hydroxyvitamin D concentrations are variable in cats with urethral obstruction, and conclusions cannot be drawn regarding its influence on iCa concentrations.[79]

CLINICAL SIGNS RESULTING FROM HYPOCALCEMIA DURING CRITICAL ILLNESS

Hypocalcemia results in a variety of clinical signs that occur as a result of increased neuronal excitability (**Box 4**). However, the signs are often undetected in critically ill patients, possibly because of factors that mask these signs, including severe acidosis, derangements in serum potassium concentrations, or administration of sedatives,

---

Box 4
Clinical signs associated with hypocalcemia

Most common

- Ataxia or staggering
- Facial rubbing/pawing (paresthesia)
- Hyperthermia
- Muscle tremors/fasciculations
- Muscle cramping/spasms
- Panting
- Restlessness/excitation
- Stiff, rigid gait
- Seizures (focal or generalized)
- Weakness (continuous or episodic)

Cardiovascular

- Decreased cardiac contractility
- Decreased cardiac output
- Decreased systemic and pulmonary vascular resistance
- Hypotension
- QT-interval and ST-interval prolongation
- Ventricular arrhythmias

---

anticonvulsants, or paralytics.[80] Cardiovascular manifestations of hypocalcemia also can occur and are more commonly observed in critically ill patients. These manifestations include ventricular arrhythmias, decreased cardiac contractility, failure to respond to drugs that act through calcium-related mechanisms (eg, digoxin, norepinephrine, dopamine), and hypotension refractory to intravenous fluids and vasopressors.[2,81] Electrocardiographic changes most often associated with hypocalcemia include QT-interval or ST-interval prolongation,[2,38,81] although wide T waves are also documented in hypocalcemic dogs.[82] The hemodynamic signs associated with hypocalcemia are not well documented in critically ill veterinary patients, but are described in dogs with experimentally induced sepsis.[83] These signs include decreased mean arterial pressure and cardiac output, as well as systemic and pulmonary vascular resistance.[83]

The severity of clinical signs is determined by the magnitude of the hypocalcemia, as well as the rate of decline in iCa concentrations. Mild hypocalcemia (iCa 0.9–1.1 mmol/L) that occurs in critically ill dogs and cats with DKA, acute pancreatitis, protein-losing enteropathies, sepsis, trauma, tumor lysis syndrome, or urethral obstruction is unlikely to result in obvious clinical signs. However, critically ill dogs and cats with acute kidney disease undergoing CRRT, eclampsia, or parathyroid disease often develop moderate (0.8–0.9 mmol/L) or severe (<0.8 mmol/L) iHCa, which is frequently accompanied by clinical signs. Approximately 25% of hypocalcemic cats (iCa 0.37–0.88 mmol/L) and dogs (iCa 0.34–0.74 mmol/L) undergoing CRRT for acute kidney disease showed clinical signs, including muscle fasciculations, muscle tremors, or tachypnea with shallow breathing.[44] Likewise, almost 80% of dogs with eclampsia show clinical signs, including seizures, trembling, twitching, shaking, and stiffness.[48] Clinical signs also occur commonly in dogs with primary hypoparathyroidism and include focal muscle twitching, generalized muscle tremors, tonic spasm of limb muscles, a stiff, rigid gait, generalized seizures, ataxia, staggering, episodic weakness, lethargy, hyperthermia, and excessive panting.[59,60] These signs also occur in approximately 25% of dogs recovering from parathyroidectomy surgery.[61–63] The clinical signs that occur in these dogs tend to manifest at higher iCa concentrations, likely because the decrease in iCa occurs within a short period (between 48 and 72 hours postoperatively).[61–63] Life-threatening signs, including cardiopulmonary arrest, can occur when the iCa concentration decreases lower than 0.5–0.6 mmol/L.[2]

TREATMENT OF HYPOCALCEMIA DURING CRITICAL ILLNESS
Recommendations

Immediate treatment of critically ill dogs and cats with clinical signs of hypocalcemia is recommended (**Table 3**). Mild hypocalcemia (iCa 0.9–1.1 mmol/L) is usually well tolerated in critically ill patients, but the threshold for development of clinical signs is variable.[2] Calcium supplementation should be considered in critically ill patients with iCa level less than 1.0 mmol/L and is recommended for patients with moderate (iCa <0.9 mmol/L) to severe (iCa <0.8 mmol/L) hypocalcemia, especially in patients requiring vasopressor or inotropic support.[2] The amount of calcium supplementation required varies among patients, but normalization of iCa concentrations is not necessary. Rather, calcium supplementation should be given to abate clinical signs or to a maximum of 1.1 mmol/L. Correction of calcium to normal or hypercalcemic concentrations can blunt the parathyroid response and predispose to urinary calculi or renal mineralization.[80] Although iHCa occurs commonly during CPR, the routine administration of calcium during CPR is not recommended.[84]

Table 3		
Treatment recommendations for critically ill patients with hypocalcemia		
Drug	**Dose**	**Comments**
Calcium gluconate 10%	0.5–1.5 mL/kg intravenously slowly (over 10–15 min) 5–15 mg/kg/h intravenously	Emergency treatment; bradycardia if given too rapidly; skin necrosis if administered perivascularly
Calcium carbonate (40% of the tablet contains calcium)	25–50 mg/kg/d orally	Most common oral form of calcium supplementation
1,25-Dihydroxyvitamin D (caltritriol)	20–30 ng/kg/d orally (first 3–4 d) 5–15 ng/kg/d orally (maintenance)	Reaches maximal effect in 1–4 d
Magnesium sulfate or magnesium chloride	0.15–0.3 mEq/kg intravenously slowly (over 5–15 min) (loading) 0.02–0.04 mEq/kg/h intravenously (maintenance)	Incompatible with calcium-containing solutions

Data from Schenck PA, Chew DJ, Nagode LA, et al. Disorders of calcium: hypercalcemia and hypocalcemia. In: DiBartola SP, editor. Fluid, electrolyte, and acid-base disorders in small animal practice. 4th edition. St Louis (MO): Elsevier; 2012. p. 120–94; and Bateman S. Disorders of magnesium: magnesium deficit and excess. In: DiBartola SP, editor. Fluid, electrolyte, and acid-base disorders in small animal practice. 4th edition. St Louis (MO): Elsevier; 2012. p. 213–30.

Rationale

Whether correction of hypocalcemia in critically ill patients provides any benefit in reducing mortality remains to be determined, and evidence-based guidelines are not available to guide treatment.[85] Arguments for the administration of calcium supplementation to critically ill patients include that hypocalcemia is associated with increased mortality in some diseases, correction of hypocalcemia can improve myocardial contractility, and calcium supplementation might reduce requirements for vasopressors or inotropic agents.[85,86] Alternatively, arguments against supplementing calcium to critically ill patients include evidence supporting that hypoxia and ischemia-reperfusion injury are associated with intracellular calcium accumulation and that mortality is increased after calcium supplementation in some experimental models of sepsis, as well as a lack of evidence proving its beneficial effects.[83,85]

Calcium Supplementation

Parenteral calcium, usually in the form of calcium gluconate 10%, is administered as a slow intravenous infusion (0.5–1.5 mL/kg) over 10 to 15 minutes. Continuous electrocardiographic monitoring is recommended during the infusion, and if the heart rate decreases or an arrhythmia occurs, the infusion should be significantly slowed or discontinued, because cardiac arrest can occur. Obvious clinical signs typically resolve within 30 minutes after the administration of intravenous calcium, but milder clinical signs can persist for 1 to 2 hours.[44,48,80] iCa concentrations should be rechecked 2 to 3 times daily to ensure adequate supplementation and to avoid iatrogenic hypercalcemia. In some critically ill patients, a constant rate infusion might be needed if signs of hypocalcemia recur or if the inciting cause of the hypocalcemia cannot be readily identified or treated (see **Table 3**). Subcutaneous administration of calcium salts is not recommended, because it results in severe skin mineralization and necrosis.[7] Oral calcium and calcitriol supplementation can also be considered for patients requiring long-term supplementation (see **Table 3**).

Magnesium Supplementation

Hypomagnesemia is a common concurrent finding in critically ill patients with hypocalcemia.[35] Magnesium is important in calcium regulation because of its effects on PTH and vitamin D activity.[34] Therefore, supplementation should be considered in critically ill patients with hypocalcemia (see **Table 3**), especially those with concurrently documented hypomagnesemia.[35] A rapid loading dose of magnesium can be administered intravenously using either the chloride or sulfate salt and can be followed with a continuous infusion during hospitalization, until the patient's dietary intake is sufficient to maintain adequate magnesium concentrations.[87] Iatrogenic hypermagnesemia is rare with appropriate supplementation, except in patients with kidney insufficiency.[35]

SUMMARY

Hypocalcemia occurs commonly in critically ill dogs and cats in association with certain medications and treatments, as well as various underlying diseases. Proposed underlying mechanisms include hypovitaminosis D, acquired or relative hypoparathyroidism, or hypomagnesemia, as well as alterations in the ionized fraction of calcium as a result of changes in chelated or protein-bound calcium. If severe or acute, hypocalcemia can cause obvious clinical signs of muscle or neurologic hyperexcitability or more subtle signs related to cardiovascular dysfunction. Emergent treatment is necessary when clinical signs are present, and supplementation of calcium, calcitriol, or magnesium should be considered for patients with moderate to severe iHCa.

REFERENCES

1. Holowaychuk MK, Hansen BD, DeFrancesco TC, et al. Ionized hypocalcemia in critically ill dogs. J Vet Intern Med 2009;23(3):509–13.
2. Zaloga GP. Hypocalcemia in critically ill patients. Crit Care Med 1992;20(2): 251–62.
3. Rosol TJ, Chew DJ, Nagode LA, et al. Pathophysiology of calcium metabolism. Vet Clin Pathol 1995;24(2):49–63.
4. Schenck PA, Chew DJ, Brooks CL. Fractionation of canine serum calcium, using a micropartition system. Am J Vet Res 1996;57(3):268–71.
5. Schenck PA, Chew DJ, Behrend EN. Updates on hypercalcemic disorders. In: August JR, editor. Consultations in feline internal medicine. 5th edition. St Louis (MO): Elsevier; 2006. p. 157–68.
6. Boden SD, Kaplan FS. Calcium homeostasis. Orthop Clin North Am 1990;21(1): 31–42.
7. Schenck PA, Chew DJ, Nagode LA, et al. Disorders of calcium: hypercalcemia and hypocalcemia. In: DiBartola SP, editor. Fluid, electrolyte, and acid-base disorders in small animal practice. 4th edition. St Louis (MO): Elsevier; 2012. p. 120–94.
8. Brown EM, Pollak M, Hebert SC. Sensing of extracellular Ca^{2+} by parathyroid and kidney cells: cloning and characterization of an extracellular Ca^{2+}-sensing receptor. Am J Kidney Dis 1995;25(3):506–13.
9. Bronner F. Mechanisms and functional aspects of intestinal calcium absorption. J Exp Zool A Comp Exp Biol 2003;300(1):47–52.
10. Schenck PA, Chew DJ. Prediction of serum ionized calcium concentration by serum total calcium measurement in cats. Can J Vet Res 2010;74(3):209–13.
11. Sharp CR, Kerl ME, Mann FA. A comparison of total calcium, corrected calcium, and ionized calcium concentrations as indicators of calcium homeostasis among hypoalbuminemic dogs requiring intensive care. J Vet Emerg Crit Care (San Antonio) 2009;19(6):571–8.
12. Schenck PA, Chew DJ. Prediction of serum ionized calcium concentration by use of serum total calcium concentration in dogs. Am J Vet Res 2005;66(8): 1330–6.
13. Slomp J, van der Voort PH, Gerritsen RT, et al. Albumin-adjusted calcium is not suitable for diagnosis of hyper- and hypocalcemia in the critically ill. Crit Care Med 2003;31(5):1389–93.
14. Byrnes MC, Huynh K, Helmer SD, et al. A comparison of corrected serum calcium levels to ionized calcium levels among critically ill surgical patients. Am J Surg 2005;189(3):310–4.
15. Schenck PA, Chew DJ. Calcium: total or ionized? Vet Clin North Am Small Anim Pract 2008;38(3):497–502.
16. Unterer S, Lutz H, Gerber B, et al. Evaluation of an electrolyte analyzer for measurement of ionized calcium and magnesium concentrations in blood, plasma, and serum of dogs. Am J Vet Res 2004;65(2):183–7.
17. Larsson L, Ohman S. Effect of silicone-separator tubes and storage time on ionized calcium in serum. Clin Chem 1985;31(1):169–70.
18. Hopper K, Rezende ML, Haskins SC. Assessment of the effect of dilution of blood samples with sodium heparin on blood gas, electrolyte, and lactate measurements in dogs. Am J Vet Res 2005;66(4):656–60.
19. Grosenbaugh DA, Gadawski JE, Muir WW. Evaluation of a portable clinical analyzer in a veterinary hospital setting. J Am Vet Med Assoc 1998;213(5):691–4.

20. Zivin JR, Gooley T, Zager RA, et al. Hypocalcemia: a pervasive metabolic abnormality in the critically ill. Am J Kidney Dis 2001;37(4):689–98.
21. Hastbacka J, Pettila V. Prevalence and predictive value of ionized hypocalcemia among critically ill patients. Acta Anaesthesiol Scand 2003;47(10):1264–9.
22. Egi M, Kim I, Nichol A, et al. Ionized calcium concentration and outcome in critical illness. Crit Care Med 2011;39(2):314–21.
23. Broner CW, Stidham GL, Westenkirchner DF, et al. Hypermagnesemia and hypocalcemia as predictors of high mortality in critically ill pediatric patients. Crit Care Med 1990;18(9):921–8.
24. Cardenas-Rivero N, Chernow B, Stoiko MA, et al. Hypocalcemia in critically ill children. J Pediatr 1989;114(6):946–51.
25. Lind L, Carlstedt F, Rastad J, et al. Hypocalcemia and parathyroid hormone secretion in critically ill patients. Crit Care Med 2000;28(1):93–9.
26. Arnson Y, Gringauz I, Itzhaky D, et al. Vitamin D deficiency is associated with poor outcomes and increased mortality in severely ill patients. QJM 2012;105(7):633–9.
27. Flynn L, Zimmerman LH, McNorton K, et al. Effects of vitamin D deficiency in critically ill surgical patients. Am J Surg 2012;203(3):379–82.
28. Lucidarme O, Messai E, Mazzoni T, et al. Incidence and risk factors of vitamin D deficiency in critically ill patients: results from a prospective observational study. Intensive Care Med 2010;36(9):1609–11.
29. McNally JD, Menon K, Chakraborty P, et al. The association of vitamin D status with pediatric critical illness. Pediatrics 2012;130(3):429–36.
30. Amrein K, Venkatesh B. Vitamin D and the critically ill patient. Curr Opin Clin Nutr Metab Care 2012;15(2):188–93.
31. Lee P. Vitamin D metabolism and deficiency in critical illness. Best Pract Res Clin Endocrinol Metab 2011;25(5):769–81.
32. Carlstedt F, Lind L, Rastad J, et al. Parathyroid hormone and ionized calcium levels are related to the severity of illness and survival in critically ill patients. Eur J Clin Invest 1998;28(11):898–903.
33. Canaff L, Zhou X, Hendy GN. The proinflammatory cytokine, interleukin-6, upregulates calcium-sensing receptor gene transcription via Stat1/3 and Sp1/3. J Biol Chem 2008;283(20):13586–600.
34. Rude RK, Oldham SB, Sharp CF Jr, et al. Parathyroid hormone secretion in magnesium deficiency. J Clin Endocrinol Metab 1978;47(4):800–6.
35. Tong GM, Rude RK. Magnesium deficiency in critical illness. J Intensive Care Med 2005;20(1):3–17.
36. Martin LG, Matteson VL, Wingfield WE, et al. Abnormalities of serum magnesium in critically ill dogs: incidence and implications. J Vet Emerg Crit Care (San Antonio) 1994;4(1):15–20.
37. Toll J, Erb H, Birnbaum N, et al. Prevalence and incidence of serum magnesium abnormalities in hospitalized cats. J Vet Intern Med 2002;16(3):217–21.
38. Kelly A, Levine MA. Hypocalcemia in the critically ill patient. J Intensive Care Med 2013;28(3):166–77.
39. Moon PF, Gabor L, Gleed RD, et al. Acid-base, metabolic, and hemodynamic effects of sodium bicarbonate or tromethamine administration in anesthetized dogs with experimentally induced metabolic acidosis. Am J Vet Res 1997;58(7):771–6.
40. Abrams KL. Hypocalcemia associated with administration of sodium bicarbonate for salicylate intoxication in a cat. J Am Vet Med Assoc 1987;191(2):235–6.

41. Jutkowitz LA, Rozanski EA, Moreau JA, et al. Massive transfusion in dogs: 15 cases (1997-2001). J Am Vet Med Assoc 2002;220(11):1664–9.
42. Niemann JT, Cairns CB. Hyperkalemia and ionized hypocalcemia during cardiac arrest and resuscitation: possible culprits for postcountershock arrhythmias? Ann Emerg Med 1999;34(1):1–7.
43. Cairns CB, Niemann JT, Pelikan PC, et al. Ionized hypocalcemia during prolonged cardiac arrest and closed-chest CPR in a canine model. Ann Emerg Med 1991;20(11):1178–82.
44. Diehl SH, Seshadri R. Use of continuous renal replacement therapy for treatment of dogs and cats with acute or acute-on-chronic renal failure: 33 cases (2002-2006). J Vet Emerg Crit Care (San Antonio) 2008;18(4):370–82.
45. Vaden SL, Levine J, Breitschwerdt EB. A retrospective case-control of acute renal failure in 99 dogs. J Vet Intern Med 1997;11(2):58–64.
46. Bruskiewicz KA, Nelson RW, Feldman EC, et al. Diabetic ketosis and ketoacidosis in cats: 42 cases (1980-1995). J Am Vet Med Assoc 1997;211(2):188–92.
47. Hume DZ, Drobatz KJ, Hess RS. Outcome of dogs with diabetic ketoacidosis: 127 dogs (1993-2003). J Vet Intern Med 2006;20(3):547–55.
48. Drobatz KJ, Casey KK. Eclampsia in dogs: 31 cases (1995-1998). J Am Vet Med Assoc 2000;217(2):216–9.
49. Aroch I, Srebro H, Shpigel NY. Serum electrolyte concentrations in bitches with eclampsia. Vet Rec 1999;145(11):318–20.
50. Thrall MA, Grauer GF, Mero KN. Clinicopathologic findings in dogs and cats with ethylene glycol intoxication. J Am Vet Med Assoc 1984;184(1):37–41.
51. Tart KM, Powell LL. 4-methylpyrazole as a treatment in naturally occurring ethylene glycol intoxication in cats. J Vet Emerg Crit Care (San Antonio) 2011; 21(3):268–72.
52. Hopper K, Epstein SE. Falsely increased plasma lactate concentration due to ethylene glycol poisoning in 2 dogs. J Vet Emerg Crit Care (San Antonio) 2013;23(1):63–7.
53. Wooldridge JD, Gregory CR. Ionized and total serum magnesium concentrations in feline renal transplant recipients. Vet Surg 1999;28(1):31–7.
54. Kimmel SE, Washabau RJ, Drobatz KJ. Incidence and prognostic value of low plasma ionized calcium concentration in cats with acute pancreatitis: 46 cases (1996-1998). J Am Vet Med Assoc 2001;219(8):1105–9.
55. Son TT, Thompson L, Serrano S, et al. Retrospective study: surgical intervention in the management of severe acute pancreatitis in cats: 8 cases (2003-2007). J Vet Emerg Crit Care (San Antonio) 2010;20(4):426–35.
56. Bishop M, Barr JW, Duff C, et al. Serum ionized calcium concentrations in dogs with and without evidence of pancreatitis. J Vet Emerg Crit Care (San Antonio) 2012;22(S2):S3.
57. Hess RS, Saunders HM, Van Winkle TJ, et al. Clinical, clinicopathologic, radiographic, and ultrasonographic abnormalities in dogs with fatal acute pancreatitis: 70 cases (1986-1995). J Am Vet Med Assoc 1998;213(5):665–70.
58. Bostrom BM, Xenoulis PG, Newman SJ, et al. Chronic pancreatitis in dogs: a retrospective study of clinical, clinicopathological, and histopathological findings in 61 cases. Vet J 2013;195(1):73–9.
59. Russell NJ, Bond KA, Robertson ID, et al. Primary hypoparathyroidism in dogs: a retrospective study of 17 cases. Aust Vet J 2006;84(8):285–90.
60. Bruyette DS, Feldman EC. Primary hypoparathyroidism in the dog. Report of 15 cases and review of 13 previously reported cases. J Vet Intern Med 1988;2(1): 7–14.

61. Rosol TJ, Chew DJ, Capen CC, et al. Acute hypocalcemia associated with infarction of parathyroid gland adenomas in two dogs. J Am Vet Med Assoc 1988;192(2):212–4.

62. Milovancev M, Schmiedt CW. Preoperative factors associated with postoperative hypocalcemia in dogs with primary hyperparathyroidism that underwent parathyroidectomy: 62 cases (2004-2009). J Am Vet Med Assoc 2013;242(4): 507–15.

63. Arbaugh M, Smeak D, Monnet E. Evaluation of preoperative serum concentrations of ionized calcium and parathyroid hormone as predictors of hypocalcemia following parathyroidectomy in dogs with primary hyperparathyroidism: 17 cases (2001-2009). J Am Vet Med Assoc 2012;241(2):233–6.

64. Sawyer ES, Northrup NC, Schmiedt CW, et al. Outcome of 19 dogs with parathyroid carcinoma after surgical excision. Vet Comp Oncol 2012;10(1):57–64.

65. Kimmel SE, Waddell LS, Michel KE. Hypomagnesemia and hypocalcemia associated with protein-losing enteropathy in Yorkshire terriers: five cases (1992-1998). J Am Vet Med Assoc 2000;217(5):703–6.

66. Mellanby RJ, Mellor PJ, Roulois A, et al. Hypocalcaemia associated with low serum vitamin D metabolite concentrations in two dogs with protein-losing enteropathies. J Small Anim Pract 2005;46(7):345–51.

67. Kellett-Gregory LM, Mittleman Boller E, Brown DC, et al. Ionized calcium concentrations in cats with septic peritonitis: 55 cases (1990-2008). J Vet Emerg Crit Care (San Antonio) 2010;20(4):398–405.

68. Luschini MA, Fletcher DJ, Schoeffler GL. Incidence of ionized hypocalcemia in septic dogs and its association with morbidity and mortality: 58 cases (2006-2007). J Vet Emerg Crit Care (San Antonio) 2010;20(4):406–12.

69. Holowaychuk MK, Martin LG. Review of hypocalcemia in septic patients. J Vet Emerg Crit Care (San Antonio) 2007;17(4):348–58.

70. Holowaychuk MK, Birkenheuer AJ, Li J, et al. Hypocalcemia and hypovitaminosis D in dogs with induced endotoxemia. J Vet Intern Med 2012;26(2):244–51.

71. Holowaychuk MK, Monteith G. Ionized hypocalcemia as a prognostic indicator in dogs following trauma. J Vet Emerg Crit Care (San Antonio) 2011;21(5):521–30.

72. Choi YC, Hwang SY. The value of initial ionized calcium as a predictor of mortality and triage tool in adult trauma patients. J Korean Med Sci 2008;23(4):700–5.

73. Calia CM, Hohenhaus AE, Fox PR, et al. Acute tumor lysis syndrome in a cat with lymphoma. J Vet Intern Med 1996;10(6):409–11.

74. Laing EJ, Carter RF. Acute tumor lysis syndrome following treatment of canine lymphoma. J Am Anim Hosp Assoc 1988;24:691–6.

75. Vickery KR, Thamm DH. Successful treatment of acute tumor lysis syndrome in a dog with multicentric lymphoma. J Vet Intern Med 2007;21(6):1401–4.

76. Arrambide K, Toto RD. Tumor lysis syndrome. Semin Nephrol 1993;13(3): 273–80.

77. Page RL. Acute tumor lysis syndrome. Semin Vet Med Surg (Small Anim) 1986; 1(1):58–60.

78. Lee JA, Drobatz KJ. Characterization of the clinical characteristics, electrolytes, acid-base, and renal parameters in male cats with urethral obstruction. J Vet Emerg Crit Care (San Antonio) 2003;13(4):227–33.

79. Drobatz KJ, Ward C, Graham P, et al. Serum concentrations of parathyroid hormone and 25-OH vitamin D3 in cats with urethral obstruction. J Vet Emerg Crit Care (San Antonio) 2005;15(3):179–84.

80. Dhupa N, Proulx J. Hypocalcemia and hypomagnesemia. Vet Clin North Am Small Anim Pract 1998;28(3):587–608.

81. Eryol NK, Colak R, Ozdogru I, et al. Effects of calcium treatment on QT interval and QT dispersion in hypocalcemia. Am J Cardiol 2003;91(6):750–2.
82. Feldman EC, Ettinger SJ. Electrocardiographic changes associated with electrolyte disturbances. Vet Clin North Am 1977;7(3):487–96.
83. Steinhorn DM, Sweeney MF, Layman LK. Pharmacodynamic response to ionized calcium during acute sepsis. Crit Care Med 1990;18(8):851–7.
84. Fletcher DJ, Boller M, Brainard BM, et al. RECOVER evidence and knowledge gap analysis on veterinary CPR. Part 7: clinical guidelines. J Vet Emerg Crit Care (San Antonio) 2012;22(S1):S102–31.
85. Forsythe RM, Wessel CB, Billiar TR, et al. Parenteral calcium for intensive care unit patients. Cochrane Database Syst Rev 2008;(4):CD006163.
86. Vincent JL, Bredas P, Jankowski S, et al. Correction of hypocalcaemia in the critically ill: what is the haemodynamic benefit? Intensive Care Med 1995;21(10): 838–41.
87. Bateman S. Disorders of magnesium: magnesium deficit and excess. In: DiBartola SP, editor. Fluid, electrolyte, and acid-base disorders in small animal practice. 4th edition. St Louis (MO): Elsevier; 2012. p. 213–30.
88. Buckley MS, Leblanc JM, Cawley MJ. Electrolyte disturbances associated with commonly prescribed medications in the intensive care unit. Crit Care Med 2010;38(Suppl 6):S253–64.
89. Atkins CE, Tyler R, Greenlee P. Clinical, biochemical, acid-base, and electrolyte abnormalities in cats after hypertonic sodium phosphate enema administration. Am J Vet Res 1985;46(4):980–8.
90. Jorgensen LS, Center SA, Randolph JF, et al. Electrolyte abnormalities induced by hypertonic phosphate enemas in two cats. J Am Vet Med Assoc 1985; 187(12):1367–8.

Diagnosis of Disorders of Iron Metabolism in Dogs and Cats

Andrea A. Bohn, DVM, PhD

KEYWORDS

- Anemia of chronic disease • Ferritin • Hemochromatosis • Inflammation
- Iron deficiency • Percent saturation • Transferrin

KEY POINTS

- Serum iron concentration is often not an accurate reflection of body iron stores.
- Serum iron concentration decreases with inflammation and iron deficiency.
- Ferritin is currently the best assay for body iron stores.
- Low ferritin indicates iron deficiency; normal ferritin does not rule it out.
- Care must be taken when interpreting levels of ferritin and transferrin because they are acute-phase proteins and inflammation can affect results.
- On a hemogram, MCV_{retic} and CH_{retic} may indicate iron deficiency before MCV and mean cell hemoglobin concentration.

REVIEW OF NORMAL IRON METABOLISM
Function

Iron is an essential element and is used by every cell in the body. Although iron is instrumental in oxygen transport and erythropoiesis, it is also necessary for numerous enzymatic reactions and is important in energy metabolism, DNA synthesis, and cellular immune responses.[1] Contrary to its importance, iron can also cause cell damage with the formation of reactive oxygen species; therefore, its regulation is tightly controlled.[2]

Location

Most total body iron is found within heme, predominantly as hemoglobin of erythroid cells and myoglobin of muscle with lesser amounts within enzymatic hemoproteins. A significant amount of total body iron can also be in storage. Within cells, the most important iron storage protein is ferritin. Much of stored iron is present within

Disclosures: The author has nothing to disclose.
Department of Microbiology, Immunology, and Pathology, College of Veterinary Medicine and Biomedical Sciences, Colorado State University, 1619 Campus Delivery, Fort Collins, CO 80523, USA
E-mail address: andrea.bohn@colostate.edu

Vet Clin Small Anim 43 (2013) 1319–1330
http://dx.doi.org/10.1016/j.cvsm.2013.07.002
0195-5616/13/$ – see front matter © 2013 Elsevier Inc. All rights reserved.

hepatocytes. Macrophages in the spleen, liver, and bone marrow can also store large quantities of iron. Hemosiderin, formed by partial degradation of ferritin, is less soluble and may become more abundant than ferritin when iron stores are high.[3]

Plasma Iron

Very little iron (<0.1% of total body iron) is actually in circulation. This iron is mostly bound to the iron transport protein, transferrin, and is turned over multiple times each day. Iron circulating in plasma is predominantly recycled iron from senescent erythrocytes that have been phagocytized by reticuloendothelial macrophages. Only a small amount of plasma iron comes from ingestion, which is the only natural route for taking iron into the body.[1] Small amounts of iron are routinely lost with the shedding of enterocytes, uroepithelial cells, and skin cells and can also occur with blood loss and sweating. Normally, the amount of iron loss about equals the amount absorbed from diet.[2]

Regulation

The regulation of body iron content occurs at the level of absorption by enterocytes because there are no known significant routes of excretion. The amount of iron that is absorbed from diet is controlled by the iron regulatory hormone hepcidin, which works as a negative regulator. It has recently been shown that the acute effect of increased hepcidin concentration is proteosomal-mediated degradation of DMT1, the apical transporter, which normally allows inorganic iron to enter the enterocyte from the intestinal lumen (**Fig. 1**).[4] Therefore, when hepcidin concentrations are elevated, less iron is able to enter the enterocyte, whereas at low hepcidin concentrations, DMT1 is available for transport.

After iron is absorbed by enterocytes from the intestinal lumen, this iron cannot be released to the systemic circulation without a different membrane transport protein on the basolateral membrane of the enterocyte, called ferroportin (see **Fig. 1**). How much ferroportin is available for transport is also dependent on hepcidin concentrations; more ferroportin is available with low hepcidin concentrations and less ferroportin with high hepcidin.

Hephaestin is a ferroxidase expressed on the basolateral membrane of duodenal enterocytes and associated with ferroportin (see **Fig. 1**). Its only known function is to mediate the reoxidation of Fe^{2+} to Fe^{3+} as iron leaves the enterocyte. Exported iron is immediately bound to transferrin for transport through the circulation. Transferrin is a glycoprotein with high affinity for one to two Fe^{3+} ions.

The general mechanism by which hepcidin has been shown to decrease ferroportin numbers has been by binding to ferroportin, which results in internalization and degradation of the membrane transport protein, although new data suggest that hepcidin may influence ferroportin expression on enterocytes by an alternative route, possibly at the level of translation.[4] In addition to enterocytes, ferroportin is also present in the membranes of hepatocytes and macrophages. Ferroportin is the only known membrane protein that exports inorganic iron from mammalian cells and hepcidin seems to be the principal factor in determining ferroportin numbers. Hepcidin, therefore, not only affects serum iron concentration through its effects on enterocytes, but also causes sequestration of iron within macrophages and hepatocytes, preventing efflux of iron into plasma (**Fig. 2**).

The factors that influence the concentration of hepcidin (and, therefore, the extracellular movement of iron) include iron status and the amount of body iron stores, tissue hypoxia, erythropoiesis, and inflammation.[5] Plentiful iron and inflammation result in increased hepcidin transcription, whereas anemia, hypoxia, and iron deficiency suppress its expression. An excellent review of hepcidin has recently been published.[5]

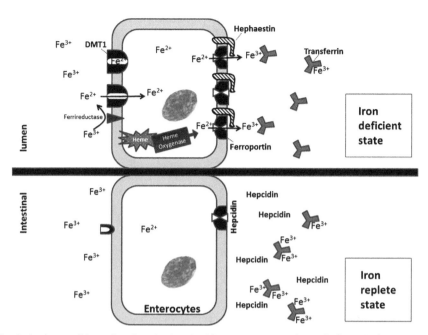

Fig. 1. In the small intestine, iron is absorbed into enterocytes through the apical transmembrane transporter, DMT-1 (*top*). Ferric iron is reduced to the ferrous state before transport. Iron is transported from the cell into circulation through a different transmembrane protein on the basolateral membrane of the enterocyte, called ferroportin. Immediately, ferrous iron is reoxidized to the ferric state by hephaestin, a multicopper feroxidase, and then bound to transferrin. In the presence of hepcidin, degradation and decreased expression of DMT-1 and ferroportin result in decreased ability of iron to enter the enterocyte and systemic circulation (*bottom*). Modifying the amount of iron absorbed by enterocytes is the primary mechanism for regulation of body iron content because no excretory pathways are known.

Understanding the homeostatic regulation of iron is important to understand the pathogenesis of diseases associated with iron metabolism and the limitations on different assays of iron status.

ASSAYS USED IN THE ASSESSMENT OF IRON STATUS

Assays to directly assess iron status include the measurement of serum iron concentration, ferritin concentration, and transferrin.

Serum Iron Concentration

In general, serum iron concentration is not an accurate indication of whole body iron status because it represents such a small fraction of total body iron (<0.1%) and is influenced by numerous other factors. This transport component of iron can increase with hemolysis, iron supplementation, recent blood transfusions, a decrease in erythropoietic uptake during hypoplastic or aplastic anemia, exogeneous administration of corticosteroids, and liver disease.[3] In addition to iron deficiency, serum iron concentration can decrease with inflammation, hypoproteinemia, hypothyroidism, and renal disease.

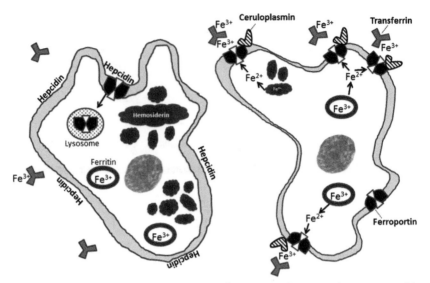

Fig. 2. The effect of hepcidin on iron transport from macrophages. In the presence of hepcidin (*left*) ferroportin is internalized and degraded by lysosomes, resulting in the sequestration of stored iron within the cell. At low concentrations of hepcidin, ferroportin is present in the cell membrane, allowing the exportation of iron (*right*). Immediately after leaving the cell, ferrous iron is reoxidized to the ferric state by ceruloplasmin, a multicopper feroxidase, and then bound to transferrin.

Ferritin

Ferritin is considered to be a better indication of total body iron content and is accurate in health. Unfortunately, it is also an acute-phase reactant and therefore levels increase with inflammation. A serum ferritin concentration below the reference interval indicates iron deficiency. Not all cases of iron deficiency, however, have a low ferritin concentration, especially if inflammation is present. Serum ferritin concentrations above the reference interval may be associated with either iron overload or with inflammation. One should consider measuring the concentration of other acute phase proteins concurrently to help with the interpretation of ferritin concentration. The ferritin assay is an enzyme-linked immunosorbent assay that is species specific; it is offered commercially by the Kansas State Veterinary Diagnostic Laboratory.

Transferrin

Transferrin is indirectly measured and reported as total iron binding capacity (TIBC). Transferrin may increase in the face of iron deficiency but is often normal. Elevated levels have been associated with iron overload and dogs with chronic liver disease.[3] Transferrin is a negative-phase reactant, so changes associated with iron deficiency can potentially be masked by inflammation. Inflammation is typically associated with decreased or low normal transferrin concentrations.

Percent Saturation

The ratio of serum iron concentration to TIBC is reported as percent saturation (%sat), which is the percentage of the TIBC that is actually occupied by iron. Normal %sat is typically between 20% and 50%. Factors that affect serum iron concentration and

TIBC also affect %sat. A %sat less than 20% is suggestive of iron deficiency. Hemochromatosis patients typically have a %sat greater than 50%.

Tissue Iron Concentration

Tissue iron concentration can be subjectively or quantitatively determined by collecting tissue from the bone marrow, liver, or spleen for cytologic or histologic examination or it can be quantitatively determined by submitting tissue to a laboratory for measurement of iron, typically on a dry-weight basis. These techniques are more invasive and are therefore less commonly performed. Cytology and histology preparations can be stained with Prussian blue stain, which highlights iron that is in the form of hemosiderin. It must be remembered that cats normally do not contain hemosiderin in their bone marrow and therefore a lack of staining is not significant in this species.

Other Assays Not Yet Available in Veterinary Medicine

In people, measuring the soluble form of the transferrin receptor 1 (sTfR1) has been very helpful in differentiating iron deficiency anemia from anemia of chronic disease. sTfR1 increases with the increased iron demand of erythropoiesis and is not affected by inflammation. It is typically used in a ratio with log serum ferritin for analysis.[2] Unfortunately, the ability to make an assay for sTfR1 for veterinary species has been elusive.

Serum hepcidin has not replaced any of the other measures of iron status in people, but its measurement in blood and urine has helped the investigation of disease pathogenesis and its central role in iron regulation could be a target for treatment of anemia and iron-overload disorders in the future.[6] Along with the other measures of iron status, hepcidin may still prove to be useful in guiding therapeutic decisions. Although hepcidin and ferritin typically respond similarly to inflammation and iron availability, changes in hepcidin concentrations occur faster than those of ferritin. In addition, aberrant response patterns may occur if an abnormality in hepcidin concentration is the cause of a disorder.[5]

ASSESSMENT OF IRON STATUS IN DISEASES ASSOCIATED WITH IRON METABOLISM

Diseases associated with iron metabolism are associated with either excess or insufficient iron availability. This could be caused by alterations in either total iron body content or in the physiologic availability of iron despite total iron body content.

Iron Deficiency

Causation

Lack of adequate body iron content (iron depletion) is uncommon, especially in cats, but can be seen in young, nursing animals that deplete their body iron stores as they grow because of the low iron content of milk.[3] Typically, the only way an adult animal on a commercial diet becomes iron depleted is because of chronic blood loss. This is most often associated with gastrointestinal bleeding (eg, bleeding tumors, such as leiomyoma, leiomyosarcoma, and carcinoma; or gastric ulceration, often from ulcerogenic drugs including corticosteroids and nonsteroidal anti-inflammatory drugs). Ectoparasites (fleas) and endoparasites (hookworms, whipworms) can also cause iron deficiency, especially in puppies and kittens. The urinary tract is another possible location for occult blood loss. Rarely, coagulopathies may lead to chronic blood loss from these sites. When iron becomes depleted, less is available for erythropoiesis, eventually resulting in anemia.

Iron assays

Expected findings associated with iron deficiency include decreased serum iron concentration, decreased ferritin concentration, normal or possibly elevated TIBC, and low %sat (**Table 1**). Results of assays for iron status must be interpreted with a patient's history, clinical findings, and other laboratory results given the potential confounding factors that can influence these values. Serum iron is often low in animals without iron deficiency, especially when inflammation is present. Ferritin concentration may be within normal limits in the face of iron deficiency if an inflammatory process is present.

Hematology

Iron deficiency anemia is often not recognized until a complete blood count reveals microcytosis or hypochromasia (**Table 2**). As a note, red blood cells from kittens and puppies are normally macrocytic or normocytic, not microcytic, at birth. Given the long half-life of erythrocytes, it takes weeks to months to accumulate a sufficient number of microcytes to shift the average erythrocyte size (mean corpuscular volume [MCV]) below the normal reference interval.[3] Red cell distribution width (RDW) is often increased because of the combination of microcytic and normocytic erythrocytes in circulation. Mean cell hemoglobin concentration (MCHC) may be normal or decreased. The overall amount of hemoglobin an erythrocyte contains may be decreased, but its concentration may be within normal limits given the cell's smaller size.

The evaluation of histograms or scattergrams from hematology analyzers can also be useful in providing evidence of iron deficiency, possibly detecting a shift toward microcytosis before the MCV becomes abnormal. Two instrument printouts demonstrating this shift are shown in **Fig. 3**.

Blood film review may also detect erythrocyte morphology that has been associated with iron deficiency anemia. Hypochromasia is caused by decreased hemoglobin concentration and is recognized when an erythrocyte contains a thin, pale red rim around an enlarged area of central pallor (**Fig. 4**). Be careful not to misinterpret "punched out" cells as hypochromic; these cells have had their hemoglobin pushed peripherally,

Table 1
Expected results in disorders of iron metabolism

Disorder	Serum Iron	TIBC	%sat	Ferritin	Bone Marrow Iron	MCV	MCHC	Hepcidin
Iron deficiency anemia	Low	N/high	Low	Low	Low	Low	N/low	Low
Anemia of chronic disease	Low	N/low	N/low	N/high	High	N	N	High
Acute inflammation	Low	N/low	N/low	N/high	N	N	N	High
Hemolytic anemia	High	N/low	High	High	N	N/high	N/low	Low
Portosystemic shunt	Low	N/low	N/low	N/high	N	Low	Low	?
Acute iron poisoning	High	N	High	N	N	N	N	High
Hemochromatosis	High	Low	High	High	High	N	N	High

Abbreviations: MCHC, mean cell hemoglobin concentration; MCV, mean corpuscular volume; N, normal (within reference interval); TIBC, total iron binding capacity; ?, unknown.

Table 2
Erythrogram from an 8-week-old Bernese mountain dog that presented with respiratory distress and anorexia[a]

Hemogram	Patient		Reference Interval
PCV	23	Low	40%–55%
RDW	18.6	High	12–15
MCV	50	Low	62–73 fl
MCHC	25	Low	33–36 g/dL
Reticulocytes	234,500	High	0–60,000/ul
CH_{retic}	15.8	Low	22.3–27.9 pg
MCV_{retic}	61	Low	77.8–100.2 fl

Hemopathology consists of hypochromasia, polychromasia, keratocytes, and schistocytes (see **Fig. 4**).

Abbreviations: MCHC, mean cell hemoglobin concentration; MCV, mean corpuscular volume; PCV, packed cell volume; RDW, red cell distribution width.

[a] The abnormalities present indicate iron deficiency anemia.

creating a larger central pallor, but with a thick, dark red rim of hemoglobin. Poikilocytosis has also been associated with iron deficiency anemia, especially keratocytes and schistocytes in dogs (see **Fig. 4**).

Reticulocyte indices

Evaluation of reticulocyte indices is known to be useful in detection of iron deficiency in people and may provide earlier recognition of iron deficiency anemia in dogs and cats. Because reticulocytes have a short life span in circulation of only approximately 2 days (compared with the life span of erythrocytes of 70 days [cats] or 120 days [dogs]), their hemoglobin content better reflects the recent functional availability of iron for erythropoiesis.[7,8] These indices are determined by the larger hematology analyzers used at reference laboratories and have shown likely value in veterinary medicine.[9–11] The hemoglobin content of reticulocytes (CH_{retic}) and average size of reticulocytes (MCV_{retic}) were associated with other indications of iron deficiency in these studies. In people, CH_{retic} seems to be the most sensitive indicator of iron deficiency.[7] Using receiver operating characteristic curve analysis, Prins and colleagues[11] found cut-off points (1.22 fmol in dogs and 0.88 fmol in cats) at which CH_{retic} was 95.2% and 93.8% sensitive and 90.5% and 76.9% specific for iron deficiency in dogs and cats, respectively. Specificity of low MCV_{retic} and CH_{retic} for iron deficiency has not been fully evaluated but observations by the author suggest that, not surprisingly, inflammatory processes can also result in decreased reticulocyte indices. Although more studies are needed to assess the use of CH_{retic} and MCV_{retic} in cats and dogs, their ability to reflect "real-time" iron availability is likely valuable and, when available in a complete blood count panel, CH_{retic} and MCV_{retic} should be monitored for possible iron-deficient states in veterinary patients (see **Table 2**).

Iron-refractory iron deficiency

Iron deficiency that is refractory to iron supplementation has been reported in humans with genetic defects in hepcidin or ferroportin. There was a recent mention of an unpublished case of a cocker spaniel with iron-refractory iron deficiency.[12] This case involved a defect in a regulatory protein (*Tmprss6*) that normally responds to iron deficiency by downregulating hepcidin.

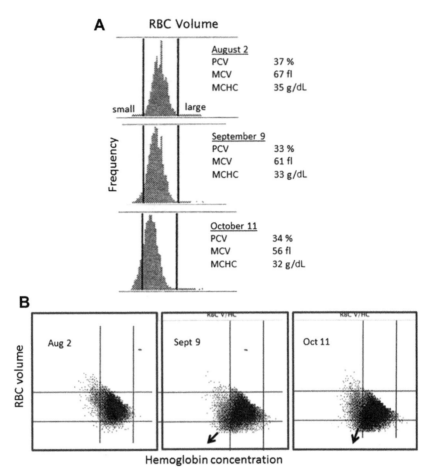

Fig. 3. Print-outs from an Advia 120 hematology analyzer showing the frequency histograms (*A*) and volume/HC scattergrams (*B*) for erythrocytes from the blood of a dog that developed iron deficiency. Samples were drawn approximately 1 month apart; values for packed cell volume (PCV), mean corpuscular volume (MCV), and mean cell hemoglobin concentration (MCHC) on each date are shown in (*A*). In (*A*), the *dark vertical lines* depict the lower and upper limits of normal erythrocyte size. As the dog becomes iron deficient, the histogram shifts to the left, indicating the presence of smaller erythrocytes. In (*B*), the *vertical lines* depict the lower and upper limits of normal hemoglobin concentration and the *horizontal lines* depict normal erythrocyte volume. As cells become smaller and contain less hemoglobin, the erythrocyte population shifts down and to the left, respectively. RBC, red blood cell.

Anemia of Inflammation (Anemia of Chronic Disease)

Causation

Lack of available iron despite adequate body stores is commonly associated with inflammation. This has been associated with the hepcidin hormone, which is increased by inflammatory cytokines. It is thought to be a protective mechanism by denying essential nutrients to infectious organisms. The increase in hepcidin causes degradation of ferroportin, which results in poor absorption of enteric iron and sequestration of stored iron within macrophages, which lead to low circulating iron concentrations (see

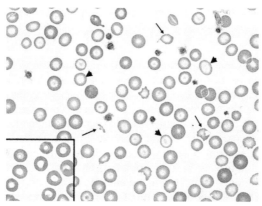

Fig. 4. Blood film from an 8-week-old Bernese mountain dog that presented with respiratory distress (probable distemper), anorexia, and diarrhea. The hemogram is indicative of iron deficiency; microcytosis is present (see **Table 2**). Hypochromasia is evident (*arrowheads*) and poikilocytosis is present, including keratocytes and schistocytes (*arrows*). The inset is blood from a dog that is not iron deficient and has "punched out" erythrocytes rather than hypochromatic cells. Note the thick, dark rim of hemoglobin with a crisp line surrounding the pale central area where hemoglobin has been pushed peripherally rather than decreased in content. The iron deficiency anemia was likely multifactorial, including poor stores caused by the dog's young age, decreased intake, and decreased gastrointestinal absorption or gastrointestinal hemorrhage caused by concurrent gastrointestinal disease.

Fig. 2, left). This gives rise to functional iron deficiency and contributes to the development of anemia.

Iron assays

Whether acute or chronic, inflammation results in low serum iron concentrations (see **Table 2**). In addition, as acute-phase proteins, transferrin decreases and ferritin increases with inflammation. Therefore, differentiating anemia of inflammation and iron deficiency anemia is often challenging because inflammation masks some of the changes typically seen with iron deficiency.

Classically, anemia of inflammation is characterized by increased iron stores, in contrast to iron deficiency anemia, which has decreased stores. Anemia of inflammation is therefore expected to have increased ferritin concentrations. TIBC and %sat are typically within normal limits or may be low.

Hemochromatosis

Causation

Iron overload can result in increased iron stores. Hemosiderosis is an increase in tissue iron stores without associated tissue damage, whereas hemochromatosis is defined as tissue damage and dysfunction from the deposition of hemosiderin in parenchymal cells.[13] Iron overload is not a common problem in small animals, but is possible with multiple blood transfusions or excess dietary iron. One case of hemochromatosis has been reported in a dog after several years of blood transfusions.[14] Hemochromatosis has also been recognized as a sequela to pyruvate kinase deficiency, likely caused by increased intestinal iron absorption associated with active hemolytic anemia.[15–17] There is a similar sequela in cats with chronic intermittent severe hemolytic anemia in which pathologic liver changes have been described.[18] Although dogs and cats seem relatively resistant to developing iron overload, the point at which too much iron causes a problem is unknown.

Iron assays

In people at risk for hemochromatosis, the standard way to monitor total iron body stores has been biopsy of the liver for iron quantification. Imaging modalities have more recently been developed to estimate liver iron concentration.[19] Ferritin has been used as a screening test for clinically significant iron overload in people, although ferritin concentrations do not correlate well with liver iron concentration and causes of elevated levels are nonspecific.[20] It has been determined, however, that cirrhosis of the liver generally does not occur in people with ferritin concentrations less than 1000 μg/L.[21] Unfortunately, ferritin concentrations have not been reported in small animal species with hemochromatosis and therefore no guidelines or cut-off values exist. It is recommended that %sat be taken into account when interpreting ferritin concentrations because %sat should also be elevated with hemochromatosis.[22] Expected abnormalities associated with hemochromatosis are shown in **Table 1**.

Portosystemic Shunt Microcytosis

Causation

The microcytosis associated with congenital or acquired portosystemic shunt is attributed to altered iron metabolism, although the exact mechanism is unknown.

Iron assays

In general, serum iron concentration is decreased, ferritin is normal to high, and TIBC is normal to low, similar to anemia of inflammation (see **Table 1**).

Copper Deficiency

Copper deficiency is associated with anemia in mammals. Typically, the anemia has been described as either microcytic or normocytic.

Causation

Copper deficiency is more of a problem in large animals, but there is one case report of suspected deficiency caused by long-term copper chelation in a dog.[23] In addition, puppies developed copper deficiency after being fed a copper-restricted diet for several months.[24] These dogs had a decrease in serum copper concentration, in ceruloplasmin oxidase activity, in hemoglobin concentration, and in PCV. Copper deficiency is thought to result in functional iron deficiency with or without iron depletion because of the importance of the copper-containing proteins hephaestin and ceruloplasmin for iron transport. Copper deficiency has been shown to result in decreased release of iron from enterocytes to plasma and from tissue iron stores.[3]

Iron assays

Presumably serum iron concentration is low as a result of copper deficiency in dogs and cats. It may be difficult to predict expected changes in iron stores because species variation exists.[3]

REFERENCES

1. Pantopoulos K, Porwal SK, Tartakoff A, et al. Mechanisms of mammalian iron homeostasis. Biochemistry 2012;51:5705–24.
2. Lawen A, Lane DJ. Mammalian iron homeostasis in health and disease: uptake, storage, transport, and molecular mechanisms of action. Antioxid Redox Signal 2013;18(18):2473–507.

3. Harvey JW. Iron metabolism and its disorders. In: Kaneko JJ, Harvey JW, Bruss ML, editors. Clinical biochemistry of domestic animals. 6th edition. Burlington (MA): Elsevier, Inc; 2008. p. 259–85.
4. Brasse-Lagnel C, Karim Z, Letteron P, et al. Intestinal DMT1 cotransporter is down-regulated by hepcidin via proteasome internalization and degradation. Gastroenterology 2011;140:1261–71.
5. Grimes CN, Giori L, Fry MM. Role of hepcidin in iron metabolism and potential clinical applications. Vet Clin North Am Small Anim Pract 2012;42:85–96.
6. Ganz T, Nemeth E. The hepcidin-ferroportin system as a therapeutic target in anemias and iron overload disorders. Hematology Am Soc Hematol Educ Program 2011;2011:538–42.
7. Urrechaga E, Borque L, Escanero JF. Erythrocyte and reticulocyte indices in the assessment of erythropoiesis activity and iron availability. Int J Lab Hematol 2013; 35:144–9.
8. Mast AE, Blinder MA, Dietzen DJ. Reticulocyte hemoglobin content. Am J Hematol 2008;83:307–10.
9. Fry MM, Kirk CA. Reticulocyte indices in a canine model of nutritional iron deficiency. Vet Clin Pathol 2006;35:172–81.
10. Steinberg JD, Olver CS. Hematologic and biochemical abnormalities indicating iron deficiency are associated with decreased reticulocyte hemoglobin content (CHr) and reticulocyte volume (rMCV) in dogs. Vet Clin Pathol 2005; 34:23–7.
11. Prins M, van Leeuwen MW, Teske E. Stability and reproducibility of ADVIA 120-measured red blood cell and platelet parameters in dogs, cats, and horses, and the use of reticulocyte haemoglobin content (CH(R)) in the diagnosis of iron deficiency. Tijdschr Diergeneeskd 2009;134:272–8.
12. Naigamwalla DZ, Webb JA, Giger U. Iron deficiency anemia. Can Vet J 2012;53: 250–6.
13. Dorland's illustrated medical dictionary. 27th edition. Philadelphia: W.B. Saunders Co; 1988. p. 747–51.
14. Sprague WS, Hackett TB, Johnson JS, et al. Hemochromatosis secondary to repeated blood transfusions in a dog. Vet Pathol 2003;40:334–7.
15. Gultekin GI, Raj K, Foureman P, et al. Erythrocytic pyruvate kinase mutations causing hemolytic anemia, osteosclerosis, and secondary hemochromatosis in dogs. J Vet Intern Med 2012;26:935–44.
16. Weiden PL, Hackman RC, Deeg HJ, et al. Long-term survival and reversal of iron overload after marrow transplantation in dogs with congenital hemolytic anemia. Blood 1981;57:66–70.
17. Zaucha JA, Yu C, Lothrop CD Jr, et al. Severe canine hereditary hemolytic anemia treated by nonmyeloablative marrow transplantation. Biol Blood Marrow Transplant 2001;7:14–24.
18. Kohn B, Goldschmidt MH, Hohenhaus AE, et al. Anemia, splenomegaly, and increased osmotic fragility of erythrocytes in Abyssinian and Somali cats. J Am Vet Med Assoc 2000;217:1483–91.
19. Joe E, Kim SH, Lee KB, et al. Feasibility and accuracy of dual-source dual-energy CT for noninvasive determination of hepatic iron accumulation. Radiology 2012; 262:126–35.
20. Majhail NS, Lazarus HM, Burns LJ. Iron overload in hematopoietic cell transplantation. Bone Marrow Transplant 2008;41:997–1003.
21. Waalen J, Felitti VJ, Gelbart T. Screening for hemochromatosis by measuring ferritin levels: a more effective approach. Blood 2008;111:3373–6.

22. Ferraro S, Mozzi R, Panteghini M. Revaluating serum ferritin as a marker of body iron stores in the traceability era. Clin Chem Lab Med 2012;50:1911–6.
23. Seguin MA, Bunch SE. Iatrogenic copper deficiency associated with long-term copper chelation for treatment of copper storage disease in a Bedlington terrier. J Am Vet Med Assoc 2001;218:1593–7.
24. Zentek J, Meyer H. Investigations on copper deficiency in growing dogs. J Nutr 1991;121:S83–4.

Making Sense of Lymphoma Diagnostics in Small Animal Patients

Mary Jo Burkhard, DVM, PhD[a],*, Dorothee Bienzle, DVM, PhD[b]

KEYWORDS

- Lymphoma • Cytology • Immunophenotyping • Flow cytometry
- PCR for clonal antigen receptor gene rearrangement (PARR)
- Immunohistochemistry/immunocytochemistry

KEY POINTS

- Cytologic assessment is diagnostic in most cases of diffuse large B-cell and diffuse lymphoblastic lymphoma in dogs.
- The cytologic diagnosis of lymphoma is more challenging in cats than in dogs.
- Although cytology is useful for staging lymphoma, histopathology is necessary for classification and grading.
- Immunophenotyping by flow cytometry allows evaluation of lymphocyte populations using a panel of antibodies, and serves as an adjunctive tool for both diagnosis and prognosis.
- Polymerase chain reaction (PCR) to detect clonal antigen receptor gene rearrangement (PARR) is a relatively new test in veterinary medicine that has strong potential for supporting the diagnosis of lymphoma. However, false-positive and false-negative results may confound the diagnosis, and PARR is less sensitive in cats than in dogs.
- Immunohistochemistry and immunocytochemistry should not be used as stand-alone diagnostic techniques, nor should an interpretation be based on a single antibody label.

INTRODUCTION

Lymphoma is the most common hemolymphatic malignancy in dogs and cats and, similar to lymphoma in people, is a heterogeneous disease with variable clinical signs and response to therapy.[1] Patient genetics, immunocompetence, location, and morphologic subtype all contribute to the heterogeneity of the disease and prognosis (**Box 1**).

Funding Sources: None.

Conflict of Interest: None.

[a] Department of Veterinary Biosciences, College of Veterinary Medicine, The Ohio State University, 1925 Coffey Road, Columbus, OH 43210, USA; [b] Department of Pathobiology, University of Guelph, 50 Stone Road East, Guelph, Ontario N1G 2W1, Canada

* Corresponding author.

E-mail address: burkhard.19@osu.edu

http://dx.doi.org/10.1016/j.cvsm.2013.07.004
0195-5616/13/$ – see front matter © 2013 Elsevier Inc. All rights reserved.
vetsmall.theclinics.com

> **Box 1**
> **Clinical evaluation of lymphoma**
>
> Several options are available for the diagnosis and characterization of lymphoma. This review helps in choosing the best test or tests for the patient.

Anatomically, lymphoma can be characterized as multicentric, alimentary, mediastinal, or extranodal. In dogs, multicentric lymphoma accounts for 80% to 85% of reported cases, and diffuse large B-cell lymphoma is the most common histomorphologic variant.[2] However, other types of B-cell lymphomas as well as T-cell lymphomas also are frequently diagnosed. The prognosis of lymphoma variants in dogs depends not only on the type of neoplastic lymphocyte but also on the location, characteristics of the cells, and the stage of disease. In cats, the diagnosis is more challenging because lymphoma more commonly affects extranodal sites, particularly the alimentary and upper respiratory tract.[3,4] Lymphoma affecting the gastrointestinal tract is common but particularly challenging to diagnose, owing to the relative inaccessibility for sampling and potential progression from lymphocytic inflammation to neoplasia. Other types of lymphoma in cats often contain a heterogeneous population of neoplastic lymphocytes plus reactive lymphocytes, plasma cells, and other inflammatory cells.

The diagnosis of lymphoma classically depended on morphologic characteristics identified by cytology and/or histopathology. In recent years, additional assays such as immunocytochemistry (ICC), immunohistochemistry (IHC), immunophenotyping by flow cytometry, and polymerase chain reaction (PCR) to detect clonal antigen receptor gene rearrangement (PARR) have been used to assist in the diagnosis of lymphoma and to classify lymphoma for prognostic purposes. Diagnostic tests are not perfectly sensitive or specific; therefore multiple assays are often used in conjunction or in sequence to enhance the accuracy of diagnosis and assist with prognosis. This article considers the utility and pitfalls of each diagnostic tool (**Box 2**).

CYTOLOGY

Cytologic examination of blood films and samples obtained by fine-needle aspiration (FNA) of tissues or fluids is commonly used in the diagnosis of lymphoma in dogs and cats. Advantages of cytology are that sample collection and slide examination are rapid and can be performed in-house with the minimal resources of glass slides, a Romanowsky stain such as Diff Quick or Wright Giemsa, and a high-quality microscope. Limitations of FNA in comparison with an incisional or excisional biopsy are that FNA does not allow assessment of tissue architecture, and material for additional studies (eg, IHC) is unavailable. Blood sampling and aspiration of superficial masses

> **Box 2**
> **Tools available for the diagnosis and characterization of lymphoma**
>
> Cytology
>
> Histopathology
>
> Immunocytochemistry and immunohistochemistry
>
> Phenotyping by flow cytometry
>
> Polymerase chain reaction to detect clonal antigen receptor gene rearrangement (PARR)

and peripheral lymph nodes are safe and simple techniques for most patients. FNA of internal organs such as the liver or spleen or abdominal or thoracic masses is more challenging, but is still commonly performed and often is diagnostically rewarding.

Lymphocyte Morphology

Lymphocyte cytomorphology is characterized by cell size, nuclear features, and cytoplasmic features (**Fig. 1**). It is important when using cytomorphology to examine only those cells that are both intact and adequately spread out on the slide.

Diagnosis of Lymphoma by Cytology

The cytologic diagnosis of lymphoma is the most straightforward if the tumor is diffuse and the entire node is replaced by a uniform population of large neoplastic lymphocytes; this is the most common type of lymphoma in dogs. Most diffuse lymphomas yield FNA that consist entirely or predominantly of large neoplastic cells. However, diffuse lymphomas composed of small or intermediate cells can be difficult to diagnose by cytology, because the cells more closely resemble benign lymphocytes. In contrast to diffuse lymphoma, follicular lymphoma, which is uncommon in dogs, may yield a heterogeneous population of benign and malignant cells of variable size and morphology, which is challenging to interpret by cytology.

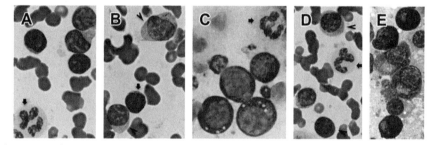

Fig. 1. Lymphocyte cytomorphology. Fine-needle aspiration (FNA) of lymph node from a dog (Wright Giemsa stain, original magnification ×1000). (*A*) One neutrophil (*lower left*) and 4 small lymphocytes: these lymphocytes are smaller than a neutrophil (*arrow*) and have a dense round nucleus that comprises the majority of the cell. Nucleoli are not seen. Cytoplasm is scant (sometimes only a very thin rim is visible). (*B*) One intermediate lymphocyte (*arrow*) and 2 small lymphocytes (*arrowheads*): intermediate lymphocytes are similar in size to neutrophils, have more abundant cytoplasm that is typically lightly basophilic, and may contain small azurophilic granules. Nuclei are often slightly eccentric within the cell and have less condensed chromatin. Indistinct nucleoli may be seen. (*C*) Four large lymphocytes and one neutrophil (*arrow*): large lymphocytes, also called lymphoblasts, are equal to or greater in size than neutrophils and contain round to oval nuclei with fine or stippled chromatin. Nucleoli are commonly seen. A rim of deeply basophilic cytoplasm surrounds the nucleus. Occasionally (especially in cats) the cytoplasm may contain punctate vacuoles, as shown in the 2 large lymphocytes at the bottom of this panel. (*D*) One reactive lymphocyte (*arrow*), 2 small lymphocytes (*arrowheads*), and 1 neutrophil: reactive lymphocytes are similar in morphology to small lymphocytes but slightly larger, and have more abundant, more deeply basophilic cytoplasm. (*E*) Several plasma cells: plasma cells are medium to large cells that contain small, round, eccentrically placed nuclei with coarsely clumped chromatin. Cytoplasm is abundant, deeply basophilic, and often contains a prominent perinuclear, clear zone that corresponds to the Golgi apparatus. The Golgi apparatus is clearly shown in the 2 plasma cells in the center.

Lymphoma in cats less commonly affects lymph nodes, and more commonly affects other tissues such as the intestine, nasal cavity, kidneys, liver, stomach, thymus, and spinal cord. In addition, those feline lymphomas that involve 1 or several peripheral lymph nodes often comprise a heterogeneous population of small and large lymphocytes as well as plasma cells and macrophages, making the diagnosis of lymphoma in cats by cytology more challenging than in dogs.

Hence, when lymph node FNA from either dogs or cats yield heterogeneous cell populations, reactive hyperplasia must be considered as a differential diagnosis (**Table 1**). Histopathology, in conjunction with ancillary diagnostic tests, should be used for additional characterization of the cell population.

Supporting Cytologic Features

There are several cytologic features (**Fig. 2**) that are more often associated with lymphoma than with benign lymphocyte proliferations, and these may be helpful in establishing a diagnosis. However, these features may be seen in both neoplastic and reactive populations and are not pathognomonic.

Staging of Lymphoma by Cytology

The World Health Organization staging scheme is based on the degree of metastasis, invasiveness, and presence of clinical signs. Cytology is useful in the staging of lymphoma by helping to identify the degree of metastasis (**Box 3**).

Limitations of Cytology

Diagnosis of small-cell and intermediate-cell lymphoma by cytology is challenging. Diagnosis in these cases may require additional supportive evidence such as generalized lymphadenopathy, identification of cells with similar cytologic features in multiple tissues, and lack of detection of infectious agents. Additional diagnostic tests such as histopathologic evaluation, flow-cytometric analysis, or PARR may be required for diagnosis.

Another cytologic diagnostic challenge is differentiating early lymphoma and reactive hyperplasia. In both processes, the percentage of lymphoblasts (large lymphocytes) will be increased within an overall heterogeneous population of lymphocytes. In these cases, examination by flow cytometry may also reveal a heterogeneous lymphocyte population, and therefore may be less specific than histopathology or PARR. Many lymphomas in cats are composed of such heterogeneous cell populations, and are therefore challenging to diagnose by cytology.

Sample Requirements

Sample collection and processing for FNA cytology of lymphoid tissue is relatively straightforward, and has been described in numerous texts and continuing education

Table 1 Differentiating lymphoma and reactive hyperplasia	
Lymphoma	**Hyperplasia**
≥50%, often >80/90% of cells are composed of homogeneous lymphoblasts or atypical lymphocytes	<50%, usually <20% lymphoblasts A heterogeneous lymphoid population that includes small lymphocytes, intermediate lymphocytes, and lymphoblasts. Plasma cells and other inflammatory cells are usually also present
Plasma cells and other inflammatory cells are rare	

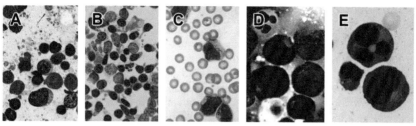

Fig. 2. Common cytologic features of lymphoma. FNA of enlarged lymph nodes from dogs with lymphoma. (*A*) Cytoplasmic fragments ("lymphoglandular bodies") are small, round, homogeneous, basophilic structures around and between cells. The presence of such fragments in cytologic preparations of lymphoid tissue is often associated with increased numbers of lymphoblasts resulting from neoplasia or hyperplasia (Wright Giemsa stain, original magnification ×1000). (*B*) Cytoplasmic pseudopodia ("uropods") may be present in some neoplastic T cells, but pseudopodia also may be present in activated T cells associated with reactive lymphoid hyperplasia (Wright Giemsa stain, original magnification ×200). (*C*) Cytoplasmic granulation is often a feature of CD8$^+$ T cells (cytotoxic T cells or CTLs) and natural killer (NK) cells. An increased proportion of granulated lymphocytes is commonly seen in rickettsial infections as well as in T-cell chronic lymphocytic leukemia (CLL) of dogs (Wright Giemsa stain, original magnification ×1000). (*D*) The Golgi apparatus is an eccentric, perinuclear clear zone often suggested as a feature of B cells and plasma cells, both reactive and neoplastic. However, the Golgi apparatus is an organelle found in most cells, including T cells and myeloid cells (Wright Giemsa stain, original magnification ×1000). (*E*) Irregular nuclear shapes such as cerebriform and flower-shaped nuclei often are present with T-cell diseases such as Sézary syndrome (a type of cutaneous lymphoma) and epitheliotropic lymphoma (a type of lymphoma that preferentially targets the cutaneous or gastrointestinal epithelium). In cats and dogs with CLL, more subtle nuclear irregularities such as small indentations and nuclear cleaves are commonly noted, and tend to be more obvious in formalin-fixed tissues. However, irregular nuclear morphology has also been described in B-cell lymphoma and leukemia (Wright Giemsa stain, original magnification ×1000).

seminars. Accurate interpretation, however, requires a representative and cellular sample of the lesion, and well-prepared and stained slides with adequate numbers of intact, spread-out, and well-stained cells for cytologic evaluation. Interpretation should always be made in the context of the signalment, history, clinical signs, and any additional diagnostic data from the patient. Samples that do not have a homogeneous population of large lymphocytes, or contain lymphocytes with cytologic atypia, should be evaluated by additional diagnostic methods.

Box 3
World Health Organization staging criteria for canine lymphoma

Stage I: Disease restricted to a single lymph node

Stage II: Regional lymphadenopathy (restricted to one side of diaphragm)

Stage III: Generalized lymphadenopathy

Stage IV: Hepatosplenomegaly (with or without lymphadenopathy)

Stage V: Bone marrow, central nervous system, or involvement of other extranodal sites

    Substage a: no clinical signs

    Substage b: clinical signs of illness

HISTOPATHOLOGY
Overview

Although both cytology and histopathology may be adequate for the diagnosis of lymphoma, histologic examination provides additional information about tissue architecture, cell distribution, and mitotic figures, and allows assessment of certain nuclear features important in the classification of lymphoma. Classification into morphologic subtypes allows comparison with published data and can provide prognostic information. Availability of paraffin-embedded tissue also allows additional studies such as IHC to be performed, and may provide a source of DNA for PARR. Histologic classification criteria include tissue involvement, the pattern of distribution of neoplastic cells within the tissue, neoplastic cell type, nuclear size, nuclear shape (cleaved vs noncleaved), presence of nucleoli, frequency of mitotic figures, presence and location of nonneoplastic cell types, and expression of surface markers (**Table 2**).[1,2]

Sample Requirements

The majority of dogs with lymphoma present with lymphadenopathy associated with diffuse effacement of lymph node parenchyma by a homogeneous population of large lymphocytes. In these cases, fine-needle biopsy typically yields sufficient numbers of cells for diagnosis. However, in the dogs with small-cell lymphoma or follicular lymphoma, and for many cats with lymphoma, excisional or Tru-Cut biopsy samples often are necessary for a definitive diagnosis. Biopsies should be placed in formalin for adequate fixation, and submitted to a veterinary diagnostic laboratory for processing and interpretation.

IMMUNOPHENOTYPING BY FLOW CYTOMETRY
Overview

One of the goals of immunophenotyping by flow-cytometric analysis is to define the types of lymphocyte in fluid samples by light-scatter characteristics and expression of phenotypic markers, thereby providing a more objective characterization of lymphocyte populations. Lymphocyte phenotyping by flow-cytometric analysis has become a relatively widely available assay to aid in the classification of benign and neoplastic lymphocytes, and in the differentiation of hematopoietic cell populations, in small animal patients.[5,6]

Flow-Cytometric Panels

Neoplastic lymphocytes often fail to express the same phenotype as their nonneoplastic counterparts, and may express antigens inappropriate for their level of differentiation. Neoplastic lymphocytes may also upregulate additional markers not typically expressed on nonneoplastic cells. Therefore, it is recommended that a panel of antibodies be used to characterize the neoplastic cell population. In both dogs and cats, several well-characterized antibodies are available for evaluation of lymphoid populations, with fewer antibodies available for examination of histiocytic, granulocytic, monocytic, erythroid, and megakaryocytic cells (**Table 3**).

Certain phenotypes, patterns of expression, or specific markers have prognostic or diagnostic utility (**Table 4**).[7–10]

Sample Requirements

Blood and nonhemorrhagic fluid samples (cerebrospinal fluid, peritoneal fluid, pleural effusion fluid, and so forth) can be placed in ethylenediaminetetraacetic acid or serum tubes, respectively, and readily processed for flow cytometry. Solid tissue aspirates

Table 2
Classification of common canine lymphoma types

Category	Typical Location and Clinical Features	Histopathologic Pattern	Cell Features	Immunophenotypic Features
Diffuse large B-cell lymphoma, NOS	LN, often generalized	Diffuse	Large cells, round nuclei, central single nucleolus, high MR	CD1, CD20, CD21, CD79, MHC II; CD18^{low}
Marginal-zone lymphoma	Nodal, splenic white pulp, or extranodal mucosal origin	Follicular	Small to intermediate cells, low MR	CD20, CD21, CD79, MHC II; CD18^{intermed}
Follicular lymphoma	LN, single to multiple	Follicular	Variable cell size, low MR	CD20, CD79
Mantle-cell lymphoma	Splenic white pulp	Follicular	Small cells, round to irregular nuclei, low MR	CD20, CD79
Peripheral T-cell lymphoma, NOS	LN, often generalized, hypercalcemia possible	Diffuse	Variable cell morphology and MR	CD3, TCRαβ, CD4 or CD8 single or dual positive or negative, CD18^{high}
Small T-cell lymphoma	LN	Paracortical, progressing to diffuse	Small to intermediate cells with variable morphology	CD3
Primary cutaneous epitheliotropic lymphoma	Mucocutaneous sites	Epitheliotropic, may form plaques	Variable cell size and morphology	CD3, CD8, TCRαβ or TCRγδ
Hepatosplenic lymphoma	Splenic red pulp origin with diffuse spread to liver and marrow. Cytopenia common	Diffuse	Cytoplasmic granulation and high MR	CD3, CD8, CD11d, CD18, TCRγδ

Abbreviations: LN, lymph node; MR, mitotic rate; NOS, not otherwise specific.

Table 3
Cell-surface markers commonly detected by flow cytometry on canine and feline leukocytes

Marker	Primary Cell Type	Additional Notes
CD1	Dendritic cells	Subpopulations of B cells and monocytes also express CD1 molecules
CD3	T cells	
CD4	Helper T cells	Canine neutrophils constitutively express CD4. Monocytes, macrophages, and dendritic cells can upregulate CD4
CD4/CD8 dual positive	Thymocytes	
CD5	T cells	In some species, CD5 is also expressed on the B-1 subset of B cells
CD8	Cytotoxic T cells	Also on a subset of natural killer cells
CD14	Monocytes	Also on some types of macrophages
CD18	All leukocytes	Greater expression intensity on granulocytes and monocytes than on lymphocytes; variable expression on different types of lymphocytes
CD21, CD22	Mature B cells	Absent on plasma cells
CD34	Hematopoietic stem cells	Present on cells in some cases of acute leukemia of either lymphoid or myeloid origin
CD45	All hematopoietic cells (except erythroid cells)	CD45 intensity varies among cell types and can be used to help differentiate cells. CD45 may be absent or reduced on neoplastic lymphocytes
CD79a or CD79b	B cells of all stages	Intracellular antigen; detection requires a directly conjugated antibody and an additional permeabilization step to allow the antibody to enter the cell. Expression is absent in plasma cells
MHC II	Antigen-presenting cells, most canine and feline lymphocytes	
Surface IgM	Immature B cells	
Light-chain expression	Antibody-producing B cells, plasma cells	λ-Light-chain expression far outweighs κ-chain expression in dogs and cats in both benign and neoplastic disorders

Abbreviation: IgM, immunoglobulin M.

also can be analyzed as long as they are processed to yield cell suspensions. FNA samples from solid tissue (eg, lymph node) should be placed into a tube containing buffered saline and a small amount of serum (bovine serum is often used) to help stabilize the cells before analysis. As there is some variation between laboratories, the collaborating laboratory should be contacted to confirm the specific submission guidelines. In general, at least 2 million cells are needed to apply a complete immunophenotyping panel for flow cytometry. Samples from different sites should not be mixed together. Samples should be shipped by express delivery, cold but not frozen,

Table 4
Flow-cytometric diagnostic and prognostic patterns

	Diagnostic Patterns	
Type of Neoplasm	**Morphologic Features**	**Common Phenotype**
Canine CLL: T-cell subtype	Small to intermediate lymphocytes often with granules	$CD3^+$ $CD5^+$ $CD8^+$
Canine CLL: B-cell subtype	Small lymphocytes	$CD21^+$ $CD79^+$, may have monoclonal gammopathy
Feline CLL	Small lymphocytes	$CD5^+$ $CD4^+$
Acute lymphoblastic leukemia	Large cells	Some are $CD45^+$ $CD34^+$
Diffuse large B-cell lymphoma	Large lymphocytes, effacement of node	$CD21^+$ $CD79^+$ $CD1^+$ $CD18^{low}$
Marginal-zone lymphoma	Small to intermediate lymphocytes	$CD21^+$ $CD79^+$ $CD1^-$, $CD18^{intermed}$
	Prognostic Patterns	
Type of Neoplasm	**Change**	**Suggested Prognostic Impact**
B-cell lymphoma	Loss of MHC II	Reduced survivability
Canine CLL	B-cell subtype	Reduced survivability compared with T-cell CLL
Canine CLL	Atypical subtype (null T cell, dual $CD4^+/CD8^+$, dual T/B lineage)	Markedly reduced survivability
ALL vs stage V lymphoma	CD34 expression	CD34 expression supports ALL rather than stage V lymphoma

Abbreviations: ALL, acute lymphoblastic leukemia; CLL, chronic lymphocytic leukemia; MHC, major histocompatibility complex.

to a laboratory that performs immunophenotyping by flow cytometry. A delay between sampling and processing can result in degradation of the cells and/or loss of marker expression or marker intensity. In general, 3 days at refrigeration temperature is the maximum period for retaining diagnostically useful samples.

An informal survey among veterinary laboratories in North America, Europe, and Asia determined that all laboratories used panels of antibodies for characterization of leukocytes. The antibody panels, fluorochromes, and instruments were variable, but similar markers were detected for classification of lymphocytes and other leukocytes. Laboratories also varied regarding the preferred anticoagulant for blood samples, the preferred additive for stabilizing cells, and the duration that samples were considered suitable for analysis after collection. Therefore, clinicians should contact individual laboratories regarding their protocols before submission of samples for flow cytometry.

PARR

Although neoplastic lymphocytes are clonal in origin, not all clonal populations of lymphocytes are neoplastic. Certain inflammatory and infectious diseases such as rickettsial infections can result in clonal lymphocyte expansions. There are no cell-surface markers that identify clonal T-cell populations in humans or veterinary species. In humans, expression of κ or λ light chain can identify clonal B-cell populations when there is uniform expression of one light chain. However, antibodies for detection of canine or feline light chains by flow cytometry are unavailable, and λ light-chain expression far outweighs κ-chain expression in dogs and cats in both benign and neoplastic disorders.[11] Therefore, the utility of light-chain expression for the diagnosis of clonal B-cell populations is limited for dogs and cats with lymphoma.

Identification of T-cell or B-cell clonality in dogs and cats requires detection of clonal receptor gene rearrangement. This detection is most typically done by PCR, and is referred to as PCR for antigen receptor gene rearrangement (PARR).[12–14] As part of their development, T cells undergo rearrangement of genes encoding the T-cell receptor (TCR), whereas B cells undergo rearrangement of genes encoding the immunoglobulin (Ig) receptor. The result is that nearly every lymphocyte has a slightly different TCR or Ig receptor. However, small stretches in the DNA coding for each receptor are similar in all lymphocytes, and allow use of primers that will amplify most receptors and yield PCR products that vary slightly in size and composition.[15] Therefore, PARR of benign lymphoid tissue detects a smear or ladder of PCR products representing the diversity of benign receptors (**Fig. 3**). Because neoplastic transformation of lymphocytes typically occurs after the cells have undergone receptor rearrangement, malignant daughter cells will have the same antigen receptor gene, which is detected on PCR as a single product and represents a monoclonal population (see **Fig. 3**). Occasionally biclonal or triclonal neoplastic populations may also be detected. Nonlymphoid neoplasms will not produce discrete PCR products, called amplicons, because gene segments for lymphocyte receptors are located too distantly from each other in nonlymphoid cells.

One of the strengths of PARR is the ability to detect a clonal population within a larger reactive process, such as might occur in early lymphoma arising amid a reactive population.

Caveats for PARR

PARR has potential to be very sensitive and specific; however, false-positive and false-negative results occur for a variety of reasons. PARR may detect lymphocytes with clonally rearranged receptor DNA, but lymphoid clonality does not always correspond to neoplasia. Oligoclonal or monoclonal expansions of reactive lymphocytes with identical gene rearrangements can be seen in chronic infections, such as with the causative agents of ehrlichiosis, anaplasmosis, Rocky Mountain spotted fever, or Lyme disease. Factors inherent to PCR amplification of DNA templates with very small sequence variation may also yield nonspecific amplicons. False-negative results can occur when the sample does not contain sufficient numbers of cells with clonal antigen receptor genes to create a visible discrete amplicon in PCR amplification, or when primers do not anneal to the particular clonal receptor genes.

In addition, PARR is substantially less sensitive in cats than it is in dogs. In dogs, the assay detects 75% to 80% of confirmed cases of lymphoma or lymphocytic leukemia. In cats, currently available protocols detect 60% to 65% of neoplastic lymphocyte samples.[14] Although a positive result is diagnostically supportive for lymphoma, a negative result in either species does not rule out lymphoma.

Sample Requirements

DNA for PCR can be harvested from blood, fluid samples, air-dried (stained or unstained) cytology slides, and histology slides or sections. The minimum number of cells needed for the assay is approximately 50,000. A unique feature of this diagnostic modality is that slides can be examined cytologically and then submitted for cell removal, DNA extraction, and PCR analysis. This process facilitates the clinical diagnosis because it ensures that the cells in question are present on the slide in adequate

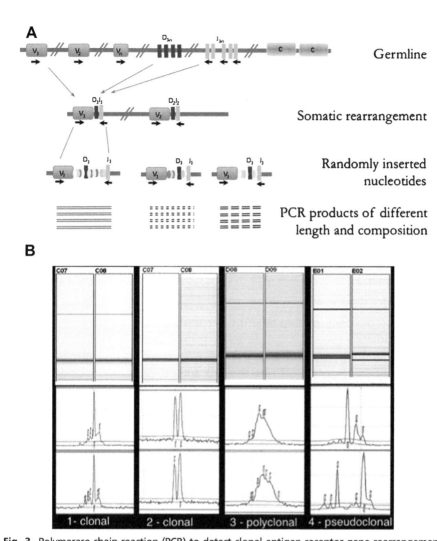

Fig. 3. Polymerase chain reaction (PCR) to detect clonal antigen receptor gene rearrangement (PARR). (*A*) Lymphocyte antigen receptor gene rearrangement. In **germline** configuration, different gene segments (V = variable; D = diversity; J = joining; C = constant) of lymphocyte antigen receptors are located distant from each other, and yield no PCR product with primers (*black arrows*) to conserved regions in different segments. During **somatic recombination** different V, D, and J regions are brought into proximity. Additional diversity is generated by **random insertion of nucleotides** (*yellow-orange*) at the joining regions. Amplification with primers to conserved regions in the V and J segment yields a **range of PCR products**. (*B*) High-resolution electrophoresis detects size variability among amplicons. Heteroduplex analysis (not shown) involves melting and reannealing of double-stranded amplicons before electrophoresis to detect sequence variability in addition to size variability. Capillary electrophoresis (*top panel*) and BioCalculator (Qiagen, Valencia, CA, USA) software analysis plots (*bottom panel*) of antigen receptor gene rearrangement PCR on DNA extracted from 4 different dogs (*1–4*). Major peaks reflect homogeneous amplicons, minor small peaks at the baseline reflect background DNA, and markers are size indicators. Dog 1 is a 7-year-old mixed breed with peripheral T-cell lymphoma, not otherwise specified (PTCL-NOS), and PARR shows a single sharp peak from a homogeneous amplicon, which confirmed clonal lymphocyte gene receptors. Dog 2 is a 1.5-year-old Dachshund with diffuse large B-cell lymphoma (DLBCL), also confirmed by detection of 2 clonal amplicons with this assay. The PCR result from dog 3 shows a range of different-sized amplicons indicating a polyclonal (reactive) result. The PCR result from dog 4 shows amplicons consisting of multiple peaks that differ in size in replicate assays, which is termed pseudoclonal, because primers likely annealed nonspecifically and the result does not reflect a clonal population. ([*B*] *Courtesy of* Dr Bill Vernau, University of California at Davis, Davis, CA.)

numbers. In addition, samples can be archived while owners consider additional diagnostic or therapeutic decisions. Fluid and blood samples should be shipped by express delivery, cold but not frozen, to a laboratory that performs PARR. Glass slides can be shipped by a variety of methods, but should be placed in a shipping container.

PARR is a relatively new test in veterinary medicine, and fewer than 10 veterinary laboratories throughout the world currently perform PARR for diagnostic purposes. There is much variation in the number and nature of primers used by different laboratories, whether amplifications are performed in single, duplicate, or quadruplicate format, whether the analysis of amplicons involves heating and reannealing of double-stranded products to increase specificity, and other test aspects. Some laboratories interpret PARR results only in conjunction with review of other laboratory data such as cytologic or histologic slides, IHC, flow cytometry, and other data, whereas other laboratories interpret PARR results as a stand-alone-test. For these reasons, until PARR becomes a more standardized test across laboratories it is best for clinicians to contact individual laboratories regarding the types of sample accepted and the nature of test interpretation.

IMMUNOHISTOCHEMISTRY AND IMMUNOCYTOCHEMISTRY
Diagnostic Utility

IHC and ICC are used to demonstrate cell antigens in tissue sections (IHC) or cytology preparations (ICC) (**Fig. 4**). In both IHC and ICC, antibodies are used to bind to specific antigens, and the binding of these antibodies is detected by a histochemical reaction

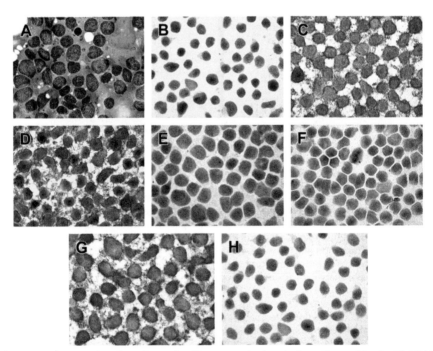

Fig. 4. Immunocytochemistry. Example of immunocytochemical results consistent with CD4 T-cell ($\alpha\beta$ TCR) lymphoma from a 5-year-old Boxer with generalized lymphadenopathy. All images were photographed at 75× and labeled as follows: (A) Wright stain; (B) negative control; (C) CD3; (D) CD4; (E) CD8α; (F) CD79a; (G) TCR$\alpha\beta$; (H). TCR$\gamma\delta$. (*Courtesy of* Dr Bill Vernau, University of California at Davis, Davis, CA.)

to produce a color change in positive cells. As in a cytology slide or histologic section, the location of this color change in cells can then be precisely determined by microscopy. Antibodies are often species specific or species limited; therefore, not all antibodies are equally suitable for dog and cat tissues.

Key Considerations for Clinical Application

When considering IHC and ICC results, diagnostic and prognostic interpretation is performed in a manner similar to that for antibody detection by flow cytometry.[16,17] In fact, some of the same antibodies (albeit with different detection labels) may be used for both flow cytometry and IHC/ICC. However, there is more often the opportunity to request a single antibody in IHC/ICC, whereas a diagnostic panel is typically performed for flow-cytometric analysis. Moreover, tissues fixed in formalin have altered expression of antigens, and are no longer suitable for evaluation with the range of antibodies that bind to unfixed cells. Given the variability of neoplastic cells to upregulate or downregulate gene expression, a single antibody label should not be considered sufficient for diagnosis. For example, confirmation of a T-cell lymphoma by CD3 expression should, at minimum, also include exclusion of B-cell type by the lack of labeling for CD79 or another B-cell antigen. IHC or ICC should never be considered stand-alone diagnostic techniques because interpretation requires expert evaluation within the context of each tumor type.[16]

In addition to classification of lymphoma type, immunostaining can be very useful for the differentiation of lymphoma from other neoplasms composed of nonlymphoid round cells. Nasal carcinomas, particularly in cats, may be morphologically similar to some lymphomas, and IHC for CD3, CD79, and cytokeratin assists in their distinction.[17]

Sample Requirements

IHC is typically performed on formalin-fixed and paraffin-embedded samples. Proper fixation is critical for consistent antigen detection, and either underfixation or overfixation may alter the ability to detect antigens. Before IHC, sections are deparaffinized and subjected to antigen retrieval. Different methods for antigen retrieval may be applied for different antibodies.

ICC may be performed on air-dried unstained, air-dried previously stained, or wet-fixed slides. Use of air-dried previously stained slides, however, is least preferred because of the potential for loss of cells, disruption of cells and cell membranes, or loss of signal detection. Cells on cytology slides progressively lose reactivity with antibodies during storage; therefore, it is best to analyze freshly prepared slides by ICC.

TUMOR BIOMARKERS

Tumor biomarkers are substances released from neoplastic cells into blood, urine, or other fluids that can be measured through specific assays. In human medicine, assessment of tumor biomarkers is increasingly performed to aid in establishing both the diagnosis and prognosis of lymphoma.

Thymidine kinase is an enzyme highly expressed by rapidly dividing cells. In both dogs and cats, serum thymidine kinase activity is increased in patients with lymphoma, and in dogs, activity was inversely associated with survival time.[18,19] However, the overall sensitivity for the test is low, owing to the lack of increased serum activity in a proportion of small animal patients with lymphoma. Therefore, as with any diagnostic test, serum thymidine kinase activity should be considered a supporting tool to be used in context with other diagnostic methods. The greatest value for serum thymidine kinase activity and other biomarkers may be for their roles in monitoring the response to treatment.

CASE STUDIES
Case 1

A 12-year-old female spayed domestic short-haired cat, presented for recheck of inflammatory bowel disease.

Numerical complete blood count results were within reference limits; however, the lymphocyte count was higher than normal (3.7 × 10⁹/L), and evaluation of the lymphocyte morphology revealed uniform cells with mild nuclear irregularities commonly seen in feline patients with chronic lymphocytic leukemia (CLL) (**Fig. 5**A). Flow cytometry (**Fig. 5**B) revealed that the lymphocyte population was composed of a heterogeneous population of T cells and B cells. However, the T cells had an abnormal phenotype and were primarily negative for both CD4 and CD8. In healthy cats, 30% to 50% of blood lymphocytes are CD4⁺ and 15% to 25% are CD8⁺. A blood sample evaluated by PARR identified a clonal T-cell receptor gene rearrangement.

Summary: Early CLL in a cat. Most feline CLL is CD4 T-cell in origin. However, null (CD4⁻ CD8⁻) as well as CD8 CLL also has been reported.

Case 2

An 8-year-old male neutered Golden Retriever with generalized massive lymph node enlargement and weight loss.

Lymph node aspirate and biopsy are shown in (**Fig. 6**A and B). The histopathologic classification was "diffuse large B-cell lymphoma of immunoblastic type."

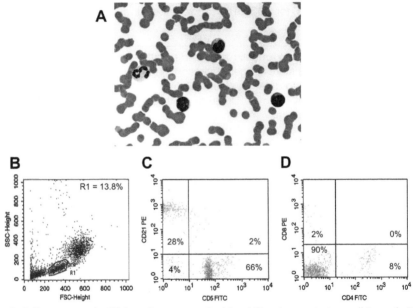

Fig. 5. Feline case study. (*A*) Lymphocytes on the blood film demonstrate small irregularities in the nuclear membrane including indentations and small nuclear cleaves (Wright stain, original magnification ×100). (*B*) Flow-cytometric analysis of blood leukocytes. The lymphocyte population (R1) was 13.8% of the total population and was gated for analysis. (*C*) Sixty-six percent of the lymphocytes were CD5⁺ T cells and 28% were CD21⁺ B cells. (*D*) The majority (90%) of lymphocytes were negative for both CD4 and CD8. Quadrant lines are set at the isotype control and the percentages of cells beyond background are listed in each quadrant.

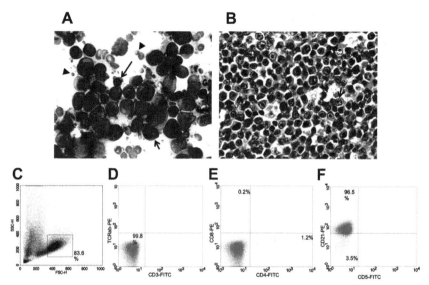

Fig. 6. Canine case study. (*A*) The cytology preparation from an FNA of an enlarged lymph node consists of numerous very large lymphocytes, many cytoplasmic fragments (*arrowheads*), occasional plasma cells (*short arrow*) and small lymphocytes (*long arrow*), and scattered red blood cells (Wright stain, original magnification ×100). (*B*) On histopathology, the lymph node architecture was replaced by a diffuse infiltrate of large lymphocytes with a single prominent central nucleolus (*arrow*) (hematoxylin-eosin stain, original magnification ×400). (*C*) Flow-cytometric evaluation of a lymph node aspirate showed a prominent population of cells with high forward and side scatter, and a few other cells with light-scatter properties of neutrophils, small lymphocytes, and red blood cells. Large gated cells lacked CD3 and TCRα/β expression (*D*) and contained a few CD4+ cells (likely neutrophils, *E*), and the majority expressed CD21 but not CD5 (*F*). These findings are consistent with diffuse large B-cell lymphoma.

Flow-cytometric analysis (**Fig. 6C–F**) was also consistent with a diffuse large B-cell lymphoma. The dog was treated with combination chemotherapy, achieved remission at 3 weeks, and remained in remission for 11 months.

SUMMARY

There is no single stand-alone assay for the diagnosis, characterization, and staging of lymphoma in small animal patients. In addition to cytology and histopathology, immunophenotyping by flow cytometry, PARR, and immunohistochemistry or immunocytochemistry all provide important diagnostic and prognostic information. However, for accurate diagnosis and staging the findings must be evaluated in concert with the clinical history, physical examination, and other ancillary data.

ACKNOWLEDGMENTS

Figs. 3B and 4 were graciously provided by Dr Bill Vernau, University of California at Davis. The following collaborators shared their protocols and provided input regarding preferred samples, standards for interpretation, and important controls for flow cytometric and PARR assays performed in their laboratories: Anne Avery (Fort Collins, Colorado); Mary Jo Burkhard (Columbus, Ohio); Stefano Comazzi (Milan,

Italy); Dorothee Bienzle (Guelph, Ontario); Jonathan Fogle, Mary Tompkins, Hiroyuki Mochizuki (Raleigh, North Carolina); Beverly Kidney (Saskatoon, Saskatchewan); Matti Kiupel (Lansing, Michigan); Casey LeBlanc (Knoxville, Tennessee); Jaime Modiano, Daisuke Ito (Minneapolis, Minnesota); Masahiko Sato, Hajime Tsujimoto (Tokyo, Japan); Tracy Stokol, Deanna Schaefer (Ithaca, New York); Masamine Takanosu (Asaka, Ohtawara, Japan); Bill Vernau, Peter Moore (Davis, California); and Melinda Wilkerson (Manhattan, Kansas).

REFERENCES

1. Bienzle D, Vernau W. The diagnostic assessment of canine lymphoma: implications for treatment. Clin Lab Med 2011;31:21–39. Available at: http://www.ncbi.nlm.nih.gov/pubmed/21295720. Accessed March 15, 2013.
2. Valli VE, San Myint M, Barthel A, et al. Classification of canine malignant lymphomas according to the World Health Organization criteria. Vet Pathol 2011;48:198–211. Available at: http://vet.sagepub.com/content/48/1/198. Accessed March 15, 2013.
3. Chino J, Fujino Y, Kobayashi T, et al. Cytomorphological and immunological classification of feline lymphomas: clinicopathological features of 76 cases. J Vet Med Sci 2013;75(6):701–7. Available at: https://www.jstage.jst.go.jp/article/jvms/advpub/0/advpub_12-0246/_pdf. Accessed March 15, 2013.
4. Little L, Patel R, Goldschmidt M. Nasal and nasopharyngeal lymphoma in cats: 50 cases (1989-2005). Vet Pathol 2007;44:885–92. Available at: http://vet.sagepub.com/content/44/6/885.full.pdf+html. Accessed March 15, 2013.
5. Sözmen M, Tasca S, Carli E, et al. Use of fine needle aspirates and flow cytometry for the diagnosis, classification, and immunophenotyping of canine lymphomas. J Vet Diagn Invest 2005;17:323–9. Available at: http://vdi.sagepub.com/content/17/4/323.long. Accessed March 15, 2013.
6. Wilkerson MJ, Dolce K, Koopman T, et al. Lineage differentiation of canine lymphoma/leukemias and aberrant expression of CD molecules. Vet Immunol Immunopathol 2005;106:179–96. Available at: http://www.sciencedirect.com/science/article/pii/S0165242705000681. Accessed March 15, 2013.
7. Williams MJ, Avery AC, Lana SE, et al. Canine lymphoproliferative disease characterized by lymphocytosis: immunophenotypic markers of prognosis. J Vet Intern Med 2008;22:596–601.http://onlinelibrary.wiley.com/store/10.1111/j.1939-1676.2008.0041.x/asset/j.1939-1676.2008.0041.x.pdf?v=1&t=hesqsixk&s=fea778825eef6f313b93d655433bb6f3381b6a6e. Accessed March 15, 2013.
8. Campbell MW, Hess PR, Williams LE. Chronic lymphocytic leukaemia in the cat: 18 cases (2000-2010). Vet Comp Oncol 2012. http://dx.doi.org/10.1111/j.1476-5829.2011.00315.x. Available at: http://www.ncbi.nlm.nih.gov/pubmed/22372648. Accessed March 15, 2013.
9. Comazzi S, Gelain ME, Martini V, et al. Immunophenotype predicts survival time in dogs with chronic lymphocytic leukemia. J Vet Intern Med 2011;25:100–6. Available at: http://onlinelibrary.wiley.com/store/10.1111/j.1939-1676.2010.0640.x/asset/j.1939-1676.2010.0640.x.pdf?v=1&t=hesqx3gu&s=43f36e809bfb6e49a5a92cbd14d320f7a42f3bf1. Accessed March 15, 2013.
10. Rao S, Lana S, Eickhoff J, et al. Class II Major histocompatibility complex expression and cell size independently predict survival in canine B-cell lymphoma. J Vet Intern Med 2011;25:1097–105. Available at: http://onlinelibrary.wiley.com/store/10.1111/j.1939-1676.2011.0767.x/asset/jvim767.pdf?v=1&t=hesqtx53&s=ea850c4b936160f27a4115195e5e86a12efa9f25. Accessed March 15, 2013.

11. Klotz FW, Gathings WE, Cooper MD. Development and distribution of B lineage cells in the domestic cat: analysis with monoclonal antibodies to cat mu-, gamma-, kappa-, and lambda-chains and heterologous anti-alpha antibodies. J Immunol 1985;134:95–100. Available at: http://www.ncbi.nlm.nih.gov/pubmed/3917286. Accessed March 15, 2013.

12. Vernau W, Moore PF. An immunophenotypic study of canine leukemias and preliminary assessment of clonality by polymerase chain reaction. Vet Immunol Immunopathol 1999;69:145–64. Available at: http://www.sciencedirect.com/science/article/pii/S0165242799000513. Accessed March 15, 2013.

13. Burnett RC, Vernau W, Modiano JF, et al. Diagnosis of canine lymphoid neoplasia using clonal rearrangements of antigen receptor genes. Vet Pathol 2003;40: 32–41. Available at: http://vet.sagepub.com/content/40/1/32.full.pdf+html. Accessed March 15, 2013.

14. Moore PF, Woo JC, Vernau W, et al. Characterization of feline T cell receptor gamma (TCRG) variable region genes for the molecular diagnosis of feline intestinal lymphoma. Vet Immunol Immunopathol 2005;106:167–78. Available at: http://www.sciencedirect.com/science/article/pii/S0165242705000632#. Accessed March 15, 2013.

15. Dongen JJ, Langerak AW, Bruggemann M, et al. Design and standardization of PCR primers and protocols for detection of clonal immunoglobulin and T-cell receptor gene recombinations in suspect lymphoproliferations: Report of the BIOMED-2 Concerted Action BMH4-CT98-3936. Leukemia 2003;17:2257–317. Available at: http://www.nature.com/leu/journal/v17/n12/full/2403202a.html. Accessed March 15, 2013.

16. Sato H, Fujino Y, Uchida K, et al. Comparison between immunohistochemistry and genetic clonality analysis for cellular lineage determination in feline lymphomas. J Vet Med Sci 2011;73:945–7. Available at: https://www.jstage.jst.go.jp/article/jvms/73/7/73_10-0528/_article. Accessed March 15, 2013.

17. Nagata K, Lamb M, Goldschmidt MH, et al. The usefulness of immunohistochemistry to differentiate between nasal carcinoma and lymphoma in cats: 140 cases (1986-2000). Vet Comp Oncol 2012. http://dx.doi.org/10.1111/j.1476-5829.2012.00330.x. Available at: http://www.ncbi.nlm.nih.gov/pubmed/22520498. Accessed March 15, 2013.

18. Von Euler H, Einarsson R, Olsson U, et al. Serum thymidine kinase activity in dogs with malignant lymphoma: a potent marker for prognosis and monitoring the disease. J Vet Intern Med 2004;18:696–702. Available at: http://www.ncbi.nlm.nih.gov/pubmed/15515587. Accessed March 15, 2013.

19. Taylor SS, Dodkin S, Papasouliotis K, et al. Serum thymidine kinase activity in clinically healthy and diseased cats: a potential biomarker for lymphoma. J Feline Med Surg 2013;15:142–7. Available at: http://jfm.sagepub.com/content/15/2/142.long. Accessed March 15, 2013.

Current Diagnostic Trends in Coagulation Disorders Among Dogs and Cats

Marjory B. Brooks, DVM*, James L. Catalfamo, MS, PhD

KEYWORDS

- Coagulopathy • Fibrinolysis • Hemorrhagic disorders • Hemostasis
- Platelet aggregometry • Platelet function • Thrombin(IIa) generation
- Thrombelastography

KEY POINTS

- Include hemostatic defects in the initial differential diagnosis of patients with signs of hemorrhage.
- Collect appropriate samples for platelet count and coagulation panel early in the diagnostic workup. Remember that sample quality is critical for valid results.
- Use results of initial screening tests and patient response to guide further testing.
- New techniques such as flow cytometry, thrombin-generation assays, thrombelastography, and anticoagulant drug monitoring are under investigation for veterinary patients; however, their ability to improve diagnosis or treatment requires further study in clinical trials.

INTRODUCTION

Hemostasis Overview

Hemostasis is a complex process involving temporospatially regulated interactions among the blood vessel wall and circulating platelets, membrane-associated tissue factor (TF), and procoagulant, anticoagulant, and fibrinolytic plasma proteins.[1] In healthy vessels, the balance favors anticoagulant reactions that maintain blood in a fluid state flowing at high pressure in a sealed compartment (**Fig. 1**). Blood vessel injury tips the balance to favor platelet and procoagulant factor activation that results in a burst of sustained thrombin (factor IIa) generation, which in turn leads to fibrin clot formation and cessation of blood loss. Thrombin-mediated feedback loops

Disclosures: The authors have nothing to disclose.
Comparative Coagulation Section, Animal Health Diagnostic Center, College of Veterinary Medicine, Cornell University, 240 Farrier Road, Ithaca, NY 13501, USA
* Corresponding author.
E-mail address: mbb9@cornell.edu

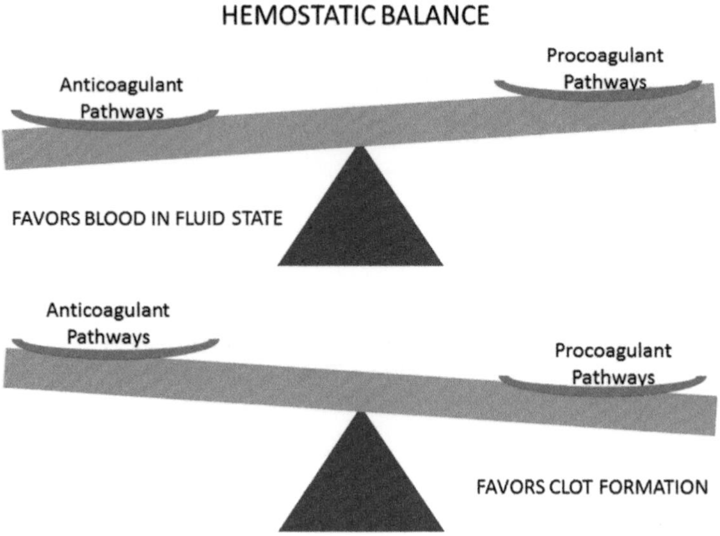

HEMOSTATIC BALANCE

Fig. 1. Hemostatic balance. Blood circulates in a fluid state because anticoagulant reactions are slightly favored. Injury tips the balance toward procoagulant pathways and clot formation. An inadequate procoagulant response caused by deficiencies or dysfunction of platelets and clotting factors, or dysregulation of fibrinolysis, causes hemostatic imbalance and clinical signs of a bleeding diathesis.

simultaneously trigger activation of anticoagulant proteins that limit clot size, with the subsequent actions of the fibrinolytic pathway promoting clot dissolution and wound healing (**Fig. 2**).

Clinical Classification of Bleeding Disorders

The diagnostic workup to differentiate hemorrhage caused by vascular injury from a systemic hemostatic imbalance typically involves a combination of broad screening tests and specific assays. The characterization of 3 overlapping phases of primary hemostasis, secondary hemostasis, and fibrinolysis provides a simple diagnostic framework for evaluating patients with clinical signs of hemorrhage (**Fig. 3**).

Primary hemostasis

Platelets play a dominant role in primary hemostasis. At the site of injury they rapidly tether, change shape, spread, and firmly anchor to exposed subendothelial proteins.[2] Platelet adhesion requires the presence of von Willebrand factor (VWF), and the exposure of collagen and other adhesive proteins in the subendothelial matrix.[3] Agonists such as thrombin, collagen, adenosine diphosphate (ADP), thromboxane, and serotonin binding to their platelet membrane receptors initiate intracellular signaling pathways leading to platelet activation.[4] Activated platelets bind fibrinogen and VWF, aggregate to each other, and release granule contents that support the formation of a stable platelet plug sufficient to control hemorrhage from small vessels and capillaries. The process is regulated by inhibitors released from activated platelets and expressed on the surface of nearby endothelial cells.[5] Primary hemostatic defects include thrombocytopenia,[5,6] platelet dysfunction,[7] and von Willebrand disease (VWD).[6]

Regulation of Fibrin Formation and Degradation

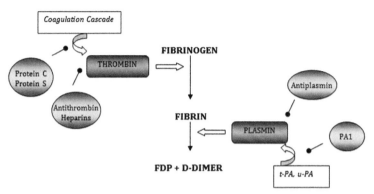

Fig. 2. Coagulation and fibrinolysis. Procoagulant and profibrinolytic reactions (*squares*) and their inhibitors (*circles*) modulate the generation and degradation of fibrin. The coagulation cascade culminates in the production of thrombin, which cleaves soluble fibrinogen to form insoluble fibrin. The actions of tissue plasminogen activator (t-PA) and urokinase (u-PA) generate plasmin, which lyses mature fibrin to form a series of degradation fragments (FDP) and the terminal lytic fragment, D-dimer. Thrombin generation is opposed by the anticoagulants Protein C and Protein S. These proteins act together to inhibit the cofactor activities of Factor V and Factor VIII. Antithrombin inhibits thrombin formation, and directly binds to and neutralizes free thrombin. Antithrombin's activity is enhanced by endogenous (or exogenous) heparin. Plasminogen activator inhibitor-1 (PA1) inhibits fibrinolysis by complexing with t-PA and u-PA to prevent their interaction with plasminogen. Antiplasmin neutralizes free plasmin.

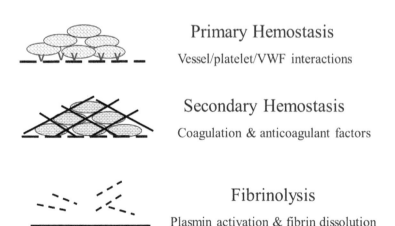

Primary Hemostasis
Vessel/platelet/VWF interactions

Secondary Hemostasis
Coagulation & anticoagulant factors

Fibrinolysis
Plasmin activation & fibrin dissolution

Fig. 3. Three phases of hemostasis. Primary hemostasis involves platelets and von Willebrand factor (VWF) at the site of vascular injury, and results in formation of a platelet aggregate. Secondary hemostasis refers to the reactions of the coagulation cascade that generate a fibrin/cellular meshwork and stable hemostatic plug. In the process of fibrinolysis, plasmin gradually degrades the mature clot to reestablish blood flow after vessel healing.

Secondary hemostasis and anticoagulant proteins

Secondary hemostasis is triggered by the exposure of TF at sites of large-vessel injury, and sustained by the procoagulant properties of platelets that promote fibrin formation. These properties include release of polyphosphates,[8] outer membrane externalization of aminophospholipids,[9] and shedding of membrane vesicles referred to as platelet microparticles (PMP).[10] Procoagulant platelets and PMP provide physiologic anchoring sites for assembly of calcium-dependent, coagulation-factor complexes that generate a large burst of thrombin, which cleaves soluble plasma fibrinogen to form a stable cross-linked fibrin clot. A cell-based model of coagulation (**Fig. 4**) describes the physiologic interactions among endothelial cells, TF-bearing cells, platelets, and the subendothelial matrix that promote fibrin formation.[11] This model illustrates the key role for the TF–Factor VIIa complex as the in vivo initiator of coagulation, amplification of thrombin generation by platelets, and the opposing actions of thrombin in promoting and inhibiting coagulation.

The classic coagulation cascade model[12] depicts the intrinsic and extrinsic pathways as 2 distinct series of activation reactions that coalesce into common terminal

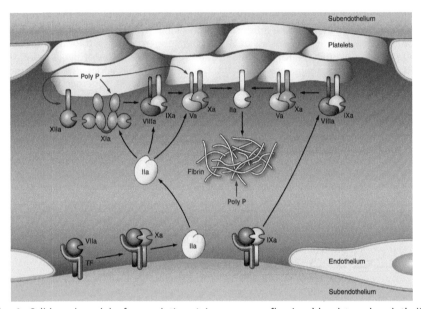

Fig. 4. Cell-based model of coagulation. Injury exposes flowing blood to subendothelial collagen and von Willebrand factor, and surrounding cells bearing tissue factor (TF). Trace amounts of circulating Factor VIIa bind TF and generate small amounts of Factor IXa and Factor Xa, which in turn activate prothrombin to thrombin (IIa). Thrombin plays a central role in amplifying and propagating coagulation through a series of reactions taking place on the surface of procoagulant platelets, formed in response to combined collagen and thrombin stimulation. These platelets also release polyphosphates (poly P) that may activate Factors XII, XI, and V, and inhibit clot lysis. Procoagulant platelets provide a phospholipid surface for assembly of the tenase complex (Factors VIIIa and IXa) and prothrombinase complex (Factors Va and Xa) that rapidly generate Factor Xa and thrombin, respectively. The resultant burst of high concentration thrombin cleaves plasma fibrinogen to form a fibrin clot. Recent murine models of coagulation suggest that collagen and neutrophil-elaborated fibrillar material (neutrophil extracellular traps, or NETs) have procoagulant actions similar to those of polyphosphates. (*From* Versteeg HH, Heemskerk JW, Levi M, et al. New fundamentals in hemostasis. Physiol Rev 2013;93:328; with permission.)

reactions, ultimately producing a fibrin clot (**Fig. 5**). These pathways represent the in vitro, fluid-phase reactions of the traditional coagulation screening tests, the activated partial thromboplastin time (aPTT) and prothrombin time (PT), as discussed later in this article.

Plasma anticoagulant proteins are critical negative regulators of coagulation (**Fig. 6**). Antithrombin (AT) and tissue factor pathway inhibitor (TFPI) are direct protease inhibitors that neutralize circulating active factors, thereby restricting fibrin formation to the site of vessel injury. The targets of AT include activated Factors IX, X, and thrombin (Factors IXa, Xa, and IIa). Protein C, with its cofactor, Protein S, binds to endothelial cell receptors and inhibits coagulation by degrading the coagulation cofactors Va and VIIIa at the endothelial cell surface.[13] Defects of secondary hemostasis that cause signs of hemorrhage include acquired and hereditary coagulation factor deficiencies and physiologic and pharmacologic coagulation inhibitors, whereas relative deficiencies of anticoagulant proteins are associated with thrombotic syndromes.

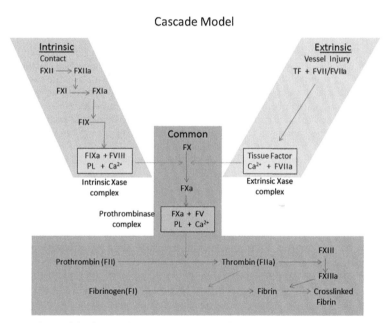

Fig. 5. Cascade model of coagulation. Coagulation factors circulate in plasma in zymogen form and are activated by a cascading series of calcium-dependent proteolytic reactions, referred to as pathways. The extrinsic pathway is initiated by the introduction of tissue factor (TF), which binds to trace levels of Factor VIIa. Factor VIIa–TF and Ca^{2+} form the extrinsic tenase (Xase) complex, which activates Factor X to Factor Xa. The intrinsic coagulation pathway is initiated by interactions among the contact group factors, prekallikrein, kininogen, and Factor XII, with a negatively charged surface. Factor XIIa activates Factor XI to Factor XIa, which in turn generates Factor IXa. Factor IXa assembles with Factor VIIIa, phospholipid (PL), and calcium to form the intrinsic Xase complex and generate Factor Xa. In the common pathway, Factor Xa generated by the extrinsic and intrinsic pathways interacts with Factor Va, PL, and calcium to form the prothrombinase complex that converts prothrombin (FII) to thrombin (FIIa). Thrombin then converts fibrinogen to fibrin, which polymerizes to form the insoluble fibrin clot. Factor XIIIa cross-links fibrin to further strengthen the clot.

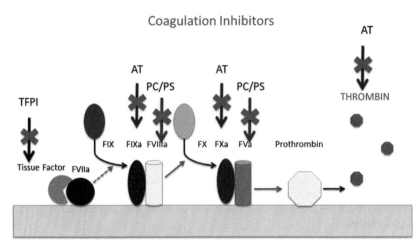

Coagulation Inhibitors

TFPI = tissue factor pathway inhibitor
AT = antithrombin
PC/PS = protein C and its cofactor protein S

Fig. 6. Coagulation inhibitors. Tissue factor pathway inhibitor (TFPI), antithrombin (AT), and Protein C (PC) are key anticoagulant plasma proteins that neutralize active clotting factors, thereby limiting the extension of a fibrin clot. TFPI binds to Factor Xa and the Factor VIIa–TF complex, and acts to rapidly neutralize Factor Xa. Protein C becomes activated at cell surfaces to form activated protein C (aPC) which, in combination with Protein S, proteolytically degrades coagulation Factor VIIIa and Factor Va. In the absence of coagulation cofactors VIIIa and Va, the tenase and prothrombinase complexes do not form, resulting in a marked decrease in thrombin formation. Antithrombin binds to and neutralizes free plasma Factor IXa, Factor Xa and thrombin. Red crosses denote inhibition.

Fibrinolytic pathway

Tissue and vascular injury initiate coagulation and fibrinolysis (see **Fig. 2**). Thrombin is the terminal enzyme of the coagulation cascade, whereas plasmin is the enzyme responsible for fibrinolysis. Tissue plasminogen activator (tPA) is the major initiator of intravascular fibrinolysis. When bound to fibrin, tPA is highly efficient in activating the proenzyme plasminogen to form plasmin, thereby localizing fibrinolysis to the mature fibrin clot. The circulating levels of tPA reflect secretion by the vascular endothelium, clearance by the liver, and its inhibition by plasminogen activator inhibitor type 1 (PAI-1).[14] Plasmin degrades cross-linked fibrin in a series of cleavage steps that generate intermediary fibrin degradation products (FDP) and terminal D-dimer fragments. Circulating free plasmin is rapidly degraded by the protease inhibitor antiplasmin. Pathologic states associated with dysregulated fibrinolysis and signs of hemorrhage include severe trauma, hepatic cirrhosis, and disseminated intravascular coagulation.

TESTING HEMOSTASIS
Primary Hemostasis Testing

Thrombocytopenia is the most common acquired hemostatic defect; therefore, platelet count is the first diagnostic test in the evaluation of primary hemostatic disorders (**Fig. 7**). Normal platelet counts for dogs and cats range from approximately 150 to 450 × 10^3 platelets/μL. Spurious low automated platelet counts are common laboratory artifacts and should be confirmed by examination of a blood smear to rule out

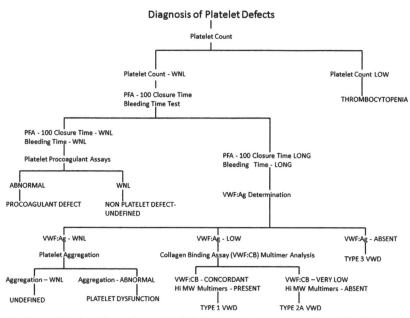

Diagnosis of Platelet Defects

Fig. 7. Diagnostic algorithm of platelet defects. Thrombocytopenia should first be ruled out in the diagnostic workup of suspect platelet defects, followed by functional screening tests, von Willebrand factor assays, and specific tests of platelet activation response. MW, molecular weight; PFA-100, platelet function analyzer 100; WNL, within normal limits; VWD, von Willebrand disease.

platelet clumping. Platelet counts (per microliter) can be estimated from the blood smear by multiplying the average number of platelets counted per 10 oil-immersion fields by 15,000.[15] Thrombocytopenia is rarely the sole cause of hemorrhage at platelets counts above 35,000/μL; however, low platelet count influences end points in functional screening tests such as in vivo bleeding time and whole blood assays.

Platelet function and VWF screening tests: bleeding time and closure time
The buccal mucosal bleeding time (BMBT) using the template system (Simplate II; Organon-Teknika, Durham, NC) and the PFA-100 closure time using the Platelet Function Analyzer (PFA-100; Siemens Diagnostics, Marburg, Germany) have been described as screening tests of primary hemostasis in dogs and cats (**Fig. 8**).[16,17] The BMBT is an in vivo assay that measures the time for cessation of blood flow from a standard incision made in the oral mucosa. Prolonged BMBT (>4 minutes) occurs in patients with platelet aggregation defects and VWD; however, the test may be prolonged in patients with anemia, thrombocytopenia, and hyperproteinemia, and is subject to interoperator variability. Bleeding-time tests are now rarely performed in medical practice because of this nonspecificity, variability, and lack of predictive value for surgical bleeding.[18,19]

The PFA-100 assay evaluates platelet function in citrated whole blood samples that are aspirated at high shear rates (5000–6000 per second) through disposable plastic cartridge assemblies. The cartridges contain a membrane coated with both collagen and epinephrine (CEPI) or collagen and ADP (CADP). As blood flows through a small aperture in the membrane, the agonists trigger platelet adhesion, activation, and aggregation, leading to occlusion of the membrane. The assay end point is reported as

Template Bleeding Time

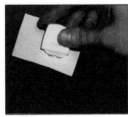
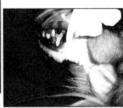
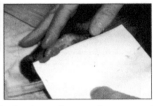

Fig. 8. Buccal mucosal bleeding time. (*Top*) A template device is used to produce a standard depth and length incision. (*Center*) The upper lip is everted and secured with gauze wrapped snugly around the muzzle. The test is initiated by triggering the template device and simultaneously starting a timer. (*Bottom*) Blood is gently blotted from below the incision. The time from incision to the cessation of blood flow is the bleeding time. After completion of the test, the gauze is removed and direct pressure applied to the wound. Tissue glue should be applied to the wound if bleeding persists beyond a 12-minute observation time or rebleeding occurs.

closure time (CT) (seconds) representing the time for cessation of blood flow. Although more readily standardized than in vivo bleeding time tests, the PFA-100 assay system is subject to preanalytical artifacts caused by improper anticoagulant, platelet activation during blood collection and transport, or prolonged (>4 hour) delays in analysis. In addition, the CT is subject to the same nonspecific influences as BMBT. Species differences in platelet epinephrine response limit the utility of the CEPI cartridge for evaluating platelet function in animals. A failure of CEPI membrane occlusion, reported as CT greater than 300 seconds, has been reported for healthy dogs (and horses) with normal platelet function.[17]

Reference ranges have been reported for canine CADP CT (approximately 60–120 seconds)[17] and feline CADP CT (60–180 seconds)[16]; however, in-house reference ranges should be established by each testing site to account for preanalytical variables. The finding of prolonged CADP CT is compatible with either VWD or intrinsic platelet aggregation defects (see **Fig. 7**). In human studies, CT has a sensitivity of greater than 98% for diagnosis of severe (types 2 and 3) VWD, and an overall sensitivity of 85% to 90% for all VWD subtypes.[20] A significant shortening of CADP CT was found in dogs with type 1 VWD treated with desmopressin[21]; however, clinical studies relating normalization of CT to positive clinical outcomes have not been reported. The PFA-100 assay system is not sensitive to defects of platelet procoagulant activity, and in human studies has not proved useful in detecting platelet-secretion defects.[19,22]

Specific Platelet Function Tests

Platelet function testing is logistically and technically challenging. Fresh blood samples are required because of platelets' short ex vivo viability, and quality assurance requires assay of paired control samples to confirm that reagent systems perform within accepted limits.[23] Preanalytical variables have a major impact on assay results. Nontraumatic venipuncture and blood-collection techniques are critical determinants for all subsequent procedures. Blood samples for platelet function testing should be withdrawn gently into premeasured anticoagulant, with no turbulent flow, and maintained at room temperature until analysis. It is of the utmost importance to confirm appropriate sample quality before any platelet function testing.

Light-transmission aggregometry

Light-transmission aggregometry (LTA) is the traditional gold-standard platelet function test, and remains a critical tool for the diagnosis of hereditary and acquired platelet function defects and the monitoring of antiplatelet drugs (**Tables 1** and **4**).[20,23] The assay end point is the amount of light transmitted through a suspension of platelets in plasma or buffer. Changes in light signal are registered electronically by the aggregometer (**Fig. 9**, inset) and displayed dynamically over time after the addition of platelet agonists. After agonist addition, responsive platelets change shape from discoid to spiny spheres, an event that causes a transient decrease in light transmission, followed by progressive increase in transmitted light that parallels ongoing platelet aggregate formation. As the size of the platelet clumps grow, more light is transmitted until a sustained plateau is reached representing maximal, irreversible platelet aggregation (see **Fig. 9**). Reversible aggregation refers to a qualitatively different profile that develops if platelets disaggregate and light transmittance decreases toward baseline after an initial increase. Low dose or weak agonist stimuli may induce biphasic aggregation, appearing as an early plateau (primary aggregation) followed by a subsequent increase to a plateau of light transmission, representing a secondary wave of irreversible aggregate formation.

Analytical variables such as platelet number, choice of agonists and agonist concentration, and reaction stir speeds all influence LTA. Traditionally, platelet numbers are adjusted to 200 to 300 $\times$ 10^3 per microliter of platelet-rich plasma (PRP) using

Table 1
Hereditary platelet disorders in dogs and cats

Disorder	Affected Breeds	Platelet Abnormalities
Glanzmann thrombasthenia	Great Pyrenees, otterhounds	GpIIb–IIIa receptor complex absent or reduced, profound aggregation and retraction defect
Macrothrombocytosis	Cavalier King Charles spaniels, Norfolk terriers	Low platelet count, large platelets, no functional defect
Procoagulant deficiency	German shepherds	Normal aggregation and retraction, failure of stimulated phosphatidylserine externalization, and microparticle release
Storage pool disorder (Chediak-Higashi)	Persian cat	Abnormal aggregation, abnormal dense granule contents and secretion
Storage pool disorder	American Cocker spaniel	Abnormal aggregation, abnormal dense granule adenosine diphosphate (ADP) content
Storage pool and thrombocytopenia	Collie	Cyclic hematopoiesis defect, abnormal aggregation to some agonists, abnormal dense granule serotonin
Thrombopathia	Basset hound, Landseer, Spitz	CalDagGEF signal transduction defect, poor aggregation to ADP, collagen, normal clot retraction

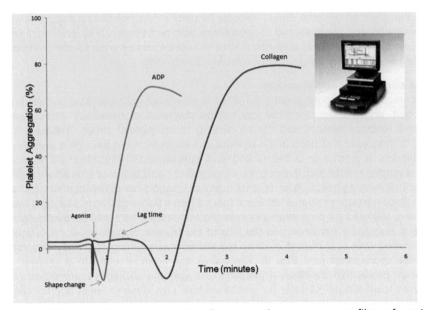

Fig. 9. Light-transmission aggregometry. Representative response profiles of canine platelet-rich plasma (PRP) activated with adenosine diphosphate (ADP; *blue tracing*) or collagen (*red tracing*). A baseline of 0% aggregation is set before agonist addition based on light transmission through turbid PRP, whereas 100% aggregation represents light transmission through platelet-poor plasma. After agonist addition, platelets change shape from flat discs to spiny spheres that block light more efficiently, resulting in a negative deflection from baseline. When platelet aggregation begins, there is a steady increase in light transmission until maxima are reached. Data collection and analyses can be semiautomated using modern instrumentation. An 8-channel platelet aggregometer, Model PAP-8E (Bio Data Corporation, Horsham, PA, USA), is shown (*inset*). Parameters of aggregometry include lag time to onset of aggregation, slope of the reaction, time to maximal platelet aggregation, maximal percent platelet aggregation, reversible aggregation, and the presence of primary and secondary waves of aggregation.

platelet-poor plasma or suspension buffer. This practice has recently been questioned as unnecessary,[24] and may actually result in a decrease in platelet function caused by inhibitory effects of substances in platelet-poor plasma.[23] The LTA reaction mixtures must be stirred at a constant speed to assure the platelets are maintained in an even suspension and to facilitate the platelet-to-platelet contact critical for aggregation. Stir speeds of 1000 rpm are often used; however, stir speeds ranging from 700 to 1200 rpm have been reported. High stir speed risks damaging platelets and inducing spontaneous secretion and aggregation.

Lumi-aggregometry
Routine LTA is an insensitive test in identifying platelet-secretion defects. However, the LTA technique has been modified for this purpose through the use of an instrument (Lumi-Aggregometer; Chrono-Log, Havertown, PA) that is capable of detecting luminescence resulting from the release of adenosine triphosphate (ATP) in the aggregation reaction mixture. In this modification, ATP released from aggregating platelets is quantified through its reaction with a chemiluminescent reagent (Chrono-lume).[25] This technique is generally restricted to specialized veterinary hemostasis laboratories

because the agonists and the chemiluminescent reagents used must be optimized to account for species differences in platelet response.[26] Complete characterization of secretion defects requires additional analyses of the platelet content of adenine nucleotides and serotonin.

Whole blood aggregometry

In contrast to LTA, impedance-based whole blood aggregometry requires minimal specimen preparation, and has been adapted for antiplatelet drug monitoring and the assessment of platelet-granule secretion in human studies. In this method, spaced-platinum electrodes are placed in whole blood warmed to 37°C and as the blood is stirred, platelets coat the electrodes with a monolayer. When an agonist is added to the reaction mixture, activated platelets, leukocytes, and red cells form an aggregate on the monolayer and impede the current between the 2 spaced electrodes.[20] The change in electrical impedance is recorded and expressed in ohms. The method has also been modified to monitor ATP release by the addition of chemiluminescent reagents. Although relatively simple, whole blood aggregometry is subject to artifacts caused by hemolysis and improper sample handling, and nonspecific influences of high or low platelet count and hematocrit.

Flow cytometry

Whereas aggregation studies assess the overall function of an entire platelet population, flow cytometry is a technique that allows examination of platelet activation on a single-cell basis.[27] Cytometric assays detect platelet activation based on changes in light scatter and labeling with fluorescent probes. Platelet studies can be performed on suspensions of washed platelets, PRP, or dilute whole blood, and assays can be configured to assess constitutive membrane receptors, basal activation status, or activation response to different agonists.[27,28] Careful attention to blood collection and processing is as important for valid cytometry assays as for other platelet function assays. The numerous parameters of platelet activation that can be evaluated with cytometry include density of outer membrane surface glycoproteins and ligands, the expression of granule proteins and neoantigens induced by receptor activation, changes in ion flux, protein phosphorylation status, the permeability of platelet cytoplasmic and mitochondrial membranes, outer membrane lipid composition, and PMP release (**Table 2**). One of the most commonly used parameters of platelet activation in animal and human studies is detection of the α-granule protein P selectin (CD62P) on the platelet outer membrane surface (**Fig. 10**, lower left). Labeling with Annexin V, a protein that binds externalized phosphatidylserine, is often used to detect procoagulant platelets and PMP (see **Fig. 10**, lower right) and is also used as a marker of platelet-storage lesion. In addition to the instrumentation and expertise required for cytometric analyses, the application of cytometric assays in veterinary medicine depends on the availability of species-specific and/or cross-reactive antibodies to identify canine and feline platelet antigens.

Von Willebrand Factor Assays

The diagnosis and subtype classification of VWD, the most common hereditary bleeding disorder in dogs and people,[6,29] is based on quantitative and functional assays of VWF protein (see **Fig. 7**; **Table 3**). Type 1 VWD is a partial quantitative VWF deficiency with concordant levels of protein concentration and function. Type 2 VWD is characterized by qualitative defects in VWF structure and function, often combined with protein deficiency. In human medicine, subtype 2A VWD refers to the specific lack of high molecular weight VWF multimers. To date, type 2A is the only type-2

Table 2
Flow cytometric measures of platelet activation

Activation Response	Markers	Process or Receptor Detected
Adhesion	CD42 (a, b, c)	VWF receptor complex (Gp Ib-V-IX)
	CD49b/CD29	Collagen receptor
	CD49e/CD29	Fibronectin receptor
	CD41/61	Fibrinogen receptor
Aggregation	CD41/61	Fibrinogen receptor
	PAC-1	Ligand induced binding site-active fibrinogen receptor
	Fibrinogen	Platelet membrane-bound fibrinogen
Degranulation	CD62P	Alpha granule release
	CD63	Lysosomal integral membrane protein
	Mepacrine	Released from dense granule after ex vivo loading
Signaling	Fluo-3	Cytosolic free calcium
	JC-1	Mitochondrial membrane potential
	TMRE	Mitochondrial membrane potential
Procoagulant activity	Annexin V	Phosphatidylserine externalization
	Lactadherin	Phosphatidylserine externalization
	Factor V	Membrane-bound Factor V
	Fibrinogen	Derivatized membrane-bound fibrinogen
Platelet microvesiculation	CD42b, CD41/61	High-density constitutive platelet membrane antigens

variant identified in dogs. Subtype 2B describes increased binding affinity of VWF to platelet GpIb, and subtype 2N is associated with impaired VWF–Factor VIII binding. Type 3 VWD, the most clinically severe form, is characterized by the virtual absence of plasma VWF (<1% VWF).

Quantitative VWF assays
Measurement of VWF protein concentration, referred to as von Willebrand factor antigen (VWF:Ag), is the first step in the diagnosis of VWD (see **Fig. 7**). Species differences in VWF antigenic structure require the use of species-specific or cross-reactive antibodies in enzyme-linked immunosorbent assays or latex-immunoassay platforms. Test results are conventionally reported in comparison with a normal, same-species standard having 100% or 100 U/mL VWF:Ag. In general, plasma VWF:Ag values of less than 50% (<50 U/mL) indicate VWF deficiency.

Functional VWF assays
Functional VWF assays measure the ability of VWF to interact with platelets, collagen, or Factor VIII. The ristocetin cofactor assay (VWF:RCo) is based on the ability of the antibiotic ristocetin to induce conformational changes in VWF that enhance its binding to platelet GpIb.[30] The application of VWF:RCo assays for canine or feline plasmas is complicated by the tendency of ristocetin to cause protein-precipitate formation that interferes with the assay end point. A reagent purified from snake venom, botrocetin, has been used as a surrogate for ristocetin in animal plasmas.[31]

Functional assays that measure VWF's collagen-binding activity (VWF:CB) have been developed and validated for use with human[32] and canine plasma.[33] In human and canine VWF:CB assays, purified bovine collagen is immobilized to the polystyrene surface of microtiter plate wells; plasma is added to allow for VWF binding; the wells are washed free of unbound VWF; and collagen-bound VWF is detected

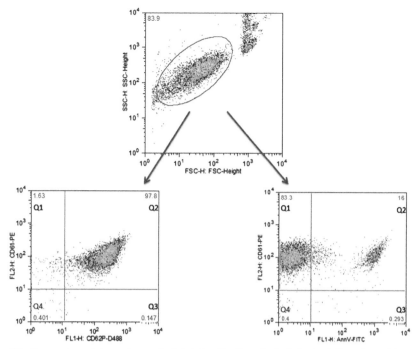

Fig. 10. Flow-cytometric analyses of platelet activation. Dot plots depicting thrombin stimulation of canine platelet-rich plasma (PRP). (*Upper panel*) Platelets are gated (*ellipse*) for analysis based on size and light-scattering properties (forward scatter [FSC-Height] and side scatter [SSC-Height]). (*Lower panels*) Fluorescence intensity of the gated population is shown on the y-axis for a constitutive platelet membrane antigen, CD61 (GPIIIa), and on the x-axis at left for a marker of P-selectin expression (CD62P) or at right, a marker of phosphatidylserine externalization (Annexin V). In each lower panel, Q1 represents nonactivated platelets and Q2 represents platelets expressing the activation marker. Fluorochrome abbreviations: D488, DyLight green; FITC, fluorescein isothiocyanate; PE, phycoerythrin.

Table 3
Subtype classification of von Willebrand disease

Type	VWF Defect	Affected Breeds
1	Low VWF concentration; residual protein has normal structure and function	Airedale, Akita, Bernese mountain dog, Dachshund, Doberman pinscher, German shepherd, Golden retriever, Greyhound, Kerry blue terrier, Manchester terrier, Mini pinscher, Papillon, Pembroke Corgi, Poodle, others Himalayan cat
2A	Low VWF concentration, selective loss of largest multimers, abnormal collagen binding	German shorthaired and wirehaired pointers
2B	Increased platelet-VWF binding	Not identified in dogs/cats
2M	Decreased platelet-VWF binding	Not identified in dogs/cats
2N	Decreased Factor VIII-VWF binding	Not identified in dogs/cats
3	Complete lack of VWF	Dutch kooiker, Scottish terrier, Shetland sheepdog, Border collie, Chesapeake retriever, Cocker spaniel, Labrador retriever, Maltese, Pomeranian Domestic short-haired cat

using VWF-specific monoclonal antibodies in a manner similar to that of VWF:Ag. Paired determinations of VWF:Ag and VWF:CB can be used to discriminate between type 1 and type 2A VWD. The ratio of VWF:Ag to VWF:CB is close to 1 for patients with type 1 VWD, whereas the disproportionate lack of VWF:CB in patients with type 2A VWD results in a VWF:Ag to VWF:CB ratio of more than 2. The VWF:CB is considered an indicator of VWF multimer structure, because VWF collagen-binding activity is a property of high molecular weight forms of VWF.[29]

Structural VWF assays

Characterization of VWF multimeric structure is technically demanding, time consuming, and difficult to standardize; however, VWF protein structure is relevant for understanding protein activity and stability, and is used to further define abnormal results obtained in functional and quantitative VWF assays.[34] To determine VWF multimeric structure, test samples are subjected to sodium dodecyl sulfate–agarose gel electrophoresis to achieve separation of VWF forms according to their molecular mass. The separated protein bands are then electrotransferred to nitrocellulose or polyvinylidene difluoride membranes and visualized using anti-VWF detector antibodies (**Fig. 11**). The full complement of VWF multimers ranges in size from 500 kDa (VWF dimer) to more than 20 million kDa for the high molecular weight forms. Multimer analyses can also discern subtle qualitative changes in VWF, including abnormal protein migration or reduced intensity, and changes in the VWF triplet structure within individual multimer bands. These changes can provide insight into the biochemical basis for abnormal VWF processing, function, or susceptibility to proteolysis.[29,34]

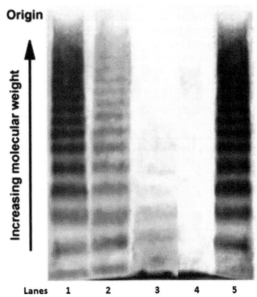

Fig. 11. Von Willebrand factor (VWF) multimer analysis. Western blot of VWF multimers from plasma samples from control dogs (lanes 1 and 5) and dogs with type 1 von Willebrand disease (VWD) (lane 2), type 2 VWD (lane 3), and type 3 VWD (lane 4). The samples were electrophoresed, blotted to nitrocellulose membranes, and immunostained to detect VWF. Type 1 VWD is characterized by a proportional reduction in all multimers, whereas type 2 VWD plasma shows specific reduction in the highest molecular weight forms, and type 3 VWD plasma lacks any detectable VWF protein.

Secondary Hemostasis Testing

Most coagulation assays are functional tests, measuring the enzyme, coenzyme, or inhibitory activity of various hemostatic proteins in samples of citrate anticoagulated whole blood or plasma. The same procedures used to collect blood samples for platelet function testing are therefore applicable to retaining hemostatic protein function.[35] The kinetics of fibrin formation and the relative activities of coagulation factors and inhibitors vary among species. Assay systems optimized for human coagulation testing may not provide accurate values for samples from other species, and different reagent and instrumentation combinations yield different clotting time values within a species.[36–38] Coagulation laboratories thus should provide species-specific reference ranges and controls to facilitate interpretation of patient values.

Coagulation screening tests

Coagulation screening tests are configured with specific reagents to differentially initiate the coagulation cascade via the extrinsic or intrinsic pathway (see **Fig. 5**).[39] Though traditionally performed on plasma samples in a testing laboratory, point-of-care instruments for use with anticoagulated whole blood are now available for veterinary practice. The PT screening test is triggered by the addition of a TF reagent and calcium to the test sample. Patients deficient in any single (or >1) factor in the extrinsic (Factor VII) or common pathways (Factors I [fibrinogen], II [prothrombin], V, and X) demonstrate prolonged clotting time in the PT. The aPTT reagent is composed of phospholipid and negatively charged contact particles. Coagulation complexes assemble during preincubation of the reaction mixture; the addition of calcium then triggers clot formation. This test is sensitive to factor deficiencies in the intrinsic (Factors VIII, IX, XI and XII) and common pathways. The activated clotting time (ACT) is a simple point-of-care test of the intrinsic and common pathway.[40] The ACT, however, is more susceptible to nonspecific prolongation because of thrombocytopenia, platelet dysfunction, hematocrit, or plasma protease activity. The thrombin clotting time (TCT) and measurement of fibrinogen concentration are performed by adding an excess of thrombin (Factor IIa) to the test plasma. These tests measure the conversion of fibrinogen to fibrin and are sensitive only to deficiency, dysfunction, or inhibition of fibrinogen. The pattern of abnormalities in coagulation screening tests thus depends on which coagulation factor or factors the patient lacks (**Fig. 12**).

Coagulation factor assays

The specific procoagulant activity of individual coagulation factors and cofactors can be measured in modified aPTT and PT screening tests, which are configured with a series of single factor–deficient plasmas.[39,41] Factor activity of the test sample should be compared with same-species standards because clotting times vary among species, and human standards generally overestimate the factor content of animal plasmas. Values are reported as percentages, U/mL, or U/dL, depending on the laboratory. In general, factor activities greater than 50% are sufficient to support in vivo fibrin formation. The clinical relevance of factor activities lower than this value depends on the identity and severity of the factor deficiency, and whether a single factor or multiple factors are involved.[41,42] In addition to modified clotting time tests, the procoagulant activities of some coagulation factors can be measured in colorimetric assays based on cleavage of chromogenic substrates. In human medicine these assays are generally reserved for pharmacodynamic studies and evaluation of factor concentrates.[43]

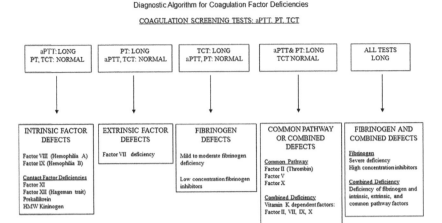

Fig. 12. Diagnostic algorithm of coagulation defects. Coagulation factor deficiencies cause distinct patterns of abnormalities in coagulation screening tests. aPTT, activated partial thromboplastin time; HMW, high molecular weight; PT, prothrombin time; TCT, thrombin clotting time.

Thrombin-generation assays

Coagulation screening tests and factor assays based on the PT and aPTT have a fibrin end point that forms from the action of approximately 10 nM thrombin in the assay system.[44] This value, however, represents only a small portion of the total thrombin potential within the plasma sample. Thrombin-generation assays (TGA) are kinetic assays that monitor thrombin formation over time based on the cleavage of a fluorogenic thrombin substrate. The assay can be performed on citrated PRP, plasma fractions free of platelets, or plasma centrifuged at high g-force to become free of cell-derived microparticles. The TGA reaction is triggered by the addition of a TF and phospholipid reagent, and proceeds through activation of the coagulation cascade and assembly of tenase and prothrombinase complexes that ultimately generate thrombin. The rate of increase and decrease in thrombin concentration over time is calculated from a thrombin calibrator and displayed as a thrombin-generation curve or thrombogram (**Fig. 13**). The resultant profile depicts different phases of coagulation representing net procoagulant and anticoagulant forces. The area under the thrombogram profile is a summary of the overall capacity for thrombin production and is referred to as endogenous thrombin potential. Additional derived parameters include lag time, slope, peak thrombin concentration, time to peak, and the total amount of thrombin generated (see **Fig. 13**).

The test principle of TGA is broadly applicable across species; however, commercially available assay reagents rely on recombinant human tissue factor (rhTF) to initiate coagulation. Species variability in response to rhTF and species differences in the contact pathway activation of Factor XII will influence the thrombogram parameters and may require adaptation of human TGA for measuring thrombin generation in animals. The potential clinical utility of TGA is still under investigation for people with hemorrhagic and thrombotic disorders, including hemophilia, sepsis, preeclampsia, and heart disease.[45]

Fibrinolytic Pathway Assays

Fibrinolysis involves the tPA-initiated formation of plasmin, which degrades fibrin to generate FDP. PAI is a major regulator of this process, and the protease inhibitor,

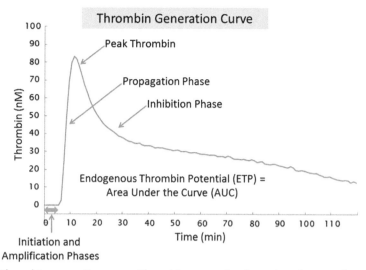

Fig. 13. Thrombin-generation curve. Thrombin generation in canine plasma activated with a tissue factor, calcium, and phospholipid reagent. The initiation and amplification phases of coagulation are measured as the parameter lag time; the propagation phase of coagulation is reflected in the parameter peak thrombin; and the net forces of thrombin generation and inhibition are summarized by the area under the thrombogram curve, also referred to as endogenous thrombin potential.

antiplasmin, further modulates fibrinolysis by neutralizing circulating free plasmin (see **Fig. 2**). The proenzyme plasminogen and its regulators can be measured in specific functional or quantitative assays; however, detection of circulating levels of FDP and the terminal fragment, D-dimer, are the most commonly used clinical tests of fibrinolysis. The D-dimer fragment consists of 2 cross-linked D domains of fibrin, and its presence is a specific indicator of plasmin's action on mature fibrin, rather than fibrinogen. The finding of high circulating FDP and D-dimer concentration indicates excessive or dysregulated fibrinolysis, and is included in the diagnostic criteria of disseminated intravascular coagulation.[46] Quantitative D-dimer assays are considered sensitive, but nonspecific, tests of pulmonary thromboembolism in people and animals.[47,48]

Viscoelastic Coagulation Assays

Thrombelastography (TEG) and rotational thrombelastometry are coagulation monitors with associated software designed to measure and display the kinetics and tensile properties of clot formation in whole blood. These tests reflect the contribution of cellular elements to clot formation, and characterize changes in clot strength and stability that occur beyond the time of initial fibrin formation.[49] In addition to a qualitative tracing, the instruments' software performs direct measurements and derived calculations that describe various parameters of clot formation and subsequent clot lysis. The routinely reported parameters using the TEG instrumentation are reaction time (R), clotting time (K), angle (α), maximal amplitude (MA), and lysis index (LY60). The R parameter is the interval from initiation of the assay until the first deviations of the tracing from baseline denoting initial fibrin formation; K is arbitrarily assigned as the time for deflection from 2 mm to 20 mm from baseline; α is the slope of a line drawn from R to K; MA is the widest vertical amplitude of the TEG tracing, reflecting maximum clot strength; and LY60 is the TEG amplitude at 60 minutes after the time of MA, denoting the extent of fibrinolysis.

The assays are influenced by preanalytical and analytical variables, such as blood-storage time and temperature, and trigger-reagent composition (**Fig. 14**). Test interpretation also requires knowledge of the patient's platelet count, hematocrit, and fibrinogen concentration. Thrombocytopenia (platelet count <50,000), high hematocrit, and low fibrinogen produce relatively poor-quality clots, manifest as prolonged time to clot formation and low clot strength (ie, hypocoagulability). By contrast, low hematocrit and hyperfibrinogenemia typically generate tracings with short clot-formation times and clots of high tensile strength, characterized as hypercoagulable. Rather than a diagnostic test, viscoelastic assays are primarily used in human practice to guide transfusion therapy in patients undergoing cardiac bypass, and patients with complex coagulopathies undergoing surgery such as orthotopic liver transplantation. Most veterinary studies have been descriptive, and the clinical utility of viscoelastic monitors for disease diagnosis, prognosis, or as guides to therapy that improve clinical outcome requires further study.

Modified thrombelastography: clot life-span analysis

After in vivo fibrin formation, the nascent clot undergoes subsequent maturation, remodeling, and gradual dissolution. These late phases of hemostasis are important for patients in perioperative settings at risk for rebleeding and/or thrombosis. A clot life-span model has been developed to characterize imbalance of the fibrinolytic pathway that might induce hyperfibrinolytic or hypofibrinolytic states.[50] Examination of clot life span uses TEG with TF-activated or contact pathway–activated coagulation, coupled with the addition of tPA to initiate fibrinolysis. In addition to amplitude measurements of clot strength, the life-span data incorporate parametric resistance units to capture the velocity of changes in clot structure as the thrombus matures and then lyses. This technique provides a system to screen for fibrinolysis defects, and to visualize the effects of pharmacologic fibrinolysis inhibitors such as ε-aminocaproic acid and tranexamic acid.

Anticoagulant Assays and Drug Monitoring

Physiologic and pathologic coagulation inhibitors

Antithrombin and Protein C are major circulating anticoagulant proteins that regulate the generation and action of thrombin (see **Fig. 6**). Functional chromogenic assays of antithrombin and Protein C, modified by the use of same-species standards, have been used in clinical veterinary studies of patients at risk for thrombosis and as biomarkers of hepatic function. Acquired antithrombin deficiency is associated with thrombosis in patients with disseminated intravascular coagulation and protein-losing disorders. Protein C deficiency has been associated with poor prognosis in dogs with septic peritonitis and liver failure,[51,52] and aids in the diagnosis of portacaval vascular shunting.[53]

Pathologic coagulation inhibitors include antibodies that bind to and neutralize clotting factors to cause signs of hemorrhage, and antibodies that bind to protein-phospholipid membrane antigens that typically cause thrombosis. Coagulation inhibitors are detected in clotting time tests configured with mixtures of patient plasma and same-species control plasma. In contrast to factor-deficient plasmas that demonstrate correction of clotting time, the presence of coagulation inhibitors results in persistent prolongation of clotting time in a mixing study.[54]

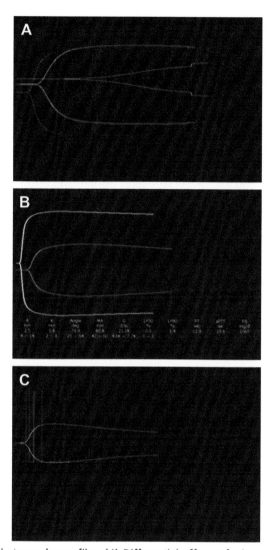

Fig. 14. Thrombelastography profiles. (*A*) Differential effects of trigger reagent composition. The 3 superimposed thrombelastograph tracings were generated from a citrated whole blood sample from a dog with hemophilia B (Factor IX coagulant activity = 3%; reference range >50%). The white tracing denotes activation with calcium alone, the green tracing activation with tissue factor and calcium, and the pink tracing activation with kaolin and calcium. Note the marked abnormality in fibrin formation in the calcium-activated sample, representing an almost complete failure of coupling between the sample cup and pin. (*B*) Thrombelastographic features of hypercoagulability. The superimposed tracings were generated from tissue factor and calcium-activated citrated whole blood samples from a control dog (green tracing) and a dog with pancreatitis and marked hyperfibrinogenemia (*white tracing*). Reference intervals for each thrombelastographic parameter are displayed below the tracing; reference interval for prothrombin time = 12.0 to17.5 seconds; activated partial thromboplastin time = 10.0 to 17.0 seconds; fibrinogen = 150 to 490 mg/dL. Angle, angle of tangent; G, clot strength; K, clot formation time; LY30, lysis at 30 minutes from MA; MA, maximal amplitude; R, reaction time. (*C*) Tissue plasminogen activator (tPA) activation to assess fibrinolysis. The tracing was generated from tissue factor and calcium-activated citrated whole blood from a control dog with the addition of tPA to the reaction mixture. The tPA activates endogenous plasminogen resulting in a relatively weak clot, with small amplitude and a rapid rate of lysis (compare with green tracing in panel *B* generated from same control dog sample with no tPA).

Antiplatelet and anticoagulant drug monitoring

Evidence-based dosage guidelines for antiplatelet and anticoagulant therapy have been established for defined clinical conditions in people, such as coronary syndromes, deep vein thrombosis, and perioperative thromboprophylaxis. Drug monitoring has been useful in establishing these guidelines (see **Table 4**). Thrombosis is also recognized as a severe complication of many common disease syndromes in animals. Pending clinical trials, drug monitoring may provide some guidance in the empirical use of these drugs to provide the benefits of appropriate antithrombotic intensity while minimizing the risks of iatrogenic hemorrhage.

Aspirin and clopidogrel

Aspirin remains the standard antiplatelet drug against which newer agents are compared.[55] Aspirin irreversibly inactivates platelet cyclo-oxygenase, thereby inhibiting the metabolism of arachidonic acid and the subsequent generation of thromboxane A_2. Thromboxane is a potent platelet agonist and acts as an amplification signal in platelet activation. Inhibition of PFA-100 CEPI CT has been advocated as a simple test to identify aspirin resistance in people; however, the CEPI cartridge is not a useful test for the monitoring of platelet function in animals, and CT has not been consistently correlated with positive clinical outcomes in people. Clinical end points such as thrombosis and hemorrhage, rather than laboratory monitoring, remain the typical means of assessing the efficacy and safety of aspirin therapy in human and veterinary practice.

Clopidogrel is a recently off-patent oral antiplatelet agent. The drug is a thienopyridine derivative that is metabolized in the liver to an active drug that binds to the platelet P2Y12 ADP receptor, thereby inhibiting the platelet release reaction and ADP-mediated activation of the platelet fibrinogen receptor.[55] The antiplatelet effects of clopidogrel vary among patients, and do not directly correlate with its plasma concentration because of differences in hepatic metabolism. Platelet ADP-induced

Table 4
Drug monitoring

Drug	Biologic Action	Monitoring Tests	TX. Target
Antiplatelet drugs			
Aspirin	Inhibit platelet COX → block TXA formation	Platelet aggregation PFA100	Variable
Clopidogrel	Inhibit platelet ADP P2Y12 receptor	Platelet ADP-induced aggregation	>50% inhibition from baseline, Residual aggregation <70%
Anticoagulants			
Heparin (unfractionated)	Enhance ATactivity → block thrombin formation and activity	ACT, aPTT Anti-Xa activity	1.5–2.5× control value 0.3–0.7 U/mL
LMW heparins	Enhance AT activity → block thrombin formation	Anti-Xa activity	0.5–1.0 U/mL

Abbreviations: ACT, activated clotting time; aPTT, activated partial thromboplastin time; AT, antithrombin, COX, cyclo-oxygenase; LMW, low molecular weight; TXA, thromboxane A_2; TX. Target, range of assay values associated with improved clinical outcome in human studies.

aggregation allows pharmacodynamic profiling of clopidogrel response; however, its routine clinical use in people is still based on fixed-dose administration and clinical end points for monitoring.[56]

Unfractionated and low molecular weight heparins

Unfractionated heparin (UFH) is a mixture of polysaccharide chains of highly variable length. Heparin exerts its anticoagulant effect indirectly, by enhancing AT's affinity for its target serine protease coagulation factors, particularly thrombin (Factor IIa) and Factor Xa.[57] A specific pentasaccharide sequence on the heparin molecule binds to AT; however, longer chain lengths mediate UFH's interactions with numerous plasma proteins (including thrombin) and intravascular cells. This extensive binding of protein and cells produces a complex pharmacokinetic profile and a wide variation in UFH anticoagulant effect among individuals. Individual patient monitoring and dosage adjustments are required to attain a desired anticoagulant intensity without causing hemorrhage.

Therapeutic targets for UFH in human medicine were first established based on prolongation of the aPTT screening test, with more recent studies defining target ranges based on in vitro inhibition of Factor Xa (anti-Xa activity).[57] Target prolongation of aPTT to 1.5 to 2.5 times the assay control (or patient baseline) or target range for anti-Xa activity of 0.3 to 0.7 U/mL have been associated with favorable clinical outcomes. Attainment of a target range of anti-Xa activity was associated with improved survival in a canine trial of immune hemolytic anemia.[58] Measurements of aPTT or anti-Xa activity are indicated for monitoring UFH therapy in animals to detect peak effect (approximately 4 hours after subcutaneous administration) to prevent iatrogenic hemorrhage in patients treated with high-dose UFH.

Low molecular weight heparins (LMWH) are produced by depolymerization of UFH and consist of short, approximately 15 monosaccharide-length chains.[57] The LMWH act via the same mechanism as UFH in enhancing AT activity; however, they demonstrate improved bioavailability and a more predictable pharmacokinetic profile. The shorter chain lengths of LMWH also reduce the formation of a ternary heparin-AT-thrombin complex, so that LMWH primarily inactivate Factor Xa. In clinical trials of human thrombotic syndromes, LMWH have proved as effective as UFH, and are generally associated with fewer bleeding complications.

Unlike UFH, therapeutic doses of LMWH do not prolong clotting times of the aPTT screening test. Pharmacokinetic studies and assessment of LMWH anticoagulant intensity are based on anti-Xa assays. A target therapeutic range of 0.5 to 1.0 U/mL anti-Xa activity is considered appropriate for human patients at risk for venous thromboembolism. Pharmacokinetic studies of LMWH in healthy dogs and cats also reveal improved bioavailability and predictability in comparison with UFH.[59,60] Species differences exist, however, in LMWH absorption and elimination. Cats demonstrate peak anti-Xa activity as early as 2 to 3 hours after subcutaneous LMWH injection, with trough values falling to baseline by 8 hours. Measurements of peak anti-Xa activity (2–3 hours after treatment for cats; 3–4 hours after treatment for dogs) can be used to gauge anticoagulant intensity for individual patients.

REFERENCES

1. Versteeg HH, Heemskerk JW, Levi M, et al. New fundamentals in hemostasis. Physiol Rev 2013;93(1):327–58.
2. Stegner D, Nieswandt B. Platelet receptor signaling in thrombus formation. J Mol Med 2011;89(2):109–21.

3. Gibbins JM. Platelet adhesion signaling and the regulation of thrombus formation. J Cell Sci 2004;117(6):3415–25.

4. Abrams CS. Intracellular signaling in platelets. Curr Opin Hematol 2005;12(5): 401–5.

5. Ruggeri ZM. Von Willebrand factor, platelets and endothelial cell interactions. J Thromb Haemost 2003;1(7):1335–42.

6. Brooks MB, Catalfamo JL. von Willebrand disease. Schalm's veterinary hematology. 6th edition. Ames (IA): Wiley-Blackwell; 2010. p. 612–8.

7. Nurdan AT. Qualitative disorders of platelets and megakaryocytes. J Thromb Haemost 2005;3(8):1773–82.

8. Muller F, Mutch NJ, Schenk WA, et al. Platelet polyphosphates are proinflammatory and procoagulant mediators in vivo. Cell 2009;139(6):1143–56.

9. Clark SR, Thomas CP, Hammond VJ, et al. Characterization of platelet aminophospholipid externalization reveals fatty acids as molecular determinants that regulate coagulation. Proc Natl Acad Sci U S A 2013;110(15):5875–80.

10. Italiano JE, Mairuhu AT, Flaumenhaft R. Clinical relevance of microparticles from platelets and megakaryocytes. Curr Opin Hematol 2010;17(6):578–84.

11. Hoffman M, Monroe DM. A cell-based model of hemostasis. Thromb Haemost 2001;85(6):958–65.

12. Macfarlane RG. An enzyme cascade in the blood clotting mechanism, and its function as a biochemical amplifier. Nature 1964;202(6):498–9.

13. Esmon CT, Vigano-D'Angelo S, D'Angelo A, et al. Anticoagulation proteins C and S. Adv Exp Med Biol 1987;214:47–54.

14. Wagner OF, de Vries C, Hohmann C, et al. Interaction between plasminogen activator inhibitor type 1 bound to fibrin and either tissue-type plasminogen activator or urokinase-type plasminogen activator. Binding of t-PA/PAI-1 complexes to fibrin mediated by both the finger and kringle-1 domain of t-PA. J Clin Invest 1989;84(2):647–55.

15. Tasker S, Cripps PJ, Mackin AJ. Estimation of platelet counts on feline blood smears. Vet Clin Pathol 1999;28(2):42–5.

16. Jandrey KE, Norris JW, MacDonald KA, et al. Platelet function in clinically healthy cats and cats with hypertrophic cardiomyopathy: analysis using the platelet function analyzer-100. Vet Clin Pathol 2008;37(4):385–8.

17. Callan MB, Giger U. Assessment of a point-of-care instrument for identification of primary hemostatic disorders in dogs. Am J Vet Res 2001;62(5):652–8.

18. Rodgers RP, Levin J. A critical reappraisal of the bleeding time. 1990. Semin Thromb Hemost 1990;16(1):1–20.

19. Brooks MB, Randolph J, Warner K, et al. Evaluation of platelet function screening tests to detect platelet procoagulant deficiency in dogs with Scott syndrome. Vet Clin Pathol 2009;38(3):306–15.

20. Harrison P. Platelet function analysis. Blood Rev 2005;19(2):111–23.

21. Callan MB, Giger U, Catalfamo JL. Effect of desmopressin on von Willebrand factor multimers in Doberman Pinschers with type 1 von Willebrand disease. Am J Vet Res 2005;66(5):861–7.

22. Quiroga T, Goycoolea M, Munoz B, et al. Template bleeding time and PFA-100 have low sensitivity to screen patients with hereditary mucocutaneous hemorrhages: comparative study in 148 patients. J Thromb Haemost 2004;2(6):892–8.

23. Cattaneo M, Cereletti C, Harrison P, et al. Recommendations for the standardization of light transmission aggregometry: a consensus of the working party from the platelet physiology subcommittee of SSC/ISTH. J Thromb Haemost 2013;11:1183–9.

24. Linnemann B, Schwonberg J, Mani H, et al. Standardization of light transmittance aggregometry for monitoring antiplatelet therapy: an adjustment for platelet count is not necessary. J Thromb Haemost 2008;6(4):677–83.
25. Feinman RD, Detwiler TC, Ingerman-Wojenski C. The lumi-aggregometer as a research and clinical tool. In: Longenecker GL, editor. The platelets; physiology and pharmacology. New York: Academic Press; 1985. p. 429–40.
26. Callan MB, Shofer FS, Wojenski C, et al. Chrono-lume and magnesium potentiate aggregation of canine but not human platelet-rich plasma. Thromb Haemost 1998;80(1):176–80.
27. Ault KA. The clinical utility of flow cytometry in the study of platelets. Semin Hematol 2001;38(2):160–8.
28. Wilkerson MJ. Principles and applications of flow cytometry and cell sorting in companion animal medicine. Vet Clin North Am Small Anim Pract 2012;42(1):53–71.
29. Favaloro EJ. Diagnosis and classification of von Willebrand disease: a review of the differential utility of various functional von Willebrand factor assays. Blood Coagul Fibrinolysis 2011;22(7):553–64.
30. Sixma JJ, Schiphorst ME, Verweij CL, et al. Effect of deletion of the A1 domain of von Willebrand factor on its binding to heparin, collagen and platelets in the presence of ristocetin. Eur J Biochem 1991;196(2):369–75.
31. Read MS, Potter JY, Brinkhous KM. Venom coagglutinin for detection of von Willebrand factor activity in animal plasma. J Lab Clin Med 1983;101(1):74–82.
32. Favaloro EJ. Collagen binding assay for von Willebrand factor (VWF: CBA): detection of von Willebrands disease (VWD), and discrimination of VWD subtypes, depends on collagen source. Thromb Haemost 2000;83(1):127–35.
33. Sabino EP, Erb HN, Catalfamo JL. Development of a collagen-binding activity assay as a screening test for type II von Willebrand disease in dogs. Am J Vet Res 2006;67(2):242–9.
34. Ledford-Kraemer MR. Analysis of von Willebrand factor structure by multimer analysis. Am J Hematol 2010;85(7):510–4.
35. Favaloro EJ, Adcock-Funk DM, Lippi G. Pre-analytical variables in coagulation testing associated with diagnostic errors in hemostasis. Lab Med 2012;43(2):1–10.
36. Karges HE, Funk KA, Ronneberger H. Activity of coagulation and fibrinolysis parameters in animals. Arzneimittelforschung 1994;44(6):793–7.
37. Mischke R. Prothrombin time standardisation in canine samples with regard to inter-batch and inter-reagent variability. Vet J 2011;188:301–6.
38. Mischke R. Activated partial thromboplastin time as a screening test of minor or moderate coagulation factor deficiencies for canine plasma: sensitivity of different commercial reagents. J Vet Diagn Invest 2000;12:433–7.
39. Triplett DA, Smith MT. Routine testing in the coagulation laboratory. In: Triplett DA, editor. Laboratory evaluation of coagulation. American Society of Clinical Pathology Press; 1982. p. 27–52.
40. See AM, Swindells KL, Sharman MJ, et al. Activated coagulation times in normal cats and dogs using MAX-ACT_ tubes. Aust Vet J 2009;87(7):292–5.
41. Brooks MB. Coagulopathies and thrombosis. In: Ettinger SJ, Feldman BF, editors. Textbook of veterinary internal medicine. 5th edition. Philadelphia: W.B. Saunders, Co; 2000. p. 1829–41.
42. Triplett DA. Coagulation and bleeding disorders: review and update. Clin Chem 2000;46(8 Pt 2):1260–9.
43. Collazo V, Alonso C, Frutos G. Validation of an automated chromogenic assay of potency of factor VIII in commercial concentrates. Int J Lab Hematol 2013;35(1):38–45.

44. Mann KG, Brummel K, Butenas S. What is all that thrombin for? J Thromb Haemost 2003;1(7):1504–14.
45. Van Veen JJ, Gatt A, Makris M. Thrombin generation testing in routine clinical practice: are we there yet? Br J Haematol 2008;142(6):889–903.
46. Taylor FB Jr, Toh CH, Hoots WK, et al. Scientific Subcommittee on Disseminated Intravascular Coagulation (DIC) of the International Society on Thrombosis and Haemostasis (ISTH). Towards definition, clinical and laboratory criteria, and a scoring system for disseminated intravascular coagulation. Thromb Haemost 2001;86(5):1327–30.
47. Huisman MV, Klok FA. Diagnostic management of acute deep vein thrombosis and pulmonary embolism. J Thromb Haemost 2013;11(3):412–22.
48. Stokol T. Plasma D-dimer for the diagnosis of thromboembolic disorders in dogs. Vet Clin North Am Small Anim Pract 2003;33:1419–35.
49. Kol A, Borjesson DL. Application of thrombelastography/thromboelastometry to veterinary medicine. Vet Clin Pathol 2010;39(4):405–16.
50. Nielsen VG. Beyond cell based models of coagulation: analyses of coagulation with clot "lifespan" resistance-time relationships. Thromb Res 2008;122(2):145–52.
51. Bentley AM, Mayhew PD, Culp WT, et al. Alterations in the hemostatic profiles of dogs with naturally occurring septic peritonitis. J Vet Emerg Crit Care 2013;23(1):14–22.
52. Dereszynski DM, Center SA, Randolph JF, et al. Clinical and clinicopathologic features of dogs that consumed foodborne hepatotoxic aflatoxins: 72 cases (2005-2006). J Am Vet Med Assoc 2008;232(9):1329–37.
53. Toulza O, Center SA, Brooks MB, et al. Evaluation of plasma protein C activity for detection of hepatobiliary disease and portosystemic shunting in dogs. J Am Vet Med Assoc 2006;229(11):1761–71.
54. Kershaw G, Orellana D. Mixing tests: diagnostic aides in the investigation of prolonged prothrombin times and activated partial thromboplastin times. Semin Thromb Hemost 2013;39(3):283–90.
55. De Meyer SF, Vanhoorelbeke K, Broos K, et al. Antiplatelet drugs. Br J Haematol 2008;142:515–28.
56. Geiger J, Teichmann L, Grossmann R, et al. Monitoring of clopidogrel action: comparison of methods. Clin Chem 2005;51:957–65.
57. Hirsh J, Raschke R. Heparin and low-molecular-weight heparin: the Seventh ACCP Conference on Antithrombotic and Thrombolytic Therapy. Chest 2004;126(Suppl 3):188S–203S.
58. Helmond SE, Polzin DJ, Armstrong PJ, et al. Treatment of immune-mediated hemolytic anemia with individually adjusted heparin dosing in dogs. J Vet Intern Med 2010;24(3):597–605.
59. Mischke R, Grebe S, Jacobs C, et al. Amidolytic heparin activity and values for several hemostatic variables after repeated subcutaneous administration of high doses of a low molecular weight heparin in healthy dogs. Am J Vet Res 2001;62:595–8.
60. Alwood AJ, Downend AB, Brooks MB, et al. Anticoagulant effects of low molecular-weight heparins in healthy cats. J Vet Intern Med 2007;21:378–87.

Molecular Diagnostics for Infectious Disease in Small Animal Medicine: An Overview from the Laboratory

Joshua B. Daniels, DVM, PhD

KEYWORDS

- Polymerase chain reaction (PCR) • Real-time PCR • Infectious disease • Diagnostics
- DNA sequencing

KEY POINTS

- The term "molecular diagnostics" refers to tests that detect nucleic acid (DNA/RNA).
- Real-time polymerase chain reaction (PCR) (ie, quantitative PCR) allows increased sensitivity and specificity compared with conventional PCR.
- Knowing the conditions under which tests are clinically validated has implications for choosing sample types and selecting transport media in which to convey the sample to the laboratory.
- There may be significant variation in the performance of quality assessment and quality control among veterinary diagnostic laboratories that offer molecular diagnostic services given the minimal regulatory oversight of veterinary diagnostic laboratories.
- Multiplex PCR tests must be interpreted with care; more information is not always better.

WHAT IS A MOLECULAR DIAGNOSTIC TEST?

Although all analytes in patient samples are technically molecules, whether a biochemical parameter or a test for an infectious agent, the use of the specific term "molecular diagnostics" implies that the analytes are nucleic acids (DNA or RNA). The methods most commonly utilized by diagnostic laboratories to detect and characterize nucleic acids are

1. Polymerase chain reaction (PCR)
2. Quantitative (qPCR) or real-time PCR
3. Reverse-transcription PCR (RT-PCR)
4. Duplex and multiplex PCR or real-time PCR
5. DNA sequencing

Disclosures: The author has nothing to disclose.
Department of Veterinary Clinical Sciences, College of Veterinary Medicine, The Ohio State University, 601 Vernon Tharp Drive, Columbus, OH 43210, USA
E-mail address: daniels.384@osu.edu

Vet Clin Small Anim 43 (2013) 1373–1384
http://dx.doi.org/10.1016/j.cvsm.2013.07.006
0195-5616/13/$ – see front matter © 2013 Elsevier Inc. All rights reserved.

PCR-based tests in infectious disease diagnostics involve detection of foreign DNA or RNA using known sequences that are specific to the infectious agent(s) in question. The most basic form of PCR uses a biochemical reaction to amplify a DNA fragment of known size. This is then compared with a laboratory positive control when the reaction is analyzed by eye using gel electrophoresis with a dye that fluoresces under ultraviolet light when bound to double-stranded DNA. The basis of the biochemical reaction is a DNA polymerase, which makes copies of the target sequence in the pathogen. The polymerase initiates the DNA copies where specific short-length oligonucleotides, referred to as primers, recognize and bind to (by base pairing) their complementary sequences in the sample DNA. The reaction is run as a series of cycles, whereby the copies of the target DNA sequence are doubled every cycle; thus the amplification of the gene target is an exponential function (**Fig. 1**). The DNA sequences chosen as targets are usually genes, but intragenic regions of DNA may also be useful for pathogen identification.

The sensitivity of PCR may be enhanced when the PCR reaction is read by a photodetector as the reaction progresses (thus the term real-time PCR) instead of using gel electrophoresis. Theoretically, if a PCR or real-time PCR reaction is 100% efficient (a perfect doubling of product each cycle), as few as 1 pathogen genomic copy (virion or bacterium) need be present for the reaction to be successful and yield a positive result. Real-time reactions commonly approach 100% efficiency when evaluated using highly purified laboratory DNA controls; however, PCR inhibitors in diagnostic samples (eg, feces or exudates) may significantly decrease efficiency (and thus assay sensitivity). Real-time PCR incorporates short pieces of DNA that specifically recognize their complementary sequences in the patient sample that are labeled with fluorophores, known as probes. These probes are detectable with photodetectors that are built into PCR thermocycler hardware. The use of probes enhances the sensitivity and specificity of PCR. The most common probe-based qPCR methods are Taqman PCR (Life Technologies Corporation, Carlsbad, California) and dual fluorescent resonance energy transfer (FRET) hybridization probes (Roche Corporation, Indianapolis, Indiana) PCR (**Fig. 2**).

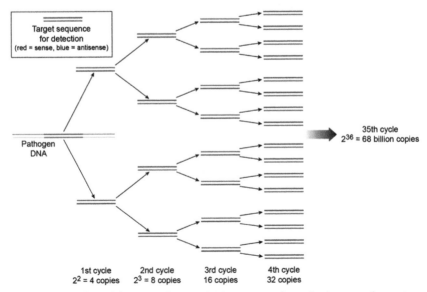

Fig. 1. Exponential amplification of target DNA sequence from single copy of target.

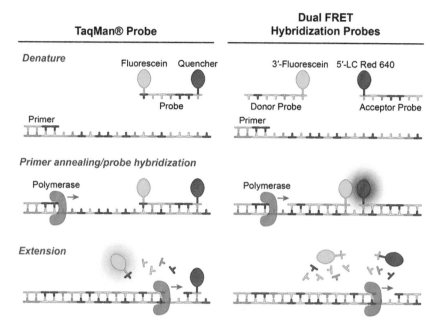

Fig. 2. Taqman and Dual Hybridization FRET probes for qPCR (real time). Fluorescence is emitted in the primer extension phase with Taqman, whereas emission occurs during the annealing phase with dual hybridization FRET probes. This feature of FRET probes enables the performance of genotyping via melting curve analysis.

The latter technology has the ability to differentiate the sequence content of target DNAs and is particularly useful when dealing with viruses that have high mutation rates.[1] The term "real-time" is used for this technology, because the PCR reaction progresses and the intensity of the emitted light from the probes increases concomitantly, which is read each cycle by the photodetectors.

Real-time PCR is also quantitative, because a laboratory has the ability to measure the number of original DNA copies in patient samples by comparing the photodetector signal from the sample to a positive control with a known number of target sequence copies. The quantitative aspect of this technology is seldom utilized clinically in veterinary diagnostics, as the interest of the laboratory is most often to state whether the sample is positive or negative for the infectious agent in question based on the lower limit of detection of the assay. However, qPCR has proved useful in human diagnostics, especially for quantifying patient viral loads in cases of human immunodeficiency virus (HIV) infection.[2] As the technology becomes more entrenched in veterinary medicine, it is reasonable to expect that the future of veterinary qPCR diagnostics will exploit the quantitative ability of these assays to inform clinicians' ability to prognosticate and alter treatment in some disease states. Recently, a qPCR assay was developed to aid in the diagnosis in feline infectious peritonitis, which remains a challenge to antemortem diagnostics. As of this writing, clinical validation data of this assay have not been made available,[3] but the assay is based on an earlier test that had high specificity in field samples.[4]

RT-PCR is used in infectious disease diagnostics to detect RNA; thus this method is used almost exclusively to detect RNA viruses. In RT-PCR, the viral genomic RNA or transcript is transcribed into a DNA copy (referred to as a complementary DNA or cDNA) using the enzyme reverse transcriptase. The DNA copy is then amplified using a PCR-based method. The first copy of cDNA synthesized in RT-PCR by reverse transcriptase is a single-stranded molecule that is complementary to the single-stranded RNA. Subsequent amplification of this strand with regular PCR primers yields regular double-stranded DNA for the exponential PCR amplification.

Duplex and multiplex PCR tests are tests that have the ability to detect 2 or more DNA sequences in the same sample in parallel.

DNA sequencing is occasionally used in clinical diagnostics, most often to identify bacterial isolates that are difficult to definitively identify using conventional biochemical methods. In this situation, a PCR product of an informative gene or intergenic sequence is generated and then sequenced after the gel electrophoresis step. The DNA sequence is compared with a large database of sequences from other bacterial isolates. DNA sequencing may also be used to add specificity to a PCR-based diagnostic test; however, this is usually not necessary if the PCR assay in question has been appropriately validated.

WHEN ARE MOLECULAR TESTS APPROPRIATE?

The appropriateness of any diagnostic test modality depends on the clinical situation at hand. The factors that influence the appropriateness of molecular technology are naturally factors that relate to the degree of sensitivity and specificity that are required to make etiologic diagnoses.

As a Substitute for Virus Isolation

PCR-based methods can be excellent substitutes for virus isolation in cell culture. Virus isolation requires maintenance of mammalian cell lines in tissue culture media that are expensive and relatively time-consuming for laboratory personnel. Virus isolation in cell culture may also be painstakingly slow to complete (several days to weeks), thus delaying diagnosis, whereas PCR-based methods take less than 1 day to arrive at a diagnosis. However, laboratories may not run individual PCR tests on a daily basis; therefore true turn-around times vary.

One advantage that virus isolation has over PCR is that virus isolation has a built-in ability to detect viruses that would not be detected by specific PCR primers that are used in any given assay. If one completely abandons virus isolation in favor of specific PCR assays, there will be missed opportunities to discover novel variants and viruses in patients.

To Obtain Diagnoses from Paraffin-Embedded Tissue

An advantage of using nucleic acid as a detection target is that the viability of infectious agents in the sample is not required. When fixed tissues are submitted for histopathology without corresponding submitted fresh tissues for ancillary bacteriology or virology, it is not uncommon to find oneself in a "hindsight is 20/20" situation once the histopathology report is in hand; the ancillary diagnostics may have nailed the etiologic diagnosis! When histopathology strongly suggests important differential diagnoses, nucleic acid can be extracted from the paraffin-embedded tissues and submitted for PCR. Such PCR assays may be directed against specific infectious agents (viral, bacterial, protozoal), or alternatively, bacteria in the sample can be identified by amplifying and sequencing informative segments of housekeeping genes, such as 16s ribosome-encoding DNA, heat-shock proteins, and RNA polymerase.[5,6] Housekeeping genes are typically highly conserved within bacterial species, but sufficiently divergent between different species to make them useful for differentiating bacteria.

The utility of individual housekeeping genes depends on the bacterial differential diagnosis, in that some housekeeping gene targets are more discriminating than others within bacterial families or genera.

However, the length of time that tissues bathe in formalin prior to paraffin embedding will impact the likelihood of successful PCR from the embedded tissues.[7] Formaldehyde causes DNA–protein and RNA–protein cross-linkages, which render the nucleic acid molecules less amenable to amplification in subsequent PCR reactions.[8] As a general rule, the sooner a tissue sample is embedded in paraffin after formalin fixation, the more likely PCR will be successful from the embedded tissue. The practical application of this rule is simple; submit formalinized tissues to the laboratory as soon as possible for histopathology, so they will be embedded in paraffin in short order.

To Detect Fastidious or Slow-Growing Bacteria in Clinical Specimens

Because relatively minute amounts of target DNA are detectable via PCR-based methods, these methods are often appropriate for detecting bacteria that are difficult or impossible to cultivate with standard bacteriology methods. *Ehrlichia* subspecies, *Anaplasma* subspecies, and hemotropic *Mycoplasma* are good examples of such agents. These organisms require mammalian cells to propagate, and it is thus laborious, expensive, and time-consuming to use culture or bioassay (as with virus isolation). Here, a positive PCR test is an excellent confirmatory diagnostic tool in a compatible clinical case with positive serology. Parallel serology and PCR for *Ehrlichia* and *Anaplasma* subspecies are particularly helpful in strengthening a diagnosis, especially if the titer is questionably significant.[9] In some acutely ill animals, DNA-based methods may actually be superior to serology, because diagnoses may be made prior to seroconversion.[9]

To Distinguish Vaccination from Natural Infection

For the majority of infectious agents for which vaccines exist, serologic diagnostic testing is fraught with low specificity. Although seroconversion between acute and convalescent sera strengthens a diagnosis, it is most often desirable to obtain a diagnosis in the acute time frame for optimal patient management and prognostication for owners. PCR methods may be useful specifically for leptospirosis, feline immunodeficiency virus, and canine distemper for distinguishing natural infection from vaccine.[10–13] However, it is important to understand that the sensitivity of PCR tests depends on several factors including pathogenesis of infection (ie, is the organism still present in the body vs continued immunopathology after infection) and patient management (eg, have antimicrobial drugs been administered in the case of bacterial disease?).[14] For example, antimicrobial therapy implemented on a patient with leptospirosis may change the PCR status of the patient's urine from positive to negative with as little as 1 dose of an antimicrobial drug (Richard E. Goldstein, DVM, personal communication, 2011). Therefore, a negative PCR result in such a situation does not rule out disease.

UNDERSTANDING WHEN TO UTILIZE MOLECULAR DIAGNOSTICS CLINICALLY

There is no one-size-fits-all solution in infectious disease diagnostics or for that matter diagnostic medicine in general. Although molecular diagnostic tests have some distinct advantages, it is essential to understand the limitations of these tests in the contexts of their respective diseases. Individual molecular diagnostic tests are thus best discussed in-depth in the context of their respective diseases, because the utility of those tests in patients will depend on when samples are taken relative to the clinical course, what samples are most appropriate for laboratory submission, and when ancillary diagnostics are desirable. Regardless of what diagnostic modality is ultimately chosen, a clinician's thought process should always begin with the mantra: "How will this result change my therapeutic and/or diagnostic plan?" It behooves the practitioner to thoroughly understand when obtaining a result on any diagnostic test will impact the management of the patient or the population of animals with which the patient cohabitates.

HOW DOES ONE KNOW HOW WELL A NEW TEST WORKS—TEST VALIDATION

The utility of a test depends on the diagnostic question that a test is being used to answer. The definition of test validation is aptly stated in the World Organisation for Animal Health (OIE) Terrestrial Manual: "a process that determines the fitness of an assay, which has been properly developed, optimized and standardized, for an intended purpose."[15] Superficially, this is intuitively obvious; however, the validation data that are made available to practitioners in order for them to evaluate the usefulness new assays offered by diagnostic laboratories may be incomplete, unpublished, or simply not made available at all. Most veterinary diagnostic testing (with the exception of regulatory disease testing for interstate or international animal movement) is unregulated. Most veterinary diagnostic tests are not required to undergo any regulatory review and approval before they are marketed by diagnostic laboratories. This is in stark contrast to virtually all tests for clinical human diagnostics in the United States, which must be approved by the US Food and Drug Administration.[16]

Because there is no regulatory validation hurdle for the marketing of most veterinary infectious disease diagnostic tests, practitioners must be smart shoppers of laboratory diagnostic tests. With all of the advantages of molecular diagnostic tests, the ultimate determination of test utility lies with positive and negative predictive values in real patient populations.

CLINICAL VALIDATION DATA VERSUS ANALYTICAL VALIDATION DATA: REAL WORLD VERSUS TEST TUBE
Clinical Validation

To estimate positive and negative predictive values, populations of gold standard-positive and-negative patients are required to first determine an assay's clinical sensitivity (Se) and specificity (Sp) (**Fig. 3**).

| | | Gold Standard | |
		POS	NEG
PCR to	POS	a	b
Validate	NEG	c	d

Sensitivity Calculation   PPV= A/A+B
Se = a/a+c

Specificity Calculation   NPV=D/D+C
Sp= d/b+d

Fig. 3. Classical 2 × 2 test validation as applied to a new PCR test and a gold-standard test. This assumes that one consider the gold standard as truth. However, the PCR test may actually be a superior detector of truth; thus as Se and Sp of the gold standard test deviate from 100% relative to truth, the PCR test will falsely appear to have inferior Se and/or Sp.

With these data in hand, and an estimate of disease prevalence in the population, given geographic location and patient demographics, a practitioner can reasonably estimate the predictive values of a new test (**Fig. 4**). However, very often, such basic clinical Se/Sp information is unavailable, because some molecular diagnostic tests are so new.

An additional complication in evaluating clinical validation data, even when they are available, is that gold standards themselves are imperfect.[17] In many instances, it is entirely possible that the PCR test has superior Se/Sp, given the technology's ability to detect miniscule quantities of DNA sequence-specific analyte. Therefore, as the sensitivity of the gold standard test decreases, the apparent specificity of the PCR

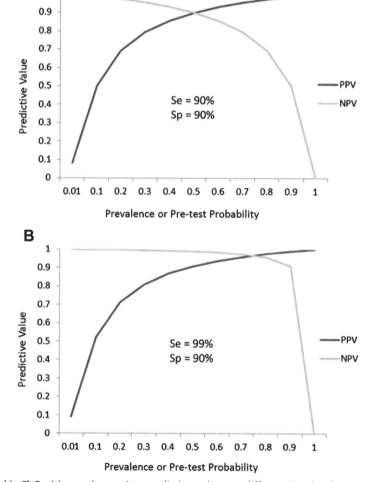

Fig. 4. (*A, B*) Positive and negative predictive values at different levels of test sensitivity, specificity, and disease prevalence. (*A*) At >50% prevalence, the positive predictive value (PPV) exceeds the negative predictive value (NPV) when Se and Sp are equal. (*B*) This figure makes clear NPV trumps PPV when Se>Sp and that very sensitive tests are excellent screening tools to rule out diseases of low prevalence.

test in the validation study decreases. As the gold standard test's specificity decreases, the apparent sensitivity of the PCR test decreases.[17]

Through advanced statistical methods, notably Bayesian Latent Class Modeling, new gold standards may be set for some infectious diseases, and in many instances those standards will be molecular tests. These methods use multiple pieces of information about populations of patients and integrate epidemiologic data and the results of multiple diagnostic tests instead of a single gold standard test. This advanced approach has gained significant traction in human medicine, where datasets with large numbers of patients are commonly available, and is just beginning to take root in veterinary medicine.[18–20]

Sample Selection and Transport

Through analytical validation studies, laboratories determine optimal protocols for nucleic acid purification from different sample types (eg, tissues, fluids, or swabs) to yield the most sensitive detection in subsequent PCR reactions. Some samples will naturally contain more target pathogen, given general knowledge of the pathophysiology of the infectious agent(s) in question. Biologic matrices may contain PCR inhibitors, a problem to some extent that has been overcome by enhancements in nucleic acid isolation technology. It is important that practitioners submitting samples for molecular diagnostics adhere to the sample type and transport media requested by their PCR laboratory. Thus, in addition to tissue/fluid selection, specimen transport media can impact the efficiency of PCR reactions.[21]

Analytical Validation

Analytical validation studies are the most basic evaluation of PCR-based tests. These studies are also referred to as limit of detection (LOD) studies. Every PCR-based test offered by diagnostic laboratories should undergo this type of validation during test development. These studies determine how many molar copies of the PCR target are minimally detected in an assay in the presence of compounds within sample matrices (eg, urine, respiratory secretions, or feces).[15] This type of evaluation is performed completely in vitro and says very little about how well an assay performs in real patient populations. Although this type of information is necessary during assay development for optimizing the efficiency of PCR reactions (many real-time PCR assays can detect as few as 1 copy of a target), it does almost nothing for the practitioner. Diagnostic laboratories may tout the analytical sensitivity of their tests in marketing materials, and it is advisable for practitioners to seek any available clinical validation data, such as from a peer-reviewed journal, when contemplating a new test.

LABORATORY QUALITY ASSURANCE AND QUALITY CONTROL

Quality assurance and control for PCR-based testing is particularly crucial, because the technology is susceptible to concerns at multiple steps in sample processing and assay performance. Foremost, the sensitivity of the technology lends itself to being susceptible to sample contamination in the laboratory. Without appropriate laboratory architecture and workflow, this issue is a constant concern.[1,22] There also are multiple factors that affect the performance and consistency of PCR-based assays, such as PCR instrument calibration, batch-to-batch variation of PCR reagents (such as enzymes), and human operator performance, to name a few. Laboratories that offer PCR as a fee-for-service should ideally have a quality management program that addresses these issues.

Human diagnostic laboratories are legally required to comply with a set of regulations known as the Clinical Laboratory Improvement Amendments (CLIA),[23] whereas veterinary laboratories may provide most diagnostic tests in an unregulated fashion. Therefore, the extent to which veterinary laboratories self-impose quality management systems is variable, and the quality control around PCR services may vary. However, the quality control may be relatively high, exemplified by laboratories that achieve accreditation from the American Association of Veterinary Laboratory Diagnosticians (AAVLD) and those that implement a quality management system developed for laboratories, such as the International Standards Organization ISO 17025 standard.[24,25] It is beyond the scope of this article to detail the components of quality management systems as they would apply to PCR; however, practitioners should be aware that not all laboratories that perform PCR do so with the same level of operational rigor and consistency.

The performance characteristics of assays will vary among laboratories for reasons related to quality management, but also because the assays themselves frequently vary, even when the same target pathogen is sought. One study demonstrated that parallel samples sent to 3 laboratories for PCR detection of feline immunodeficiency virus yielded wildly discordant results.[11]

PCR (OR REAL-TIME PCR) PANELS VERSUS INDIVIDUAL TESTS

More often than not, a differential diagnosis of infectious disease will include the possibility of 2 or more potential infectious agents. The workflow of PCR in a diagnostic laboratory, in which the purification of nucleic acid from the patient specimen is the first process step, renders testing for multiple agents from the same purified nucleic acid sample to be highly efficient. In addition, 2 or more PCR or real-time PCR reactions (Taqman and hybridization probe) can be run in the same tube with appropriate analytical validation. Given this win-win: multiple differentials tested for the practitioner on 1 sample and minimal additional effort for the diagnostic laboratory after the nucleic acid purification step, the use of PCR panels has become very popular, as they are offered by private service laboratories, university laboratories, and state diagnostic laboratories alike.

Although these panels are appealing to practitioners (and to diagnostic laboratories) for the reasons mentioned previously, they are relatively expensive and may contain differential diagnoses that have no meaningful bearing on treatment planning in an individual patient. The ability to test for everything with this technology should not mean that an etiologic diagnosis need be sought in every single case. Moreover, the high sensitivity of these methods increases the likelihood of red herring diagnoses, especially if the results of these tests are considered in a vacuum. It is critical that practitioners consider all available information when evaluating a result for a test with high analytical sensitivity. This caveat goes double for tests with no available clinical validation data.

EXAMPLES OF MULTIPLEX PCR UTILITY AND LACK THEREOF

An illustrative pitfall of multiplex PCR is the application of a real-time PCR panel for feline upper respiratory disease (URD). Such panels often include: Feline Herpesvirus 1 (FHV-1), Feline Calicivirus (FCV), *Bordetella bronchiseptica, Mycoplasma felis,* and *Chlamydophila felis.* In a household with 1 cat with a typical outpatient acute upper respiratory syndrome, there is little justification for such testing. Such infections are typically self-limiting, and there is no population management issue. Individual cats require almost identical supportive care regardless of etiologic agent(s) involved in their upper respiratory infection (URI) complex. Moreover, because feline herpes virus is essentially endemic, and vaccination does not induce a sterile immunity, many cats tested are positive for that agent regardless of the presence of other pathogens.[26,27]

A contrasting situation, in which such testing would be beneficial in managing cats with URD is an outbreak involving testing of multiple cats, such as in a shelter or cattery. The identification of persistent calicivirus shedders and the involvement of *Bordetella bronchiseptica* and/or *Chlamydophila felis* would logically impact population management, antimicrobial therapy, disinfection, and perhaps vaccination protocols in the face of the outbreak. In this situation, information garnered from a PCR panel, if carried out on a representative sample of diseased cats, could prevent substantial additional morbidity in a population.

Given the frequency of diarrhea as a presenting complaint to the small animal practitioner, it is only logical that PCR panels directed against enteropathogens for the differential diagnosis of infectious diarrhea in dogs and cats have been readily marketed by commercial diagnostic laboratories. Because enteropathogenic bacteria are frequently present in the feces of healthy patients, the application of such sensitive methodology increases the likelihood of making red herring diagnoses, especially in a patient species population that is naturally prone to diarrhea related to dietary indiscretion (dogs). *Salmonella enterica*, *Campylobacter* subspecies, *Clostridium perfringens, and Clostridium difficile*, all of which are components of such PCR panels, may be recovered in double-digit percentages from healthy dogs.[28,29] Therefore utilization of these panels to make definitive etiologic diagnoses in cases of diarrhea could lead to false conclusions, which in turn could lead to suboptimal patient management. In the case of *Salmonella*, it is also desirable to obtain an actual bacterial isolate in culture for antimicrobial susceptibility testing and serotyping, information that may be valuable in case management and infection control; this is information that is not provided by real-time PCR technology. Diagnosis of enteric disease is a challenge, and often requires multiple diagnostic modalities.[29]

In addition, it is not advisable to use these panels as zoonotic screens in healthy nondiarrheic animals (such as for therapy dogs going into hospitals and eldercare facilities), because there may be concerns with assay sensitivity if the assay in question has not been specifically validated to detect the presence of these organisms in healthy animals.[29] Finally, variation exists among infection control requirements for therapy dogs, and screening may be required for bacteria not included on these panels that are intended to diagnose infectious diarrhea in dogs and cats. Human clinical microbiologists involved in therapy dog programs may be extremely thorough in screening these dogs and include uncommon human opportunistic pathogens such as *Plesiomonas shigelloides* and *Edwardsiella tarda* that are not included on these veterinary diagnostic panels (Michael Kubera, DVM, personal communication, 2009).

REFERENCES

1. Espy MJ, Uhl JR, Sloan LM, et al. Real-time PCR in clinical microbiology: applications for routine laboratory testing. Clin Microbiol Rev 2006;19(1):165–256.
2. Doyle T, Geretti AM. Low-level viraemia on HAART: significance and management. Curr Opin Infect Dis 2012;25(1):17–25.
3. Auburn College of Veterinary Medicine. Feline infectious peritonitis virus. 2011. Available at: http://www.vetmed.auburn.edu/feline_infectious_peritonitis_virus2. Accessed March 27, 2012.
4. Simons FA, Vennema H, Rofina JE, et al. A mRNA PCR for the diagnosis of feline infectious peritonitis. J Virol Methods 2005;124(1–2):111–6.

5. Dai J, Chen Y, Lauzardo M. Web-accessible database of hsp65 sequences from *Mycobacterium* reference strains. J Clin Microbiol 2011;49(6):2296–303.

6. Ghebremedhin B, Layer F, Konig W, et al. Genetic classification and distinguishing of *Staphylococcus* species based on different partial gap, 16S rRNA, hsp60, rpoB, sodA, and tuf gene sequences. J Clin Microbiol 2008;46(3):1019–25.

7. Okello JB, Zurek J, Devault AM, et al. Comparison of methods in the recovery of nucleic acids from archival formalin-fixed paraffin-embedded autopsy tissues. Anal Biochem 2010;400(1):110–7.

8. Gilbert MT, Haselkorn T, Bunce M, et al. The isolation of nucleic acids from fixed, paraffin-embedded tissues-which methods are useful when? PLoS One 2007; 2(6):e537.

9. Neer TM, Breitschwerdt EB, Greene RT, et al. Consensus statement on ehrlichial disease of small animals from the infectious disease study group of the ACVIM. American College of Veterinary Internal Medicine. J Vet Intern Med 2002;16(3): 309–15.

10. Bolin CA. Finds fault with implications of PCR assay conclusions. J Am Vet Med Assoc 2003;223(2):178 [author reply: 178–9].

11. Crawford PC, Slater MR, Levy JK. Accuracy of polymerase chain reaction assays for diagnosis of feline immunodeficiency virus infection in cats. J Am Vet Med Assoc 2005;226(9):1503–7.

12. Harkin KR, Roshto YM, Sullivan JT. Clinical application of a polymerase chain reaction assay for diagnosis of leptospirosis in dogs. J Am Vet Med Assoc 2003; 222(9):1224–9.

13. Leutenegger CM, Crawford C, Levy J, et al. Canine distemper virus quantification by real-time PCR allows to differentiate vaccine virus interference and wild-type infection. Presented at: ACVIM Forum. Denver, June 15-18, 2011.

14. Sykes JE, Hartmann K, Lunn KF, et al. 2010 ACVIM small animal consensus statement on leptospirosis: diagnosis, epidemiology, treatment, and prevention. J Vet Intern Med 2011;25(1):1–13.

15. Jacobson RH, Wright P. OIE terrestrial manual. Principles and methods of validation of diagnostic assays for infectious diseases. Paris, France: World Organization for Animal Health (OIE); 2010. p. 1–18.

16. United States Food and Drug Administration. Medical devices. 2012. Available at: http://www.fda.gov/MedicalDevices/ProductsandMedicalProcedures/InVitro Diagnostics/LabTest/ucm126079.htm. Accessed March 28, 2012.

17. Limmathurotsakul D, Turner EL, Wuthiekanun V, et al. Fool's gold: why imperfect reference tests are undermining the evaluation of novel diagnostics: a reevaluation of 5 diagnostic tests for leptospirosis. Clin Infect Dis 2012;55(3):322–31.

18. Hartnack S, Budke CM, Craig PS, et al. Latent-class methods to evaluate diagnostics tests for echinococcus infections in dogs. PLoS Negl Trop Dis 2013; 7(2):e2068.

19. Mainar-Jaime RC, Andres S, Vico JP, et al. Sensitivity of the ISO 6579:2002/Amd 1:2007 standard method for detection of *Salmonella* spp. on mesenteric lymph nodes from slaughter pigs. J Clin Microbiol 2013;51(1):89–94.

20. Pinches MD, Diesel G, Helps CR, et al. An update on FIV and FeLV test performance using a Bayesian statistical approach. Vet Clin Pathol 2007;36(2):141–7.

21. Gibb AP, Wong S. Inhibition of PCR by agar from bacteriological transport media. J Clin Microbiol 1998;36(1):275–6.

22. Jacobson RH, Wright P. OIE terrestrial manual. Validation and quality control of polymerase chain reaction methods used for the diagnosis of infectious diseases. Paris, France: World Organization for Animal Health (OIE); 2008. p. 11.

23. Centers for Medicaid and Medicare Services. Clinical Laboratory Improvement Amendments (CLIA). 2012. Available at: http://www.cms.gov/Regulations-and-Guidance/Legislation/CLIA/index.html. Accessed March 27, 2013.

24. International Standards Organization. ISO 17025 general requirements for the competence of testing and calibration laboratories. 2009. Available at: http://www.iso.org/iso/home/store/catalogue_tc/catalogue_detail.htm?csnumber=39883. Accessed August 1, 2013.

25. American Association of Veterinary Laboratory Diagnosticians. Requirements for an accredited veterinary medical diagnostic laboratory. 2012. Available at: http://www.aavld.org/assets/Accreditation/aavld%20requirements%20v6%201%206-1-12%20final.pdf. Accessed March 28, 2012.

26. Gaskell R, Dawson S, Radford A, et al. Feline herpesvirus. Vet Res 2007;38(2):337–54.

27. IDEXX Laboratories. IDEXX Feline Upper Respiratory Disease (URD) RealPCR Panel. Diagnostic update 2010. Available at: http://www.idexx.com/pubweb resources/pdf/en_us/smallanimal/reference-laboratories/diagnostic-updates/realpcr-feline-urd-panel.pdf. Accessed March 25, 2012.

28. Goldstein MR, Kruth SA, Bersenas AM, et al. Detection and characterization of *Clostridium perfringens* in the feces of healthy and diarrheic dogs. Can J Vet Res 2012;76(3):161–5.

29. Marks SL, Rankin SC, Byrne BA, et al. Enteropathogenic bacteria in dogs and cats: diagnosis, epidemiology, treatment, and control. J Vet Intern Med 2011;25(6):1195–208.

Using Cytology to Increase Small Animal Practice Revenue

Joanne Hodges, DVM

KEYWORDS

- Cytology • Practice building • Staining techniques • Cytology artifact

KEY POINTS

- Cytology is a readily available, practical test for use in general and specialty practice.
- Most tissues are amenable to routine sampling methods.
- Knowledge about specific tissue-sampling or lesion-sampling methods can improve specimen quality for cytology interpretation.
- Cytology generates revenue whether performed in-house or sent to reference laboratory for expert evaluation.
- Clear client communication about goals, expectations, and plans for using cytology in the diagnosis and treatment of each patient is important.
- Microscopic review of each cytology specimen should be performed in an organized fashion with assessment for cellularity, quality, and any potential artifacts.

Cytology is often acclaimed for ease of obtaining of samples, swift results, and lower cost when compared with other diagnostic tests in veterinary practice. Many samples for cytology can be obtained without anesthesia or even sedation, with minimal risk in both healthy and critical patients.[1,2] With the increasing availability of ultrasonography, many more internal organs and tissues can be evaluated than previously were accessible. Therefore, cytology has become a cornerstone for confirming initial clinical impressions and thereby guiding early client communication and treatment plans. Tissue aspirates and fluid samples provide a definitive diagnosis in many cases but also can indicate the need for additional testing such as molecular diagnostics, special stains, or histopathology. Cytology is most commonly used in general and specialty practice as a guide to direct additional testing, initially screen and rule out specific diseases, and for staging purposes.[3]

Character of the lesion and tissue sampled play pivotal roles in the diagnostic value of cytology. Familiarity with preferred sampling methods and reported accuracy is critical for veterinary practitioners. The diagnostic performance of cytology in comparison

The author has nothing to disclose.
VDx Veterinary Diagnostics, 2019 Anderson Road, Suite C, Davis, CA 95616, USA
E-mail address: jhodges@vdxpathology.com

Vet Clin Small Anim 43 (2013) 1385–1408
http://dx.doi.org/10.1016/j.cvsm.2013.07.007
0195-5616/13/$ – see front matter © 2013 Elsevier Inc. All rights reserved.

with histopathology is reported by organ system and tissue type to guide diagnostic expectations.[4] A sample of good quality is also imperative. Reviews of sampling techniques to increase diagnostic yield are available.[4–6] In addition, detailed, active communication between practicing veterinarians and clinical pathologists is important for diagnostic accuracy of cytology.[3] In many cases, veterinarians and owners can make confident decisions about the next step for the patient via the use of cytologic examination.

OVERVIEW

Topics covered in this review focus on the clinical use of cytology in building small animal practice. In-house and reference laboratory analyses are discussed, followed by: (1) tips for improving sample quality and staining; (2) use and techniques of skin/otic cytology for in-house diagnosis and therapy monitoring; and (3) recent information regarding sample acquisition and correlation studies for certain tissue types.

IN-HOUSE VERSUS REFERENCE LABORATORY TESTING

Cytology samples are obtained for both in-house review and interpretation by a trained clinical pathologist often in association with a reference laboratory. Both in-house and send-out cytology samples generate revenue. The decision to submit a sample to a veterinary diagnostic laboratory may depend on multiple variables including sample type and source, experience and expertise of the veterinarian, cost, and differential diagnosis. Depending on skill and technique, many common lesions can be primarily diagnosed in a practice setting. A recently surveyed coterie of general and specialist veterinarians revealed that approximately 48% of cytology samples were reviewed in-house only, 30% were directly submitted to a diagnostic laboratory, and 22% were first reviewed in-house and then sent to a diagnostic laboratory.[3]

Benefits of in-house cytology include direct generation of practice revenue, ease of preparation without special or expensive equipment, and rapid results to allow direction of further actions. Certain samples, such as skin and ear preparations, semen, and urine sediment, often require rapid evaluation or "wet" slide preparations. In these cases, sample instability may alter some features of the sample over time.[7,8] "Wet" slide preparations are often stained with a vital stain such as new methylene blue. Once stained in this way, these samples should not be sent to a reference laboratory because they dry shortly after staining, causing cellular distortion that is nonreversible even when restained.

Potential pitfalls of solely reviewing samples in-house include: limited experience, causing uncertainty in diagnosis; misinterpretation; and incomplete evaluation of the entire specimen. Initial review of the sample often will indicate that evaluation by a clinical pathologist is the best approach for the patient. Specific tips for submitting samples to and communicating with a reference laboratory are discussed at the end of this article.

Expert opinion by a trained clinical pathologist is helpful in confirming initial impressions in many cases. Diagnostic laboratories, with rapid turnaround times for results and quality reporting, are readily available to veterinarians. Because human medicine relies on specialist opinions, veterinary clients can relate to the need to involve pathologists and seek expert advice. Moreover, if the sample has high quality and provides a definitive diagnosis, clients may be more likely to approve additional cytology evaluations in the future. Initial in-house microscopic review is recommended to assess sample quality before submitting samples to a reference laboratory. Samples should be reviewed for cellularity, adequacy of preparation, and presence of artifacts. High-quality, diagnostic cytology specimens can streamline achievement of a definitive diagnosis and/or prioritize additional diagnostic tests to enhance patient care and build practice income. This article discusses common artifacts and optimal sample qualities. With practice, many preanalytical problems can be detected while the patient is still in hospital. Resampling can then be attempted.

MAXIMIZING THE DIAGNOSTIC AND PRACTICAL YIELD OF CYTOLOGY

In an effort to continually improve the quality of cytology specimens and interpretation, staining methods and tips to prevent cytology artifacts are discussed. With cytology, it is the clinician's responsibility to both collect the specimen appropriately and adequately prepare the sample to be examined. Learning to evaluate each case for diagnostic quality may decrease the incidence of poor-quality or low-cellularity samples that often result in an "inconclusive" interpretation when evaluated by a clinical pathologist.

Of note, poor cellularity and/or sample quality are the most common barriers to a definitive diagnosis with aspiration cytology.[9] Overinterpretation of cytology samples of poor cellularity has also resulted in diagnostic errors reported in malpractice suits involving human medical pathologists.[10] Some lesions, despite appropriate sampling and slide preparation, require assessment of tissue architecture with histopathology. Lesions that often fall into this category include cystic or fibrous masses, cytology samples with multiple cell types, and cell proliferations without striking criteria of malignancy.

CYTOLOGY SAMPLES AND RECOGNIZING COMMON ARTIFACTS

Decreasing the number of sample artifacts can improve the diagnostic accuracy of cytology. Artifacts often indicate the need for resampling or alteration of technique before sending the sample on to a reference laboratory. A checklist for consultation when acquiring cytology samples is provided here.

Sample Acquisition for Cytology

- Evaluate what method of sampling is best for that type of lesion based on evidence-based literature or personal experience (**Box 1**). Consultation with a clinical pathologist may also be helpful before sampling if questions arise.
- If preparing impression smears, try to decrease the chances of hemodilution by gently blotting surface blood from superficial skin lesions, and biopsy tissue samples before preparing the imprint. Wipe excess lubricant or ultrasound gel from the lesion or skin surface before fine-needle sampling (**Fig. 1**).
- If the lesion is cavitary or cystic, consider sampling in multiple locations including any more solid aspect or the wall of the lesion, which may yield more tissue cells.
- Prepare multiple smears. If sampling only yields small amounts of material, it should be spread within the middle of the slide. A permanent marker, grease pencil, or etching pen can be used to indicate the area of cellular material.
- A cell monolayer is ideal. Smears that are too thick can obscure cell detail and staining quality. Even with restaining, smears that are too thick often do not have adequate stain penetration (**Fig. 2**).
- Air-dry slides at room temperature.
- Stain one of the slides with in-house stain for screening sample quality. When submitting cytology samples to a reference laboratory, it is often helpful to submit 1 stained and multiple unstained smears. Staining before transport can improve cellular preservation and decrease sensitivity to environmental artifacts.

Box 1
Methods of sampling commonly used to acquire cytology specimens

1. Fine-needle aspirates. The method most commonly used for sampling of masses, lymph nodes, parenchymal organs, and fluid samples, among others. Techniques vary but commonly involve a small-gauge (≤20 gauge) needle of appropriate length attached to a 6–20-mL syringe. The needle is directed into the area/lesion and approximately 6–8 mL of suction pressure is applied; the needle is redirected a few times without release of suction. Suction is released before removing the needle.

2. Fine-needle nonaspirates (also known as the woodpecker method). A method that can be used in (1) vascular lesions or tissues and (2) masses or tissues (such as lymph nodes) that may contain fragile cells. A small-gauge (≤20 gauge) needle of appropriate length with or without an attached air-filled syringe is gently inserted in and out of the tissue several times, often with redirection, without applied suction. The attached syringe is solely for the purpose of expelling the sample onto the glass slide.

3. Impression smears. A method used for ulcerative or exudative superficial skin lesions or cytologic assessment of biopsy specimens (often intraoperatively). Superficial crusts and exudates should be gently removed or blotted away from the lesion first. Samples are collected by pressing a clean glass slide directly onto the lesion. This type of sample is often not representative of deeper tissue but may be good for diagnosis of superficial infections and inflammatory responses.

4. Swabs. A method commonly used for sampling the ear canal, vagina, and cornea, among others. Samples are collected by either inserting a sterile cotton swab into or rolling over the area to be sampled. If the area is dry the swab can be premoistened with sterile saline. Once obtained, the swab should be gently rolled over a clean glass slide. It is important to roll, not wipe, the swab.

5. Scrapings. Scrapings are used for superficial skin lesions and may be more representative of deeper abnormality than impression smears of similar lesions. Superficial crusts and exudates should be gently removed or blotted away from the lesion first. Samples are then collected by scraping a scalpel blade across the surface of the lesion, followed by transfer of the material from the blade to a clean glass slide.

6. Tape preparations. A method for evaluation of skin disease, particularly for detecting *Malessezia* dermatitis and skin mites. A piece of clear, pressure-sensitive tape (Scotch 3M) is placed on the skin lesion. The tape strip is removed and fixed on a microscopic slide containing a drop of blue (counter) stain.

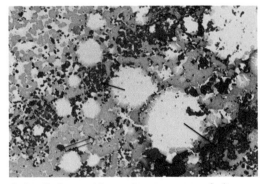

Fig. 1. Nucleated cell detail obscured by copious amounts of ultrasound gel precluding a definitive diagnosis. Solid arrows indicate aggregates of gel. Open arrow indicates few intact neutrophils. Intact tissue cells are not visible (kidney; Wright-Giemsa, HP oil, original magnification ×50).

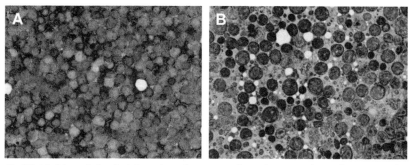

Fig. 2. (*A*) Highly cellular but too densely prepared cytology specimen from an enlarged lymph node. (*B*) In comparison, a highly cellular preparation allowing adequate staining and detailed cytomorphologic evaluation, owing to adequate cell dispersion (lymph node; high-grade lymphoma; Wright-Giemsa, HP oil, original magnification ×100).

- Evaluate the stained smear for cellularity and quality. Are the cells intact with a defined rim of cytoplasm (**Fig. 3**)? Certain tissue types, for example, endocrine tissue, commonly yield many free nuclei on aspiration cytology. However, cellular disruption can result from either excessive pressure applied to either the syringe with the aspiration technique or the spreader slide in the case of squash or smear preparations (**Table 1**). Neoplastic cells can also be more fragile and prone to lysis. If lysis is a recurring problem, try using the nonaspiration technique (see **Box 1**). A coverslip can also be used to make the preparation by laying it on top of the aspirated material and then quickly making a squash preparation. Coverslips are lighter and tend to cause less cell disruption.
- Evaluate the stained smear for other artifacts previously mentioned. If present, resampling is strongly encouraged.

Specimen Staining for Cytology

Many diagnostic laboratories routinely use robust methanol-based Romanowsky-type stains for cytologic specimens. Standard rapid-type dip stains, such as Diff-Quik (Siemens Healthcare Diagnostics, Tarrytown, NY, USA), Hema 3 (Fisher Diagnostics, Middletown, VA, USA), and Dip Quick (Jor-Vet, Loveland, CO, USA), are most commonly used in veterinary practices, because of their ease of use. These stains are water-based (aqueous) stains despite the initial methanol fixation step. When

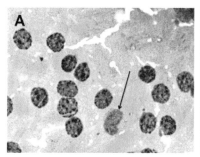
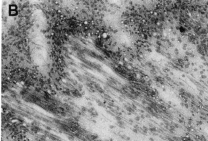

Fig. 3. (*A*) Free nuclei resulting from cellular lysis. One round cell remains intact with a distinct rim of blue cytoplasm (*arrow*) (spleen; Wright-Giemsa, HP oil, original magnification ×100). (*B*) Streams of disrupted cellular material resulting from excessive pressure when preparing the smear (kidney; Wright-Giemsa, HP oil, original magnification ×50).

Table 1 Methods commonly used for preparation of cytology slides	
Method	**Description**
Squash or compression preparation	Collected material is placed toward the end of one clean glass slide. A second slide angled perpendicularly to the first slide is allowed to rest on the slide containing the cellular material. The second slide is then gently and smoothly drawn over the length of the first slide while concurrently rotating the two slides from perpendicular to parallel. Both slides can be stained
Needle or starfish preparation	Collected material is placed at the center of a clean glass slide and the needle is used to gently move material outwards in multiple directions
Blood-smear technique	A small drop of bloody aspirate material or fluid can be placed toward the end of one clean glass slide. The short edge of a second slide is placed 1–2 mm in front of the sample, tilted to 45°, and pulled backward into the cellular material. The material disperses along the short edge and this spreader slide is then smoothly, uniformly, rapidly, and evenly slid forward

appropriately maintained, these rapid stains can provide adequate quality for routine blood smear and cytology staining, but longer staining time is likely to be needed for thicker cytology specimens. Maintaining separate stain sets for superficial skin/ear preparations and tissue-aspiration samples is recommended, as bacteria, yeast, lipid, and cellular debris from skin and ear preparations may "float" off the samples during staining and then become deposited on tissue-aspiration slides, creating artifacts and diagnostic concerns. An individualized hospital protocol for routine filtering and complete changing of stains and fixative should also be implemented based on usage and microscopic evaluation of stain quality. Stain and fixative jars should not be not simply "topped off" by adding fluid to partially depleted jars.

Staining quality and intensity of cytoplasmic granules is variable between aqueous and methanol-based stains. Mast-cell, granular lymphocyte, and basophil granules can stain poorly or not at all with aqueous stains, leading to misdiagnosis of these lesions if only an aqueous stain is used (**Fig. 4**).[11]

In addition, mast-cell granule staining did not improve with fixation times up to 2 minutes before staining with rapid, aqueous-based stains.[12] It is uncertain why certain

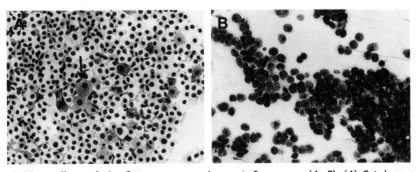

Fig. 4. Mast-cell neoplasia. Cutaneous mass in a cat. Same case (*A, B*). (*A*) Cytology preparation stained with rapid stain. Note that most cells have clear cytoplasm whereas others have faint cytoplasmic granules (*arrow*) (HP oil, original magnification ×50). (*B*) Methanol-based Romanowsky staining allows vibrant staining of the highly granulated mast cells (Wright-Giemsa, HP oil, original magnification ×50).

mast-cell granules do not stain. Nonetheless, these studies emphasize the necessity of preparing both stained and unstained smears for submission to a reference laboratory. Submission of a single previously stained slide for review by a trained clinical pathologist may simply indicate the need for resampling because the slide was not stained adequately.

CYTOLOGY OF CUTANEOUS LESIONS

Skin lesions are easily available for cytologic sampling. This review focuses on tips for preparing samples in-house, and recent information found on literature review. Readers are referred to a comprehensive review on the cytology of cutaneous lesions for additional information beyond the scope of this article.[13,14]

Methods of Skin Sampling for Cytology

Sampling methods of the ear and skin are numerous. The ideal method of sampling for cytology may vary with the type and location of the lesion, differential diagnostic list, and patient temperament. Sample types for cytologic evaluation include swabs, impression smears, scrapings, tape preparations, and needle aspirates (see **Box 1**). By obtaining high-quality samples using current techniques, the diagnostic yield will increase and thereby build comfort, expand use, and ultimately lead to practice revenue. Serial sampling of skin lesions and ear canals assists in monitoring the response to therapy. Communicating the expectation and importance of serial sampling may increase client compliance, generate income, and improve the quality of patient therapy.

Acetate (clear) tape preparation is an established method for evaluation of skin disease, particularly for detecting *Malessezia* dermatitis and extrafollicular mite infections.[15,16] In this method, a piece of clear, pressure-sensitive tape (Scotch 3M) is placed on the skin lesion. The tape strip is removed and fixed on a microscope slide containing a drop of blue (counter) stain for immediate review. Many reference laboratories do not include standard procedures for receiving tape preparations. It is important to call and find out whether these can be accepted. In-house evaluation is often the best recourse. Review of the entire slide is imperative for evaluation of the number and stage of any organisms (one or multiple types) and whether inflammatory cells are present. Skin biopsy and even deep skin scrapings are often negative in canine *Malessezia* dermatitis, emphasizing the critical importance of superficial sampling in suspected cases (**Fig. 5**).[16]

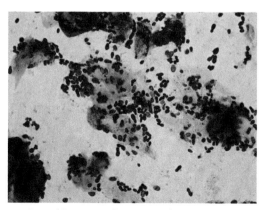

Fig. 5. *Malessezia* organisms. (*Courtesy of* Lynette Cole, DVM, MS, DACVD, Ohio State University, Columbus, OH.)

- Acetate tape impression while squeezing the skin has been found to be a sensitive method for the diagnosis of *Demodex canis* in dogs, and often detects more adult and larval mites than deep skin scraping (**Fig. 6**).[17] The tape method may be better tolerated by patients and easier to perform than deep scrapings, depending on location.

Utility of Special Stains

Infectious agents causing skin disease can be present in low numbers. Organisms do stain with typical Romanowsky stains, but special cytologic stains are also available through reference laboratories. These stains can confirm the findings of the Romanowsky-stained slide (**Figs. 7** and **8**) and/or be particularly helpful in detection of low numbers of organisms (**Table 2**).

Cytologic Features of Some Common Cutaneous Masses

Many comprehensive cytology resources are available with detailed descriptions of specific inflammatory, proliferative, and neoplastic lesions.[13,14] A brief review of some common tissue types and proliferative lesions is provided here.

- Epithelial. Many types of epithelial lesions and tissues are seen in cytology samples. Epithelial tissue commonly exfoliates readily on aspiration, and cells are often present in cohesive clusters and sheets (**Fig. 9**). Individual cells are round, cuboidal, or polygonal. Many epithelial cells have well-defined cell borders. Tissue cells can be present along with inflammatory cells or infectious agents (**Fig. 10**). Sheets of keratinocytes and keratin debris are commonly seen with aspiration of epithelial inclusion–type cysts or cystic epithelial tumors (**Fig. 11**). Cells should be critically evaluated for cytologic criteria of malignancy (see **Fig. 10**; **Fig. 12**, **Table 3**).
- Mesenchymal. Tissue cells tend to exfoliate in low numbers. Cells are typically seen as individual cells that sometimes are present in loose aggregates or groups, sometimes with associated extracellular matrix. Individual cells are usually spindle shaped but can appear more ovoid and plump (**Fig. 20**A, B). Caution is required in interpretation of cytology specimens containing both inflammatory and spindled cells. Reactive spindled cells (often fibroblasts) can become quite

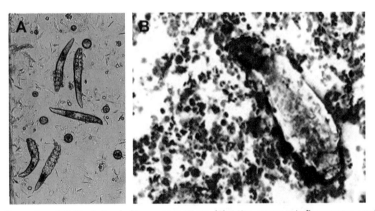

Fig. 6. Demodex. (*A*) Unstained skin preparation. (*B*) Mite among inflammatory cells in a Wright-Giemsa–stained cytology preparation. (*Courtesy of* [*A*] Gwendolen Lorch, DVM, PhD, DACVD, Ohio State University; and [*B*] Sonjia Shelly, DVM, DACVP, VDx Pathology, Davis, CA.)

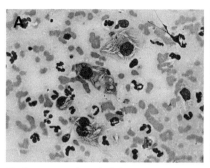
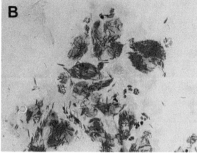

Fig. 7. Same case (A, B). (A) Nonstaining intracellular linear structures (Wright-Giemsa, HP oil, original magnification ×100). (B) Special staining confirms mycobacterial organisms (Ziehl-Neelsen/Fites, HP oil, original magnification ×100).

pleomorphic and mimic neoplasia. However, a high number of stromal/spindled cells without inflammation raise suspicions for neoplasia. In some cases, definitive diagnosis is achieved based on cytology (**Fig. 13**). Biopsy with histopathology is often needed to confirm and fully classify these lesions. Lipomas can be readily diagnosed with in-house cytology when the clinical features are consistent (**Fig. 14**). Careful evaluation for other cell types among the adipocytes is critical.

- Round-cell. Round-cell lesions tend to exfoliate readily, although cells can be fragile, requiring gentle preparation for cytology. Cells are discrete with well-defined cell borders. Common cells of this category include lymphocytes, histiocytes, mast cells, and plasma cells, as well as cells of transmissible venereal tumors (see **Fig. 2B**; **Figs. 15** and **18**).

CYTOLOGY OF THE EAR

Ear-canal cytology is perhaps one of the most commonly performed in-house cytologic examinations for initial diagnosis and monitoring of otitis externa. Most cytology specimens from dogs with otitis are mixed infections.[18,19] Each slide should be closely evaluated for both bacteria and yeast. Detection of organisms is imperative for determining the need for culture(s), guiding initial treatment, and monitoring response to

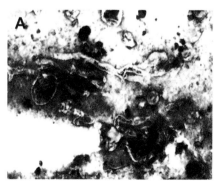
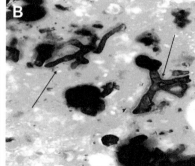

Fig. 8. Same case (A, B). (A) Pale to nonstaining hyphenating structures (Wright-Giemsa, HP oil). (B) Special staining confirms fungal organisms indicated by arrows (Gomori-Grocott methenamine silver, HP oil). (*Courtesy of* Sonjia Shelly, DVM, DACVP, VDx Pathology, Davis, CA.)

Table 2
Commonly used special stains in cytology and histopathology for detection of infectious agents

Stain	Infectious Agents
Giemsa	Many bacteria and protozoa
Gomori-Grocott methenamine silver (GMS)	Fungi, algae, *Pneumocystis*
Ziehl-Neelsen or Fites	Acid-fast bacteria (*Mycobacteria, Actinomyces,* some *Nocardia*); some histoplasma
Periodic acid-Schiff (PAS)	Fungi, yeast

Data from Ramos-Vara JA, Avery AC, Avery PR. Advanced diagnostic techniques. In: Raskin RE, Meyer DJ, editors. Canine and feline cytology: a color atlas and interpretation guide. 2nd edition. St Louis (MO): Saunders; 2010. p. 395–437.

therapy. Samples should also be evaluated for abnormal exfoliative tissue cells and inflammatory responses.

Methods of Ear Sampling for Cytology

Cotton-tip applicator swabs are most often used for acquiring samples from the ear canal. If the lesion is not moist, the swab should be moistened in sterile saline before collection to help minimize cell disruption. In many instances, swabs of the ear canal are taken for both cytology and culture during the same visit. Sterile swabs should be used for culture. In dogs, it has been shown that there is no significant difference in the number of microorganisms detected in 2 sequentially obtained swab samples taken from the same canal.[18] This study reports only moderate agreement in the type of organisms present in 2 serially obtained cytology samples. This finding emphasizes the importance for close monitoring and repeat cytologic examination, particularly in cases that are not responding to therapy.

When preparing smears for cytologic evaluation, gentle yet even rolling of the swab in serial horizontal lines over the glass slide is recommended. Smearing or swiping of the swab often leads to cellular disruption.

Preparation of Ear-Swab Specimens for Cytology

- Heat fixation. A recent study compares fixation and staining methods for the diagnosis of canine otitis externa using cotton swabs for sample acquisition.[20]

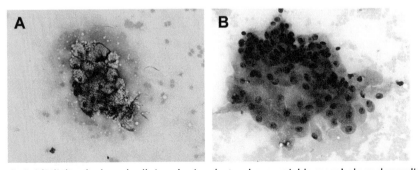

Fig. 9. Epithelial and adnexal cells in cohesive clusters have variable morphology depending on tissue type. (*A*) Sebaceous cells (sebaceous adenoma; Wright-Giemsa, HP oil, original magnification ×50). (*B*) Perianal gland type cells (perianal adenoma; Wright-Giemsa, HP oil, original magnification ×50).

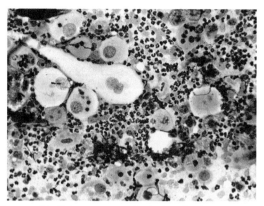

Fig. 10. Aspirates from epithelial tumors can include mixed tissue and cell types. Atypical squamous epithelial cells are admixed with inflammatory cells (squamous cell carcinoma; Wright-Giemsa, HP oil, original magnification ×50).

Fig. 11. Sheets of anucleated keratinocytes are commonly aspirated from inclusion cysts or cystic epithelial tumors (benign keratinizing acanthoma; Wright-Giemsa, HP oil, original magnification ×50).

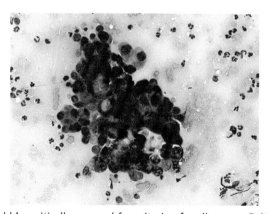

Fig. 12. Cells should be critically assessed for criteria of malignancy. Epithelial cells exhibit anisocytosis, anisokaryosis, high nuclear to cytoplasmic ratio, visible nucleoli, cluster crowding, and cellular/nuclear molding (mammary carcinoma; Wright-Giemsa, HP oil, original magnification ×50).

Table 3
Cytologic criteria of malignancy

Feature	Criterion
Specimen	Increased exfoliation for tissue type
Cellular elements	Anisocytosis: variation in cell size Cellular crowding Cellular molding Large cell size Increased nuclear to cytoplasmic ratio
Nuclear elements	Anisokaryosis: variation in nuclear size Immature or irregular chromatin Nucleoli: prominence, multiple, angular Anisonucleosis Mitotic figures ± aberrant figures Multinucleation Karyomegaly: giant nuclei

Heat fixation before staining did not increase sample quality or cellularity in comparison with air-drying. Another independent study of dogs with *Malessezia* otitis also reports no benefit to heat fixation of ear-swab samples.[21]

- Staining. Comparison of ear-cytology slides stained with rapid 3-step modified Wright stain (Dip Quick; Jorgensen Laboratories Inc, Loveland, CO, USA) according to the manufacturer's instructions, and slides stained with a 1-step dip for 10 to 20 seconds in the blue counterstain, did not significantly alter cytologic findings (**Box 2**).[20] Keratinocytes, yeast, and bacteria were all readily detected in all slides using both 1-step and 3-step methods with and without heat fixation. Eliminating these extra steps did not decrease the sensitivity of disease detection, and will reduce the time required in evaluating samples from patients with otitis.

Methods of Ear-Mass Sampling for Cytology

Patients with refractory and atypical otitis cases should be subjected to complete and thorough ear-canal evaluation. Evaluation for and sampling of any ear masses associated with nonresponsive or chronic otitis may help guide therapy and any further

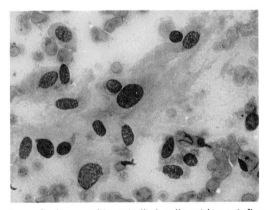

Fig. 13. A population of pleomorphic spindled cells without inflammation (sarcoma; Wright-Giemsa, HP oil, original magnification ×100).

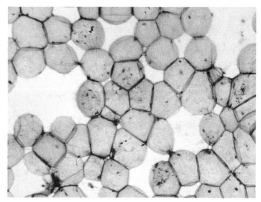

Fig. 14. Adipocytes present in cohesive clusters from a soft subcutaneous, encapsulated mass (lipoma; Wright-Giemsa, HP oil). (*Courtesy of* Connie Wu, DVM, Antech Diagnostics, Chesterfield, CA.)

surgical planning. Swab samples are less likely to be representative of any underlying mass lesion. Direct visual or endoscopically guided fine-needle aspiration (FNA) technique with a 23-gauge needle has been shown to yield highly cellular and diagnostic samples.[22] With this method the nonaspiration technique is preferred; that is, suction is not applied to the syringe.

Diagnostic Correlation

Review of the literature yields limited reports comparing superficial impression smear, scraping, or swab cytology diagnosis with dermatopathologic diagnosis involving large numbers of cases. Often these cytology specimens represent superficial inflammatory or infectious conditions that may or may not reflect histopathology results.

Fine-needle aspirates of ear-canal masses in cats have been reported to have good correlation with histology, with sensitivity of approximately 86% and specificity of 80%.[22] Cytology can be used to distinguish between inflammatory, benign, and neoplastic processes in many cases. Agreement for differentiation between inflammatory polyps and neoplasia was high. Histopathology is often required, and is

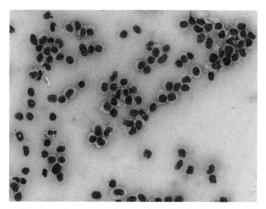

Fig. 15. Histiocytes present as large numbers of individualized round cells (benign cutaneous histiocytoma; Wright-Giemsa, HP oil, original magnification ×50).

Box 2
Proposed 1-step rapid staining method for ear-swab cytology

1. Roll preparation of cotton tip applicator swab sample of the external ear canal onto a clean glass slide free of keratin debris

2. No heat fixation step

3. 1-step dip in blue counterstain for 10–20 seconds

4. Gentle tap water rinse followed by air-drying

5. Microscopic review

Adapted from Toma S, Cornegliani L, Persico P, et al. Comparison of 4 fixation and staining methods for the cytologic evaluation of ear canals with clinical evidence of ceruminous otitis externa. Vet Clin Pathol 2006;35(2):194–8; with permission.

---

recommended for differentiating between benign and malignant ceruminous-gland neoplasms in cats.

RECENT INFORMATION REGARDING SAMPLE-ACQUISITION AND CORRELATION STUDIES FOR CERTAIN TISSUE TYPES
Urinary Tract

Cells suspended within urine degenerate relatively quickly.[23,24] Therefore, immediate preparation of samples taken from the urinary tract is recommended to best preserve cell morphology. At least 1 to 2 slides should be promptly prepared from urine sediment, bladder-tissue aspirates, prostatic washes, and samples taken by traumatic catheterization; any remaining fluid can be used for additional slide preparation or testing. In brief, prostatic wash fluid or urine concentration by sedimentation is achieved by centrifugation at 165 $\times$ g to 360 $\times$ g for 5 minutes followed by removal of the supernatant (urine supernatant can be used for biochemical urinalysis). The sediment is resuspended with 1 to 2 drops of supernatant, and a drop of the resulting fluid is used to prepare smears for cytology.[5] Cytospin preparations of low-cellularity urine (and fluid) samples can also be a helpful tool, and is often used in reference laboratories. Newer-generation cytospin centrifuges are available and may be practical for use in some veterinary practices. Remaining urine or fluid should be placed in ethylenediaminetetraacetic acid (EDTA) for best cellular preservation and/or a sterile tube without additives if culture is indicated.

Transitional-cell carcinoma (TCC) is the most common bladder neoplasm in dogs. Definitive cytologic diagnosis of carcinoma is often possible if a quality high-cellularity sample is obtained. In the case of bladder masses in dogs and cats, evaluation of urine or urine sediment cytology rarely results in diagnostic numbers of well-preserved tumor cells. Many urine sediment samples submitted are nondiagnostic because of low cellularity and cell degeneration (**Fig. 16**). Traumatic urethral catheterization can be a useful technique for obtaining higher numbers of cells for cytology evaluation (**Fig. 17**). False negatives are still possible, and cells yielded from this method may represent superficial, reactive, or polypoid tissue. Direct ultrasound-guided fine-needle aspirates of mass lesions can also be practical.[23] Rare cases of abdominal-wall tumor seeding are reported in a low number of dogs with TCC, including a recent retrospective case series of 24 dogs.[25,26] Significantly, most cases of abdominal-wall TCC are associated with laparotomy and cystotomy, not percutaneous sampling alone.[25] Nonetheless, the investigators recommend exercising caution in percutaneous/transabdominal sampling of bladder masses. If the bladder

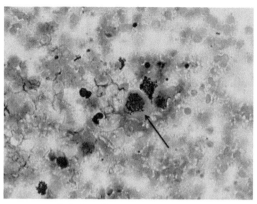

Fig. 16. Few degenerate epithelial cells (*arrow*) within a low-cellularity canine urine sediment preparation. Diagnosis: inconclusive (Wright-Giemsa, HP oil, original magnification ×100).

mass is amenable to sampling by traumatic catheterization, this sampling method is recommended.

Spleen

FNA of the spleen is a safe procedure with a low risk of complication.[2] There is significant overlap between sonographic appearance and histopathologic diagnosis,[2,27] emphasizing the importance of performing tissue cytology or biopsy. Recent information is available regarding sampling techniques, pathologic correlation, and staging of mast-cell neoplasia.[28–30]

Methods of spleen sampling for cytology
Various techniques for FNA of the spleen have been used. The nonaspiration (also known as woodpecker) technique has recently been reported to yield samples of higher cellularity with less hemodilution and better preservation of cellular morphology when compared with samples obtained using aspiration in dogs and cats.[31] The nonaspiration method involves a 22-gauge needle guided into the spleen followed by

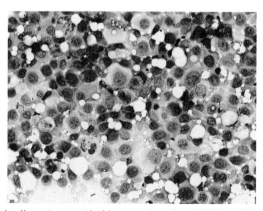

Fig. 17. Transitional cell carcinoma. Bladder mass in a dog. Highly cellular cytology preparation from a sample obtained with the traumatic catheterization technique (Wright-Giemsa, HP oil, original magnification ×50).

gentle movement up and down along the needle tract; no negative pressure is applied to the attached 6- or 12-mL syringe while obtaining the sample. After withdrawing the needle, the material aspirated is then rapidly expelled onto 1 or more clean glass slides and dispersed by various preparation methods (see **Table 1**). Preloading air into the syringe before obtaining the sample permits rapid slide preparation before the sample clots. If the sample is allowed to clot, a well-spread smear is not possible.

Splenic aspiration may yield low-cellularity samples despite careful technique, owing to the vascular nature of splenic parenchyma. For example, mesenchymal neoplasms often exfoliate poorly when sampled by FNA. Needle guidance into more solid portions of a cavitary lesion may be more likely to yield representative cells, and sampling multiple sites may increase overall cellularity.

Diagnostic correlation

Complete cytologic and histopathologic agreement of samples from the splenic aspirates from dogs and cats is reported to be between 51% and 61%.[2,27] A recent study comparing results obtained by 22-gauge spinal needle aspiration and 18-gauge Tru-Cut formalin-fixed biopsy reported fewer false-negative results for the aspiration technique than for biopsy samples.[2] The 40 cases included neoplastic, inflammatory, and benign lesions, and normal splenic tissue from dogs with diffuse splenomegaly or focal parenchymal lesions. Poor-quality friable tissue samples led to inconclusive diagnoses for some needle biopsies (12% of cases) in this study, whereas all FNA samples were considered diagnostic. Cytology and incisional biopsy assist in formulating the initial diagnoses in many cases. It is noteworthy that diagnostic splenectomy remains the gold standard for the evaluation of some splenic lesions, such as benign and malignant lesions of endothelial origin, and for more fully differentiating lesions that have previously been grouped into the diagnosis of fibrohistiocytic nodules.[32]

Splenic sampling for staging of mast-cell neoplasia

Results of multiple recent studies conclude that routine splenic aspiration is important for staging mast-cell neoplasia of dogs (most reported cases) and cats.[28–30] Although many spleens infiltrated with neoplastic mast cells have detectable ultrasonographic abnormalities, ranging from splenomegaly to increased echogenicity to a nodular pattern, affected spleens also can appear normal on ultrasonography. Visceral involvement with mast-cell neoplasia is known to decrease survival times. FNA sampling of the spleen (and liver) despite "normal" ultrasonographic findings should be considered in the staging of mast-cell neoplasia (see **Fig. 18**).

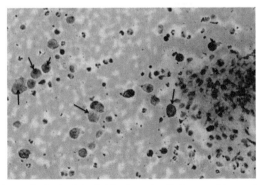

Fig. 18. Large numbers of atypical, individual mast cells (*arrows*) in a splenic aspirate from a dog with high-grade disseminated mast-cell neoplasia (Wright-Giemsa, HP oil, original magnification ×50).

It must be borne in mind that low numbers of mast cells are commonly seen in normal splenic aspirates (**Fig. 19**). Detailed, consensus cytologic criteria for the diagnosis of splenic mast-cell neoplasia are not established when low numbers of mast cells are present, but several cytologic criteria are proposed (**Table 4**).[28] Expert evaluation of these cases is suggested.

Bone

FNA cytology of bone is a cost-effective diagnostic test in the evaluation of primary osseous lesions.[33] FNA is less invasive and less expensive than incisional or excisional biopsy for histopathology. There is also minimal disruption of bone integrity and less severe patient morbidity.[33,34] Osteomyelitis and bone neoplasia can be difficult to distinguish based on imaging findings alone, thus necessitating tissue evaluation.[35] In addition, rapid and definitive diagnosis of osteosarcoma is important for defining prognosis in dogs with bone neoplasia.

Sampling of the bone marrow is also a valuable and sometimes crucial diagnostic tool in canine and feline hematologic disorders. Indications for bone marrow aspiration, sampling method and slide preparation, and cytologic evaluation are reviewed elsewhere.[6]

Methods of bone sampling for cytology

Lytic lesions of bone can vary in exfoliation characteristics. Correlation between cytology and histopathology diagnosis increases significantly in concordance with cellularity of the cytology specimen.[36] Image guiding of FNA samples has been suggested to improve diagnostic samples from bone.[37–40] While advanced imaging modalities such as computed tomography, fluoroscopy, and magnetic resonance imaging have been used for guiding acquisition of both aspiration and biopsy samples, ultrasound guidance to sample lytic bone lesions can also be used.[37,40] Ultrasound is typically more readily available and less expensive than other needle-guiding imaging methods. With this technique, ultrasonography is used to identify the region with either the most cortical destruction or periosteal reaction. Once the area to be sampled is identified, a 20-gauge needle attached to a 12-mL syringe is inserted for aspiration. In lesions with cortical destruction, the needle is directed into the medullary cavitary before applying suction to the attached syringe (aspiration method). When the cortex is intact, ultrasound is used to direct the needle into the region of the most severe

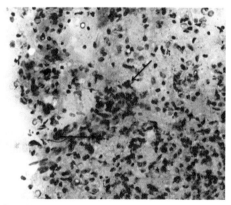

Fig. 19. Low numbers of well-granulated mast cells (*arrows*) embedded within stromal tissue from a dog with splenic reactive lymphoid hyperplasia (spleen; Wright-Giemsa, HP oil, original magnification ×50).

Table 4	
Proposed criteria for evaluation and staging of mast-cell neoplasia in the liver and spleen	
Cytologic Evidence in Support of Tissue Involvement with Mast Cell Neoplasia	Cytologic Evidence Not Indicative of Tissue Involvement with Mast-Cell Neoplasia
Aggregates of well-differentiated mast cells	No mast cells detected
Large numbers of well-differentiated mast cells	Low numbers of scattered, individualized, well-differentiated mast cells
Presence of mast cells with immature and/or atypical morphology	Well-differentiated mast cells primarily associated with stromal elements

Adapted from Stefanello D, Valenti P, Faverzani S, et al. Ultrasound-guided cytology of spleen and liver: a prognostic tool in canine cutaneous mast cell tumor. J Vet Intern Med 2009;23(5):1051–7; with permission.

periosteal reaction. Using this method, FNA resulted in a diagnostic cytology sample in 89% of cases.[37] This result is based on a study in which a majority of lesions were neoplastic, thus increasing the positive predictive value reported. Future studies using this method in larger numbers of patients and with a larger variety of bone lesions will be needed to further assess its sensitivity and specificity.

A novel method of using a bone marrow biopsy needle, termed core aspirate (CA) cytology, has been compared with traditional FNA in canine lytic and/or proliferative bone lesions.[41] Core aspirate samples were obtained using a 16-gauge bone marrow biopsy needle with removable stylet (Jor-Vet; Jorgensen Laboratories Inc). Although the CA technique resulted in higher overall diagnostic accuracy compared with the traditional FNA technique using histopathology as the gold standard, the difference in diagnostic accuracy was not statistically significant. The CA technique may be most beneficial in those cases where traditional FNA yields a low cellularity sample, in lesions with intact cortical bone and minimal soft-tissue involvement, and for sampling lesions with a calcified matrix.

Diagnostic correlation

Cytology is reported to correctly identify the primary pathologic process involving bones in 69% to 95% of cases.[36,41–43] Cytologic diagnosis of osseous neoplasia and high-cellularity samples are more likely to correlate with histopathology than are nonneoplastic processes or less cellular samples, respectively.[36] In this study, cytology correlated with histopathology in 92% of cases involving neoplasia and in 27% of nonneoplastic lesions.[36] Poor-cellularity samples and samples with artifacts precluding interpretation were excluded from this study. The exclusion of samples introduces potential bias and increases the percentage of agreement between cytology and histology.

Utility of special stains

Bone-aspirate samples diagnosed as neoplastic, but lacking differentiating features, can also be additionally evaluated by applying an alkaline phosphatase (ALP) stain directly to cytology preparations at some reference laboratories (see **Fig. 20**). ALP is a biochemical marker that has been used to differentiate between osteosarcoma and other mesenchymal bone neoplasms, including chondrosarcoma, fibrosarcoma, hemangiosarcoma, histiocytic sarcoma, and amelanotic melanoma.[44,45] A recent study evaluated the ability to apply this method to cytology slides previously stained with Wright-Giemsa.[44] Sensitivity of ALP expression by this method for osteosarcoma is reported at between 88% and 100%,[41,44] with a specificity of 94% reported in one study.[44] Of importance, both neoplastic and reactive osteoblasts express the ALP isoenzyme, and thus will not help to differentiate between reactive and neoplastic

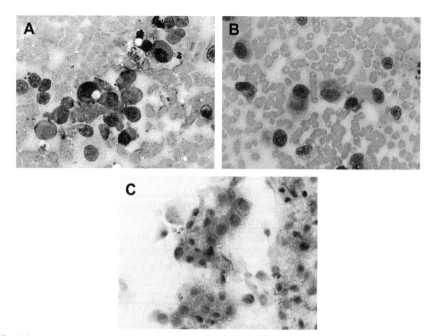

Fig. 20. Osteosarcoma. Bone aspirate from a dog. (*A, B*) Canine sarcoma cells from 2 FNA aspirates of lytic, productive bone lesions (Wright-Giemsa, HP oil, original magnification ×50). (*C*) ALP-positive staining of the sarcoma cells seen in *A* (ALP stain, HP oil). ([*A, C*] Courtesy of Andrew Burton, DVM, University of California, Davis, CA.)

bone lesions. Moreover, positive ALP staining has been reported in nonosteosarcoma neoplasms. A combination of ALP staining and immunophenotyping may be most helpful. Immunocytochemical differentiation of 103 primary and 14 metastatic mesenchymal neoplasms demonstrates the usefulness of an antibody panel in the diagnosis of poorly differentiated neoplasia, including tumors of muscle, endothelium, fibrocytes, melanocytes, histiocytes, and others (**Table 5**).[46,47]

PACKAGING CYTOLOGY SAMPLES FOR THE REFERENCE LABORATORY

Artifacts related to inappropriate sample handling are frustrating for all involved. A checklist is provided here to help decrease the incidence of this occurring.

- Cytology smears should be packaged separately from biopsy samples submersed in formalin. Formalin or formalin fumes coat unstained cytology smears, permanently interfering with the ability of Romanowsky-type stains to penetrate cells and thus rendering the sample unreadable (**Fig. 21**). Even exposure to formalin fumes emitted from an open biopsy jar can sometimes result in this artifact.
- Smears should be completely air-dried before packaging. If the sample is not completely dried before packaging, cellular degeneration and artifact can occur.
- Slides should be kept out of the refrigerator and away from ice packs (even in the "overnight" laboratory container). In geographic areas prone to cold winter temperatures, providing additional protection in outdoor sample-holding containers may be beneficial. Cool temperature causes moisture condensation and cell lysis (**Fig. 22**).

Table 5
Select advanced diagnostic stains available for undifferentiated mesenchymal neoplasms

Immunophenotyping Markers and Chemical Stains	Common Use in Diagnostics
von Willebrand factor, CD31 (PECAM-1)	Hemangiosarcoma, primary or metastatic; hemangioma
Desmin	Muscle tumors; rhabdomyoma (sarcoma), leiomyoma (sarcoma)
Myoglobin	Skeletal muscle tumors; rhabdomyoma (sarcoma)
CD18	Leukocyte tumors, including histiocytic tumors
CD11d	Macrophage differentiation (hemophagocytic histiocytic sarcoma)
CD1/CD11c	Dendritic cells (malignant histiocytosis, histiocytic sarcoma)
Melan A, S100	Melanocytic tumors
Vimentin	General mesenchymal tumor marker; also reported with mesothelioma and other tissues
ALP	Osteoblasts; positive staining also reported with amelanotic melanoma, chondrosarcoma
Fontana-Masson	Melanin; pigment-containing melanocytic tumors

The sensitivity and specificity of each marker is variable.

Data from Höinghaus R, Hewicker-Trautwein M, Mischke R. Immunocytochemical differentiation of canine mesenchymal tumors in cytologic imprint preparations. Vet Clin Pathol 2008;37(1):104–11; Ramos-Vara JA, Avery AC, Avery PR. Advanced diagnostic techniques. In: Raskin RE, Meyer DJ, editors. Canine and feline cytology: a color atlas and interpretation guide. 2nd edition. St Louis (MO): Saunders; 2010. p. 395–437; and Moore PF. Canine histiocytosis. Available at: http://www.histiocytosis.ucdavis.edu. Accessed August 30, 2013.

COMMUNICATION WITH THE CLINICAL PATHOLOGIST

Clear, concise, and complete communication about the patient's signalment, pertinent clinical history, physical examination findings, and diagnostic test results, as well as sample source, is crucial when sending a cytology sample to a reference laboratory. Details about the duration of a lesion (if known), method of collection, and

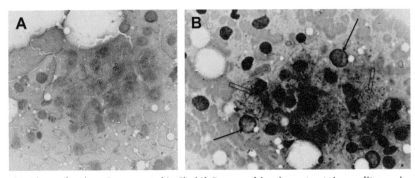

Fig. 21. Liver of a dog. Same case (*A, B*). (*A*) Poor and inadequate stain quality, owing to formalin exposure. Unstained cytology smears were shipped in a bag also containing a formalin biopsy jar (Wright-Giemsa, HP oil, original magnification ×100). (*B*) Resubmitted slides. Note the population of large lymphocytes (*arrows*) among the hepatocyte population (*open arrows*). Diagnosis: high-grade lymphoma (Wright-Giemsa, HP oil, original magnification ×100).

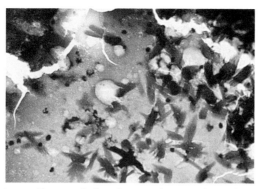

Fig. 22. Crystallization artifact rendering the sample inconclusive because of exposure to cold and moisture (subcutaneous mass; Wright-Giemsa, HP oil, original magnification ×50).

description of the lesion or imaging characteristics are other important pieces of information that can help the pathologist provide a more specific diagnosis and comments about the case. If questions arise regarding a pathologist's report, open and direct communication with the pathologist is encouraged.

SUBMISSION OF CYTOLOGY SAMPLE FOR ADVANCED MOLECULAR DIAGNOSTICS

Many reference laboratories offer advanced molecular techniques, including immunophenotyping, clonality assays, and flow cytometry. Readers are referred to the article on lymphoma diagnostics by Burkhard and Bienzle elsewhere in this issue for further detail. Careful case selection and correlation with cytologic or histologic evaluation is imperative for accurate interpretation of these tests. A pathologist can help determine if and when these tests may be appropriate and helpful.

- Immunophenotyping has become one of the most commonly used ancillary tests in diagnostic pathology. Immunophenotyping by immunocytochemistry (ICC) requires multiple high-quality smears; the ultimate number required depends on the number of stains to be applied, but usually varies from 3 to 6 unstained cytology slides.[48] If the need for immunophenotyping is anticipated, such as lymphoma in dogs, preparation of extra unstained cytology smears at the time of initial sampling and before therapy can result in more rapid results. In addition, a high-quality, representative sample is imperative for accurate interpretation of immunocytochemistry stains. ICC must be correlated with findings from the Romanowsky-stained slide.
- Clonality assessment also is becoming more readily available for use in veterinary practice to evaluate for the presence of monoclonal or polyclonal lymphocyte populations corresponding to neoplastic or reactive cells, respectively. Polymerase chain reaction (PCR) testing can determine whether a single neoplastic clone of B or T lymphocytes is present in many cases. Clonality by PCR, as a compliment or in some cases an alternative to ICC, can be performed on previously stained high-quality cytology slides. Clonality assays vary between laboratories, and results should always be interpreted along with cytologic and/or histologic evaluation.

ACKNOWLEDGMENTS

The author wishes to thank Dr Sonjia Shelly for her critical review of this article, and Drs Andrew Burton and Mary Jo Burkhard for assistance with photomicrographs.

Appreciation is also extended to all of the clinical pathologists at the University of California, Davis and IDEXX, West Sacramento, for supportively sharing their years of experience in our field.

REFERENCES

1. Leveille R, Partington BP, Biller DS, et al. Complications after ultrasound-guided biopsy of abdominal structures in dogs and cats: 246 cases (1984-1991). J Am Vet Med Assoc 1993;203(3):413–5.
2. Watson AT, Penninck D, Knoll JS, et al. Safety and correlation of test results of combined ultrasound-guided fine-needle aspiration and needle core biopsy of the canine spleen. Vet Radiol Ultrasound 2011;52(3):317–22.
3. Christopher MM, Hotz CS, Shelly SM, et al. Use of cytology as a diagnostic method in veterinary practice and assessment of communication between veterinary practitioners and veterinary clinical pathologists. J Am Vet Med Assoc 2008; 232(5):747–54.
4. Sharkey LC, Dial SM, Matz ME. Maximizing the diagnostic value of cytology in small animal practice. Vet Clin North Am Small Anim Pract 2007;37(2):351–72, vii.
5. Menkoth JH, Cowell RL. Sample collection and preparation in cytology: increasing diagnostic yield. Vet Clin North Am Small Anim Pract 2002;32(6): 1187–207.
6. Grindem CB, Neel JA, Juopperi TA. Cytology of bone marrow. Vet Clin North Am Small Anim Pract 2002;32(6):1313–74.
7. Albasan H, Lulich JP, Osborne CA, et al. Effects of storage time and temperature on pH, specific gravity, and crystal formation in urine samples from dogs and cats. J Am Vet Med Assoc 2003;222(2):176–9.
8. Root Kustritz MV. The value of canine semen evaluation for practitioners. Theriogenology 2007;68:329–37.
9. Christopher MM, Hotz CS. Cytologic diagnosis: expression of probability by clinical pathologists. Vet Clin Pathol 2004;33(2):84–95.
10. Troxel DB, Sabella JD. Problem areas in pathology practice. Am J Surg Pathol 1994;18:821–31.
11. Allison RW, Velguth KE. Appearance of granulated cells in blood films stained by automated aqueous versus methanolic Romanowsky methods. Vet Clin Pathol 2010;39(1):99–104.
12. Jackson DE, Selting KA, Spoor MS, et al. Evaluation of fixation time using Diff-Quik for staining of canine mast cell tumor aspirates. Vet Clin Pathol 2013; 42(1):99–102.
13. Shelly SM. Cutaneous lesions. Vet Clin North Am Small Anim Pract 2003;33(1): 1–46.
14. Raskin RE. Skin and subcutaneous tissues. In: Raskin RE, Meyer DJ, editors. Canine and feline cytology: a color atlas and interpretation guide. 2nd edition. St Louis (MO): Saunders; 2010. p. 26–76.
15. Bond R. *Malessezia* dermatitis. In: Greene CE, editor. Infectious diseases of the dog and cat. 4th edition. St Louis (MO): Elsevier Saunders; 2012. p. 602–6.
16. Gross TL. Diseases of the epidermis. In: Gross TL, Irkhe PJ, Welder EJ, et al, editors. Skin diseases of the dog and cat: clinical and histopathologic diagnosis. 2nd edition. Ames (IA): Blackwell; 2005. p. 142–6.
17. Pereira AV, Pereira SA, Gremial ID, et al. Comparison of acetate tape impression with squeezing versus skin scraping for the diagnosis of canine demodecosis. Aust Vet J 2012;90(11):448–50.

18. Lehner G, Sauter Louis C, Mueller RS. Reproducibility of ear cytology in dogs with otitis externa. Vet Rec 2010;167:23–6.
19. Graham-Mize CA, Rosser EJ Jr. Comparison of microbial isolates and susceptibility patterns from the external ear canal of dogs with otitis externa. J Am Anim Hosp Assoc 2004;54:424–7.
20. Toma S, Cornegliani L, Persico P, et al. Comparison of 4 fixation and staining methods for the cytologic evaluation of ear canals with clinical evidence of ceruminous otitis externa. Vet Clin Pathol 2006;35(2):194–8.
21. Griffin JS, Scott DW, Erb HN. *Malessezia* otitis externa in the dog: the effect of heat-fixing otic exudate for cytologic analysis. J Vet Med A Physiol Pathol Clin Med 2007;54(8):424–7.
22. De Lorenzi D, Bonfant U, Maserdotti C, et al. Fine-needle biopsy of external ear canal masses in the cat: cytologic results and histologic correlations in 27 cases. Vet Clin Pathol 2005;34(2):100–5.
23. Borjesson DL, DeJong K. Urinary tract. In: Raskin RE, Meyer DJ, editors. Canine and feline cytology: a color atlas and interpretation guide. 2nd edition. St Louis (MO): Saunders; 2010. p. 249–73.
24. Ahmed HG, Tom MA. The consequence of delayed fixation on subsequent preservation of urine cells. Oman Med J 2011;26(1):14–8.
25. Higuchi T, Burcham GN, Childress MO, et al. Characterization and treatment of transitional cell carcinoma of the abdominal wall in dogs: 24 cases (1985-2010). J Am Vet Med Assoc 2013;242(4):499–506.
26. Nyland TG, Wallace ST, Wisner ER. Needle-tract implantation following us-guided fine-needle aspiration biopsy of transitional cell carcinoma of the bladder, urethra, and prostate. Vet Radiol Ultrasound 2002;43:50–3.
27. Ballegeer EA, Forrest LJ, Dickinson RM, et al. Correlation of ultrasonographic appearance of lesions and cytologic and histologic diagnosis in splenic aspirates from dogs and cats: 32 cases (2002-2005). J Am Vet Med Assoc 2007;230(5):690–6.
28. Stefanello D, Valenti P, Faverzani S, et al. Ultrasound-guided cytology of spleen and liver: a prognostic tool in canine cutaneous mast cell tumor. J Vet Intern Med 2009;23(5):1051–7.
29. Sato AF, Solano M. Ultrasonographic findings in abdominal mast cell disease: a retrospective study of 19 patients. Vet Radiol Ultrasound 2004;45:51–7.
30. Book AP, Fidel J, Wills T, et al. Correlation of ultrasound findings, liver and spleen cytology, and prognosis in the clinical staging of high metastatic risk canine mast cell tumors. Vet Radiol Ultrasound 2011;52(5):548–54.
31. LeBlanc CJ, Head LL, Fry MM. Comparison of aspiration and nonaspiration techniques for obtaining cytologic samples from the canine and feline spleen. Vet Clin Pathol 2009;38(2):242–6.
32. Moore AS, Frimberger AE, Sullivan N, et al. Histologic and immunohistochemical review of splenic fibrohistiocytic nodules in dogs. J Vet Intern Med 2012;26:1164–8.
33. Layfield L, Dodd LG, Hirschowitz S, et al. Fine-needle aspiration of primary osseous lesions: A cost effectiveness study. Diagn Cytopathol 2010;38(4):239–43.
34. Layfield L, Dodd LG. Fine needle aspiration of bone and joint neoplasms. In: Helliwell TR, editor. Pathology of bone and joint neoplasms. Philadelphia: WB Saunders; 1999. p. 129–56.
35. Wrigley RH. Malignant versus nonmalignant bone disease. Vet Clin North Am Small Anim Pract 2000;30(2):315–7, vi–vii.

36. Berzina I, Sharkey LC, Matise I, et al. Correlation between cytologic and histopathologic diagnoses of bone lesions in dogs: a study of the diagnostic accuracy of bone cytology. Vet Clin Pathol 2008;37(3):332–8.

37. Britt T, Clifford C, Barger A, et al. Diagnosing appendicular osteosarcoma with ultrasound-guided fine-needle aspiration: 36 cases. J Small Anim Pract 2007; 48:145–50.

38. Vignoli M, Ohlerth S, Rossa F, et al. Computed tomography-guided fine-needle aspiration of tissue-core biopsy of bone lesions in small animals. Vet Radiol Ultrasound 2004;45:125–30.

39. Saifuddin A, Mann BS, Mahroof S, et al. Dedifferentiated chondrosarcoma; use of MRI to guide needle biopsy. Clin Radiol 2004;59:268–72.

40. Samii VF, Nyland TG, Werner LL, et al. Ultrasound-guided fine-needle aspiration biopsy of bone lesions: a preliminary report. Vet Radiol Ultrasound 1999;40:82–6.

41. Neihaus SA, Locke JE, Barger AM, et al. A novel method of core aspirate cytology compared to fine-needle aspiration for diagnosing canine osteosarcoma. J Am Anim Hosp Assoc 2011;47(5):317–23.

42. Cohen M, Bohling M, Wright JC, et al. Evaluation of sensitivity and specificity of cytologic examination; 269 cases (1999-2000). J Am Vet Med Assoc 2003;222: 964–7.

43. Loukopoulos P, Rozmanec M, Sutton RH. Cytological versus histopathologic diagnosis in canine osteosarcoma. Vet Rec 2005;157(24):784.

44. Ryseff JK, Bohn AA. Detection of alkaline phosphatase in canine cells previously stained with Wright-Giemsa and its utility in differentiating osteosarcoma from other mesenchymal tumors. Vet Clin Pathol 2012;41(3):391–5.

45. Barger A, Graca R, Bailey K, et al. Utilization of alkaline phosphatase to differentiate canine osteosarcoma from other vimentin-positive tumors. Vet Pathol 2005; 42(2):161–5.

46. Höinghaus R, Hewicker-Trautwein M, Mischke R. Immunocytochemical differentiation of canine mesenchymal tumors in cytologic imprint preparations. Vet Clin Pathol 2008;37(1):104–11.

47. Ramos-Vara JA, Avery AC, Avery PR. Advanced diagnostic techniques. In: Raskin RE, Meyer DJ, editors. Canine and feline cytology: a color atlas and interpretation guide. 2nd edition. St Louis (MO): Saunders; 2010. p. 395–437.

48. Valli V, Peters E, Williams C, et al. Optimizing methods in immunocytochemistry: one laboratory's experience. Vet Clin Pathol 2009;38(2):261–9.

Index

Note: Page numbers of article titles are in **boldface** type.

A

N-Acetyl-β-D-glucosaminidase (NAG)
  in advanced renal function testing in dogs and cats, 1202
Acid(s)
  bile
    overview of, 1217–1218
Acid-base disturbances
  identification of, 1273
Acid-base homeostasis
  in veterinary patients, 1274–1275
Acid-base interpretation
  in veterinary patients, **1273–1286**
    acid-base homeostasis, 1274–1275
    equipment and sample collection, 1275
    metabolic acidosis, 1277–1278
    metabolic alkalosis, 1278–1280
    methods of, 1273–1274
    mixed disturbances, 1282–1284
    respiratory acidosis, 1280–1282
    respiratory alkalosis, 1282
    traditional interpretation, 1275–1277
Acidosis
  lactic. *See* Lactic acidosis
  metabolic
    in veterinary patients, 1277–1278
  respiratory
    in veterinary patients, 1280–1282
Acute kidney disease
  hypocalcemia of critical illness in dogs and cats related to, 1307
Alanine aminotransferase (ALT)
  overview of, 1210–1212
Alkaline phosphatase (ALP)
  overview of, 1213
Alkalosis
  metabolic
    in veterinary patients, 1278–1280
  respiratory
    in veterinary patients, 1282
ALP. *See* Alkaline phosphatase (ALP)
ALT. *See* Alanine aminotransferase (ALT)
Ammonia
  overview of, 1218–1219

Vet Clin Small Anim 43 (2013) 1409–1423
http://dx.doi.org/10.1016/S0195-5616(13)00189-7
0195-5616/13/$ – see front matter © 2013 Elsevier Inc. All rights reserved.

vetsmall.theclinics.com

United States Postal Service

Statement of Ownership, Management, and Circulation
(All Periodicals Publications Except Requestor Publications)

1. Publication Title
Veterinary Clinics of North America: Small Animal Practice

2. Publication Number
0 0 3 - 1 5 0

3. Filing Date
9/14/13

4. Issue Frequency
Jan, Mar, May, Jul, Sep, Nov

5. Number of Issues Published Annually
6

6. Annual Subscription Price
$294.00

7. Complete Mailing Address of Known Office of Publication *(Not printer) (Street, city, county, state, and ZIP+4®)*
Elsevier Inc.
360 Park Avenue South
New York, NY 10010-1710

Contact Person
Stephen Bushing

Telephone *(Include area code)*
215-239-3688

8. Complete Mailing Address of Headquarters or General Business Office of Publisher *(Not printer)*
Elsevier Inc., 360 Park Avenue South, New York, NY 10010-1710

9. Full Names and Complete Mailing Addresses of Publisher, Editor, and Managing Editor *(Do not leave blank)*

Publisher *(Name and complete mailing address)*
Linda Belfus, Elsevier, Inc., 1600 John F. Kennedy Blvd. Suite 1800, Philadelphia, PA 19103-2899

Editor *(Name and complete mailing address)*
John Vassallo, Elsevier, Inc., 1600 John F. Kennedy Blvd. Suite 1800, Philadelphia, PA 19103-2899

Managing Editor *(Name and complete mailing address)*
Barbara Cohen-Kligerman, Elsevier, Inc., 1600 John F. Kennedy Blvd. Suite 1800, Philadelphia, PA 19103-2899

10. Owner *(Do not leave blank. If the publication is owned by a corporation, give the name and address of the corporation immediately followed by the names and addresses of all stockholders owning or holding 1 percent or more of the total amount of stock. If not owned by a corporation, give the names and addresses of the individual owners. If owned by a partnership or other unincorporated firm, give its name and address as well as those of each individual owner. If the publication is published by a nonprofit organization, give its name and address.)*

Full Name	Complete Mailing Address
Wholly owned subsidiary of	1600 John F. Kennedy Blvd., Ste. 1800
Reed/Elsevier, US holdings	Philadelphia, PA 19103-2899

11. Known Bondholders, Mortgagees, and Other Security Holders Owning or Holding 1 Percent or More of Total Amount of Bonds, Mortgages, or Other Securities. If none, check box   ☐ None

Full Name	Complete Mailing Address
N/A	

12. Tax Status *(For completion by nonprofit organizations authorized to mail at nonprofit rates) (Check one)*
The purpose, function, and nonprofit status of this organization and the exempt status for federal income tax purposes:
☐ Has Not Changed During Preceding 12 Months
☐ Has Changed During Preceding 12 Months *(Publisher must submit explanation of change with this statement)*

PS Form 3526, September 2007 (Page 1 of 3 (Instructions Page 3)) PSN 7530-01-000-9931 PRIVACY NOTICE: See our Privacy policy in www.usps.com

---

13. Publication Title
Veterinary Clinics of North America: Small Animal Practice

14. Issue Date for Circulation Data Below
September 2013

15. Extent and Nature of Circulation

		Average No. Copies Each Issue During Preceding 12 Months	No. Copies of Single Issue Published Nearest to Filing Date
a. Total Number of Copies *(Net press run)*		1,491	1,290
b. Paid Circulation (By Mail and Outside the Mail)	(1) Mailed Outside-County Paid Subscriptions Stated on PS Form 3541. *(Include paid distribution above nominal rate, advertiser's proof copies, and exchange copies)*	938	855
	(2) Mailed In-County Paid Subscriptions Stated on PS Form 3541 *(Include paid distribution above nominal rate, advertiser's proof copies, and exchange copies)*		
	(3) Paid Distribution Outside the Mails Including Sales Through Dealers and Carriers, Street Vendors, Counter Sales, and Other Paid Distribution Outside USPS®	217	196
	(4) Paid Distribution by Other Classes Mailed Through the USPS (e.g. First-Class Mail®)		
c. Total Paid Distribution *(Sum of 15b (1), (2), (3), and (4))* ▶		1,155	1,051
d. Free or Nominal Rate Distribution (By Mail and Outside the Mail)	(1) Free or Nominal Rate Outside-County Copies Included on PS Form 3541	102	99
	(2) Free or Nominal Rate In-County Copies Included on PS Form 3541		
	(3) Free or Nominal Rate Copies Mailed at Other Classes Through the USPS (e.g. First-Class Mail)		
	(4) Free or Nominal Rate Distribution Outside the Mail (Carriers or other means)		
e. Total Free or Nominal Rate Distribution *(Sum of 15d (1), (2), (3) and (4))* ▶		102	99
f. Total Distribution *(Sum of 15c and 15e)* ▶		1,257	1,150
g. Copies not Distributed *(See instructions to publishers #4 (page #3))* ▶		234	140
h. Total *(Sum of 15f and g)* ▶		1,491	1,290
i. Percent Paid *(15c divided by 15f times 100)* ▶		91.89%	91.39%

16. Publication of Statement of Ownership
☐ If the publication is a general publication, publication of this statement is required. Will be printed in the November 2013 issue of this publication.   ☐ Publication not required

17. Signature and Title of Editor, Publisher, Business Manager, or Owner

Stephen R. Bushing *(signature)*

Stephen R. Bushing –Inventory Distribution Coordinator

Date
September 14, 2013

I certify that all information furnished on this form is true and complete. I understand that anyone who furnishes false or misleading information on this form or who omits material or information requested on the form may be subject to criminal sanctions (including fines and imprisonment) and/or civil sanctions (including civil penalties).

PS Form 3526, September 2007 (Page 2 of 3)

Printed and bound by CPI Group (UK) Ltd, Croydon, CR0 4YY

03/10/2024

01040409-0004